Lactation

A Foundational Strategy for Health Promotion

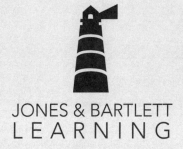

JONES & BARTLETT
LEARNING

Lactation

A Foundational Strategy for Health Promotion

Suzanne Hetzel Campbell, PhD, RN, IBCLC, CCSNE
Associate Professor
Applied Science | School of Nursing
The University of British Columbia | Vancouver Campus

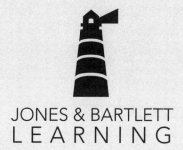

JONES & BARTLETT
LEARNING

World Headquarters
Jones & Bartlett Learning
5 Wall Street
Burlington, MA 01803
978-443-5000
info@jblearning.com
www.jblearning.com

Jones & Bartlett Learning books and products are available through most bookstores and online booksellers. To contact Jones & Bartlett Learning directly, call 800-832-0034, fax 978-443-8000, or visit our website, www.jblearning.com.

Substantial discounts on bulk quantities of Jones & Bartlett Learning publications are available to corporations, professional associations, and other qualified organizations. For details and specific discount information, contact the special sales department at Jones & Bartlett Learning via the above contact information or send an email to specialsales@jblearning.com.

Production Credits

VP, Product Management: Christine Emerton
Director of Product Management: Matthew Kane
Product Manager: Tina Chen
Product Specialist: Melina Leon-Haley
Project Specialist: Roberta Sherman
Digital Project Specialist: Rachel DiMaggio
Sr. Marketing Manager: Lindsay White
Product Fulfillment Manager: Wendy Kilborn
Composition: S4Carlisle Publishing Services
Project Management: S4Carlisle Publishing Services

Cover Design: Michael O'Donnell
Senior Media Development Editor: Troy Liston
Media Development Editor: Faith Brosnan
Rights Specialist: Maria Leon Maimone
Cover and Title Page Images: © Jose Luis Pelaez Inc/
    DigitalVision/Getty Images; Courtesy of Erica Miller;
    © Hadynyah/E+/Getty Images; © Johner Images -
    Nyman, Fredrik/Brand X Pictures/Getty Images
Printing and Binding: McNaughton & Gunn

Library of Congress Cataloging-in-Publication Data

Names: Campbell, Suzanne Hetzel, author.
Title: A foundational strategy for health promotion / Suzanne Hetzel
    Campbell.
Description: First edition. | Burlington, Massachusetts : Jones & Bartlett
    Learning, [2022] | Includes bibliographical references and index.
Identifiers: LCCN 2020041894 | ISBN 9781284197167 (paperback)
Subjects: MESH: Breast Feeding | Lactation | Health Promotion | Social
    Determinants of Health
Classification: LCC RJ216 | NLM WS 125 | DDC 613.2/69--dc23
LC record available at https://lccn.loc.gov/2020041894

6048

Printed in the United States of America
25 24 23 22 21   10 9 8 7 6 5 4 3 2 1

Dedication

This book is dedicated to all those who have supported, mentored, and taught me along the way. This includes, most especially, my husband Gerry Campbell and our children Lilly and Greg, who continue to believe in me and inspire me to be a better partner, parent, nurse, teacher, and researcher. My journey to motherhood and lactation came from my ancestors—Great Grandma Raffaella Astarita Parlato, a lay midwife in New York City in the early 1900s; my grandmother Phillomena Parlato Ruffolo; and my mother Anne Cecilia Ruffolo Hetzel, whose heartbreaking story of mastitis and "failed" breastfeeding with my older brother inspired in me the desire to "succeed." My mother's story of a "natural birth" with me inspired and empowered me for that experience that helped to lay the foundation for lactation. I dedicate this book to all those who do not meet their infant-feeding goals—who somehow feel they have "failed"—in the hope of educating the next generation of health care professionals, teachers, parents, and policy makers to be present and helpful; to end the judgment; and to support each family where they are to where they are going. I dedicate this to my children, their partners, nieces and nephews, present and future grandchildren and great-grandchildren, and all the present, past, and future parents so that they may be brave and courageous in protecting the precious gift of human milk for infants and children.

Suzanne Hetzel Campbell

Brief Contents

Contents

PART 1 The Context and Foundations of Lactation as Health Promotion 1

PART 2 Breastfeeding as Developmental Health Promotion   91

PART 3 Lactation as Health Promotion Under Challenging Circumstances 149

CHAPTER 11 Breastfeeding: An Essential Link in Healthy Weight Promotion and Obesity Prevention 151

Cecilia Jevitt

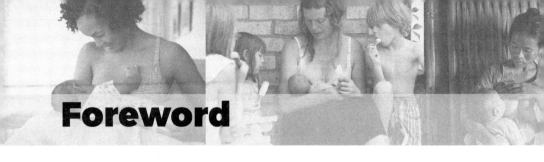

Foreword

Many times during my career as a clinician and educator, I have looked for a book like this one and found nothing that came close. The fields of lactation and health promotion have needed this book for a long time. It fills a gap within the field of lactation support and promotion that is long overdue. Many books have been written about the clinical aspects of lactation for learners at both the public and professional levels. Breastfeeding families have an array of educational materials that present the how-to aspects of feeding. Professionals of all levels have texts aimed at providing the specialized clinical knowledge appropriate for their roles. However, there has been no single book providing the broader public health approach, which focuses on the socio-cultural grounding required to develop, plan, implement, and evaluate the community-based programs needed by the diversity of breastfeeding families.

For public health interventions to be successful, more than expert clinically focused knowledge is required. Previously, texts for students or teachers to use when focusing on lactation-specific health education, program planning, and community-based interventions, which inherently have advocacy as a fundamental component, did not exist. Advocacy has been at the heart of all the positive changes that have occurred in public health policy and interventions within the lactation field; yet, it is seldom taught. This book addresses all these issues from a multidisciplinary approach that is sensitive to the major issues in our field.

The field of lactation support and promotion is unlike many specialty areas in the health sciences; it is very dependent on socio-cultural contexts. I would suggest that there are very few other fields that draw on so many varied disciplines (e.g., biological sciences, social sciences, health education, public health), making clinical practice and study in this field more complicated than most. My academic colleagues were always amazed at the 4+ shelves of books about lactation and breastfeeding I had in my office, frequently stating, "I didn't know there was so much to write about in lactation." Ours is a field that is both broad and deep—characteristics well developed in this book.

Breastfeeding is one of the most important preventative and cost-effective health measures that can be implemented in any region, country, or globally. The World Health Organization considers breastfeeding to be one of the few child survival strategies that is essential globally for saving lives. Breastfeeding is an essential primary prevention activity that facilitates better health outcomes throughout infancy and for years beyond. Supporting and promoting breastfeeding has been a priority within the international public health arena for over 50 years, and yet there is still much that needs to be done. A real strength of this book lies in its international scope and its multidisciplinary approach, making it a useful teaching tool for anyone who has an interest in a community-based approach to promoting and supporting breastfeeding families.

Joan E. Dodgson, PhD, MPH, RN, FAAN
Editor in Chief, Journal of Human Lactation

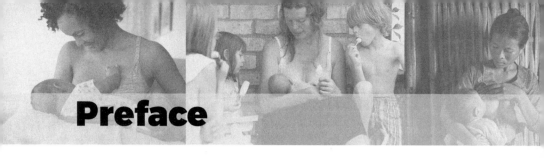

Preface

Overview

Evidence to support the maternal and infant health benefits, societal benefits, and economic benefits of lactation throughout the world has steadily increased over the years. Although progress has been made since the early 1980s, exclusive breast-feeding in the developing world and on the global level has need for improvement. Lactation support providers across disciplines are well positioned to promote breastfeeding as an overall health strategy, impacting the health of families throughout the lifespan. Global organizations have worked to break societal barriers where artificial feeding is the norm. Support, protection, and advocacy of the breastfeeding parent are essential for all countries to make progress toward global breastfeeding targets, thereby improving the overall health of the world.

Background

In the past 30 years of teaching I have focused on educating undergraduate and graduate nursing students and interprofessional health care providers on maternal–infant health and lactation—the concept of breastfeeding as a health behavior and health promotion possibility for all families has always been in the back of my mind. In teaching health promotion to graduate students in nursing (family nurse practitioners and advanced practice), I realized that breastfeeding is not acknowledged or represented in the literature specific to health promotion. Further, the most likely impediments to parents in meeting their infant feeding goals include a lack of societal, peer, family, and physician or health care professional support for breastfeeding parents. This text places lactation in a global context as a health promotion strategy given the strong and cumulative evidence of its impact on women, children, and society specifically related to health (Brown, 2017; Victora et al., 2016). My strong belief is that this specific topic—Lactation as Health Promotion— is of great significance for public health as we commit to prolonging life and promoting health through organized societal efforts (Acheson, 1988; WHO, 2018). Everyone has a role to play in supporting new parents in their infant feeding decisions, and health care professionals have unique opportunities in communicating positively with new parents around intimate health decisions such as infant feeding.

The Text

The authors have incorporated many key factors throughout the text in how we approach lactation as health promotion. We have endeavored wherever possible to keep an international perspective, with inclusive terminology and trauma-informed attention to practices; to reflect the current state of practice (e.g., global and political code of ethics, human rights); to ensure that content is evidence based and practice informed; to focus on what students need to know and instructors need to teach; and to align with the Academy of Breastfeeding Medicine protocols. Other factors that you will find incorporated include patient-centered care, shared decision making, mutual goal setting, cultural sensitivity, trauma–violence informed care, interprofessional teams, and reflective practice.

Lactation can be situated as "intimate care behavior" related to the societal stigma placed on intimate body parts (such as the breast) and the controversies that lie behind social representation of lactation as a gender-related and feminist issue. Not surprisingly, the topic of infant feeding, specifically breastfeeding, often creates societal taboos related to discussing it. Regardless of breastfeeding's placement as the biological norm for infant feeding, it exists within a social construct (Cattaneo, 2012). The rate and practice of breastfeeding are determined by the same social determinants of health that shape other health inequalities and inequities. In addition, examining lactation as a simply "biological/physiological" function of the breasts deemphasizes the importance of the social, cultural, and psychological components required for its success. Parents' confidence in their body's ability to produce sufficient milk to contribute to the growth and development of their newborns is paramount in their minds. Lack of confidence in that ability to produce the right amount and composition of milk for their infants can lead to "perceived insufficient milk supply" and can affect parents' ability to meet their infant feeding goals. Other social determinants of health, including the effects of racism, poverty, housing insufficiency, food insecurity, trauma–violence, substance use, and mental and physical health, can all affect parents' ability to meet their goals.

Our focus on social determinants of health for this text (e.g., related to poverty, health literacy, lack of housing and sustainable food sources, and the effects of racism and trauma–violence) is important to contextualize the global issues faced by parents worldwide, knowing that breastfeeding can be a "solution" for the health and safety of the family. (See Chapter 12: Infant Feeding Emergencies). Women and their families lack support from health care providers, their communities, and their governments/countries to meet their lactation goals and infant feeding needs. Health care professionals can be hesitant to support new families due to concerns about pressuring already overburdened parents.

As part of your journey through this text, we hope you will consider the broader ramifications of supporting families to breastfeed. In an age of global catastrophes, such as the most recent pandemic, and protests related to systemic racism, we hope to outline some of the basic premises of the "natural" aspect of feeding babies from the breast, which is biologically the way mammals provide food for their offspring. We have framed the text so that you will consider the unique components of lactation: both the product of human milk and the process of breastfeeding (e.g., the parent–infant relationship). First, human milk is individually suited and created for each child at the moment they are born. We are learning more everyday about the microbiome, the genetic components, and the living factors within human milk that are individually suited between the parent and infant. These factors should humble us toward the miraculous qualities of human milk, which are dose dependent (e.g., enhanced benefits with duration and exclusivity of breastfeeding), with research demonstrating the health benefits of breastfeeding to both the mother/parents and the infant (Gomez-Gallego et al., 2016; Victora et al., 2016). We recognize that hormonal components of prolactin and oxytocin lay down receptors in breast and brain tissue of both mother and infant during lactation. So the breastfeeding experience is passed on through generations. My lived experience includes being born into a society in North America where parents do not trust their bodies for birth or lactation, and we accept human milk substitutes (e.g. infant formula) as safe in place of lactation. It's no wonder that low milk supply and breast pain (nipple damage and trauma) are two of the most common reasons women give for not continuing breastfeeding. The perception of low milk supply is often passed down from generations, like it is in our DNA. Parents have said to me "Oh, women in my family cannot make enough milk to feed their children, so it's not surprising to me that I need to use formula (a human milk substitute)." While there certainly may be a genetic component, more recent research speaks to the effects of social determinants of health, especially trauma and adverse childhood events (ACEs) on an individuals' physical and mental health, which in turn affects their pregnancies, deliveries, and ability to meet their infant feeding goals of lactation (Kendall-Tackett, 2007). Add to this the systemic effects of racialization that sustain and exacerbate social and health inequities (Browne, 2017), and it is not surprising that there are gaps between groups on breastfeeding initiation and duration rates globally.

The terms 'human milk substitutes' and 'formula' will be used interchangeably throughout the text recognizing the power of language. Although 'formula' is universally understood, framing it as a 'human milk substitute' to new parents struggling with supply issues may cause feelings of shame. Reminding parents of options for human milk substitution with donor milk rather that seeing infant formula as their only option is worth considering. The intent is to help you, the reader, recognize that human milk is the gold standard and to remove some of the 'magical quality' of formula as 'good enough' or 'superior' to human milk. It is not.

As a society, specifically health care providers and others who interact with pregnant and breastfeeding families, we can learn to communicate with new parents about intimate health decision making, such as infant feeding within the context of strengths-based health promotion that empowers new parents. Our hope for this text is that it will provide a way to frame breastfeeding and lactation as health promotion and provide you ways to move forward in protecting this global resource of human milk while considering the context of parents' goals and life. This text will provide concrete resources, skills, and conversation starters to help all health care professionals feel confident in their knowledge and skills. We will outline the benefits of lactation, the risks associated with the use of human milk substitutes, and how to be respectful and supportive of parents in meeting their infant feeding goals as they transition to parenthood. This book will reflect a postmodern society that values and respects the diversity of families. Taking a socio-ecological perspective using a person-centered care framework with the dyad and family at the center, this text will provide practitioners and students a way forward that is culturally sensitive and provides holistic care within a therapeutic relational practice model. Our hope is that it will help us all reflect on our implicit biases such that we are able to take a critical view of the health care system we are working in, the communities in which we live, and our own position to be ally, steward, or champion depending on the context. Ultimately our goal is the same: a healthy world, healthy citizens, and systems that are socially just and in the best interest of all.

There are three parts to the text. The first section includes the foundation for general knowledge and definition of health promotion, behavioral theories relevant to the use of health promotion, and examining lactation from a local, regional, national, and global perspective incorporating global health policies and best practices. Part 1 provides the context and foundations of examining lactation as a health promotion strategy starting with the historical context of infant feeding. Chapter 1 incorporates industrialization and the complex factors that have contributed to the increased use of human milk substitutes and the overall effect on public health of changes in infant feeding practices. Chapter 2 provides the key concepts to examine lactation as health promotion, and Chapter 3 outlines behavioral theories used in the examination of lactation as health behavior. Chapter 4 explores the important role of social policy and its impact globally on the initiation, promotion, and support of lactation. Chapter 5 describes key concepts related to relational practice theory and incorporates them into a framework for professional practice that integrates humility, cultural sensitivity, trauma–violence informed practice, and reflection on practice by health care professionals.

Part 2 dives more deeply into the specific areas of Baby-Friendly Initiatives (BFIs), globalization, and equitable lactation health promotion. Chapter 6 reviews the Baby-friendly Hospital Initiative (BFHI) and key roles of health care professionals (HCPs) in protecting, promoting, and supporting breastfeeding families. Chapter 7 explores more deeply the developmental processes core to lactation as health promotion including the impact of pregnancy and birth interventions on breastfeeding. Chapter 8 incorporates a global perspective with a case study from Brazil and sociopolitical factors that affect lactation as health promotion given the impact of globalization. Chapter 9 provides examples of successful breastfeeding programs from an international perspective and methods of scaling up public policy, research, and practice for health promotion. The last chapter in Part 2, Chapter 10, outlines equitable lactation health promotion, considering incorporation of the social determinants of health and briefly examining interprofessional health care professional education related to lactation.

Part 3 provides specifically more challenging situations we face in promoting health with our patients and advocating for an interprofessional team approach. Specific chapters focus on the role of breastfeeding in healthy weight promotion and obesity prevention (Chapter 11), infant feeding in emergencies (Chapter 12), breastfeeding for people experiencing criminalization and incarceration (Chapter 13), the use of domperidone for low milk supply (Chapter 14), and the role of the physiotherapist (Chapter 15). In addition to being a foundational text for all pre-licensure health care professional students, this text also provides guidance and outlines for health care professional providers, administrators, policy makers, and government officials. Recognizing the possible enhanced health and well-being that promoting lactation and supporting parents and families in meeting their infant feeding goals can provide, this approach also contributes to the emotional, physical, and spiritual health of all global citizens.

Throughout each chapter, where appropriate, you will find chapter objectives, key terms, key points to remember, a case study with questions based on the scenario, and lists of additional resources, such as suggested reading, videos, and websites.

Thank you for being on this journey with us. We look forward to feedback regarding how we can improve this text and enhance its usefulness for interdisciplinary colleagues in all areas who have an interest in supporting families in their transition to new parenthood and incorporating key components to define and meet their infant feeding goals.

Some of the outstanding features of this text include:

- Framing breastfeeding as the ultimate health promotion option (strategy) globally
- Addressing intricacies of relational practice, patient-centered care, and mutual goal setting
- Providing theoretical frameworks to support health care practitioners' education of new parents
- Specific guidelines of international models that have worked
- Policy making and global perspectives that promote, initiate, and support breastfeeding
- Empowerment of health care practitioners to advocate for, support, and be present for new parents

Some pedagogical features of the chapters include the following:

- Chapter objectives
- Key terms and definitions
- Examples of research, policy, and programs
- Chapter summaries
- Questions for further learning
- Websites and accessible learning materials

In addition, chapters may include boxed items with key information, interdisciplinary applications, and evidence-informed practice: what current research indicates is needed for further research. Some chapters have also incorporated tables, illustrations, and assessment and evaluation instruments. In addition, where appropriate, teaching/learning points, counseling/clinical implications, and authors' real-life stories are incorporated.

Suzanne Hetzel Campbell
PhD, RN, IBCLC, CCSNE

References

Acheson, D. (1988). Public health in England: The Report of the Committee of Inquiry into the Future Development of the Public Health Function. London, UK: HMSO.

Brown, A. (2017). Breastfeeding as a public health responsibility: A review of the evidence. Journal of Human Nutrition and Dietetics, 30(6), 759–770. doi:10.1111/jhn.12496

Browne, A. J. (2017). Moving beyond description: Closing the health equity gap by redressing racism impacting indigenous populations. Social Science & Medicine, 184, 23–26. https://doi.org/10.1016/j.socscimed.2017.04.045

Cattaneo, A. (2012). Academy of breastfeeding medicine founder's lecture 2011: Inequalities and inequities in breastfeeding: An international perspective. Breastfeeding Medicine, 7(1), 3–9.

Gomez-Gallego, C., Garcia-Mantrana, I., Salminen, S., & Collado, M. C. (2016). The human milk microbiome and factors influencing its composition and activity. Seminars in Fetal and Neonatal Medicine, 21(6), 400–405. https://doi.org/10.1016/j.siny.2016.05.003

Kendall-Tackett, K. A. (2007). Violence against women and the perinatal period: The impact of lifetime violence and abuse on pregnancy, postpartum, and breastfeeding. Trauma, Volence, & Abuse, 8(3), 344–353.

Victora, C. G., Bahl, R., Barros, A. J. D., França, G. V. A., Horton, S., Krasevec, J., Murch, S., Sankar, M. J., Walker, N., & Rollins, N. C. (2016). Breastfeeding in the 21st century: Epidemiology, mechanisms, and lifelong effect. The Lancet, 387(10017), 475–490. doi:10.1016/S0140-6736(15)01024-7

WHO. (2018). Breastfeeding. Nutrition. http://www.who.int/nutrition/topics/exclusive_breastfeeding/en

Acknowledgments

No work is done in isolation, especially the completion of a book containing a life-time of experience, pain, and joy. First and foremost, thank you to the creative, passionate, and wise women who authored the chapters and shared their wisdom with our readers, as well as the reviewers who supported our goal to create this book.

The inspiration for this book comes from an adult lifetime of wise women; grandmothers; mothers; aunts; sisters (Kathy) and sisters-in-law (Carole, Pamela, Susie, and Lisa); women and men friends (Cathy, Nicky, Aimee & Phil); leaders; teachers; nurses; doctors; midwives; dieticians; social workers; pharmacists; and dare I say, so many health care professionals and other academic colleagues who have challenged me and my thinking. It is hard when completing a book such as this, which harnesses a life's journey that has been formulating and growing in me for so long, to find the right words and identify just who to thank and acknowledge... so many who I encountered, worked alongside, volunteered and served with, practice and taught (or was taught by) influenced my thinking and perceptions on lactation, parenthood, and health promotion.

I want to acknowledge the wise women at Mansfield Center's La Leche League International (Mary, Jan, and Pat), who sustained, role-modeled for, taught me while holding space for that "village" of support in my early days as a new parent, and mentored me into becoming a leader. Marilyn, my labor nurse with my daughter, who helped me nurse right after birth with baby skin-to-skin wisdom 30 years ago! My LLLI friends Gail and Denise who became family, and my BFF Donna who was a role model and sounding board. Without them, I'm certain my lactation experience would have ended prematurely. Next was my nutrition colleague Pat, at Willimantic WIC, who saw potential in me and helped create a similar safe space for breastfeeding support for WIC parents at that office, which led to engagement at the state level thanks to Susan Jackman, and eventually nationally thanks to Cathy Carothers and all the incredible WIC staff and clients in Connecticut and across the United States. Over almost a decade, I served alongside colleagues in the Connecticut Breastfeeding Coalition with Michelle Griswold, Jennifer Matranga, and so many others—Dr. Christina Smillie, Susan Iwinski, and the team at Breastfeeding Resources in Connecticut; my colleagues and friends at Fairfield University, especially in the School of Nursing; the International Lactation Consultant Association and colleagues; the brilliant board of directors I served with from 2006–2009 (especially Becky Mannel, Liz Brooks, Roberta Graham-Escobar, and Kathy Parkes); and the Lactation Education Approval and Accreditation Committee (Judi Lauwers, Becky Spencer, and Cheryl Benn) for their national and global leadership on behalf of lactation professionals and educators. These names include my co-editors of the *Core Curriculum for Interdisciplinary Lactation Care*, but acknowledgment of the authors and reviewers for that text is needed as well.

Since immigrating to Canada, my lactation colleagues and confidants have included the BC Lactation Consultants Association, especially Tina Revai, and the Baby-Friendly Network, especially Lea Geiger. At the University of British Columbia, I need to acknowledge the support and mentoring of the Faculty of Applied Science and School of Nursing, financial support for research and scholarship, support for innovative teaching, and global connections. Importantly, I want to thank all my colleagues in the UBC School of Nursing for the lens, wisdom, patience, and support they have given me to persevere—a special thank you to Sally Thorne, Wendy Hall, Colleen Varcoe, John Oliffe, Annette Brown, Elizabeth Saewyc, and Maura MacPhee for guiding me in the art of being curious, socially just, and mindful of equity and health promotion and for helping me find the words to present it through much of their own amazing scholarship. I want to acknowledge my graduate students Janet Currie, Damaris Grunert, and Thayanthini Tharmaratnam—part of my Lactation Research Team at UBC—and my visiting international research scholars Dr. Flaviana Vieira and Dr. Nicole Bernardes. Other mentors include Dr. Kerstin Hedberg Nyqist, who informed my knowledge and my student helper Caris Tin who supported me with proofing the book chapters and understanding of BFHI and Neo-BFHI in Brazil and Sweden; Dr. Joan Meek; and Dr. Laura N. Haiek. Thanks to Anna Sadovnikova and Sam Chuisano for making my dream of a lactation-simulation model come true with their LiquidGoldConcept. A shout out to my research committee from the University of Rhode Island School of Nursing; Dr. Jacqueline Fortin, and Dr. Susie Hesook-Kim, who supported me in my first exploration of health promotion theory, self-efficacy, and lactation; and Dr. Cheryl Beck and Dr. Peggy Chinn, who inspired me as a new faculty at the University of Connecticut and continue to inspire me as nurse researchers, theorists, philosophers, and scholars whose knowledge of nursing and emancipatory theories set me on the path to visualizing lactation as a foundational strategy for health promotion. We come full circle—from child to student to faculty and supervisor!

Sincere thanks to the team at JBL - Theresa for inspiring me to take on this project, Melina for continued support, and Pal and team who have made the editing and copy-editing happen. So many invisible hands behind the scene to reach this finished project!

Finally, and not least, I acknowledge all the parents, mothers, babies, children, students (nursing and interprofessional), national (United States and Canada), and international friends and colleagues who, along with my own children, have taught me "everything I needed to know about breastfeeding." To those family members, friends, and wise women in my lives (including new supports Dori, Nikki, and Cat and members of the White Raven Collective) and to all those I'm sure I have left out but did not mean to slight ... thank you!

PART 1

The context and Foundations of Lactation as Health Promotion

CHAPTER 1

Infant Feeding, Industrialization, and History

Jacqueline H. Wolf, Professor,
Department of Social Medicine, Ohio University

LEARNING OBJECTIVES

1. Describe the factors that have contributed historically to the use of artificial food for infants.
2. Outline the unique contributions of mothers, physicians, and infant food companies to the move away from breastfeeding and human milk and toward the use of bottles and animal milk.
3. Explain the effect on public health of changing infant feeding practices.

KEY WORDS

*   Breastfeeding, formula, artificial food, history, industrialization, infant feeding, infant food companies, formula industry, mothers, pediatricians, public health, urbanization

Overview

Isaac Abt, a Chicago pediatrician practicing in the late 19th and early 20th centuries, examined thousands of sick, bottle-fed infants during his long career. He described them as "so emaciated that they looked like ancient, wrinkled dwarfs." Distressingly, he had no effective treatment to offer them. As he explained, the babies did not lack food. Rather, "they lacked the right food. Some of them rallied when they were put on breast milk, but the majority died" (Abt, 1944, p. 43).

The **artificial foods** sickening bottle-fed infants at the end of the 19th century were varied. They included raw cows' milk; homemade concoctions consisting of puréed table scraps, cows' milk, and water; and the commercial infant foods (to be mixed with cows' milk or water) that had become increasingly available in the

United States since the end of the Civil War; during the war, canned cows' milk had been provided to soldiers. In their advertising, the manufacturers of these "foods" focused on denigrating the other commercially prepared infant products rather than claiming that their particular creation was superior to human milk. Indeed, all the advertising consistently paid homage, either directly or indirectly, to mother's milk.

Lactated Food (wheat, partially predigested barley malt, phosphate of lime, and milk sugar) "Brought [babies] Past the Danger Time" when they were not breastfed. The Nestlé's Food company advised, "Nurse your baby if you can. If you can't, give it the nearest thing to mother's milk—Nestlé's Food." An ad for Eskay's Albumenized Food (eggs, barley, oats, wheat, and milk sugar) described what was likely to befall an artificially fed infant who consumed any product other than Eskay's: "From three weeks to four months about every artificial food but ESKAY's was tried and utterly failed, and the child wasted away to a shadow. Whooping cough, Meningitis and Pneumonia followed, and finally, when almost dying of Cholera Infantum [the 19th-century term for infant diarrhea], all hope of recovery was given up. He had to be carried on a pillow, and his little bones were almost through his skin. At five months he weighed less than six pounds" (Wolf, 2001, pp. 162–166, quotes on 164 and 165).

Pediatricians Respond to the Crisis

Artificially fed infants contributed heavily to the 13% infant mortality rate in the United States in 1900. That year, more than 50% of the children who died before their first birthday died of diarrhea (Wolf, 2001). The Chicago Department of Health estimated that artificially fed infants died at a 15-to-1 ratio when compared to breastfed infants (Davis, 1910). **Pediatricians** responded to the crisis, in part, by spearheading what they called "the certified milk movement" to provide free, unadulterated cows' milk to the sick, bottle-fed babies they were seeing daily in their medical practices. Certified milk, by definition, was pasteurized milk produced according to the strict standards set by certified milk commissions. Pediatricians and **public health** workers regularly inspected these certified dairy farms and established "certified milk stations" in large cities to distribute the product in sterilized bottles (Wasserman, 1972).

Beginnning in the 1890s, pediatricians also created urban "milk laboratories" where chemists "humanized" cows' milk according to the unique mathematical formula written by a pediatrician for a particular baby. These 19th-century mathematical formulas are the source of the word **formula** as used today to refer to standardized human milk substitutes. Doctors based each formula on variables that included, but were not limited to, an infant's age, height, weight, "energy expenditure," pallor, texture of stools, color of stools, and medical diagnoses such as "protein digestion weak." Each formula dictated the ratio of fat, protein, and sugar deemed optimal in a particular baby's food (Allen, 1908).

A mother would bring her infant's formula, written on paper by a pediatrician, to a chemist at the local milk laboratory; the chemist would then tweak cows' milk according to the instructions conveyed by the formula. Each formula was dizzyingly complex. "W12, P5, R7¼, whole milk r = 4¼ E = 5 x 7¼ = 36¼ Milk = 12 × 5/4 = 15 oz. Sugar = 12 × 5 × 3 = 1.8 oz. Water = 12 × 2.5 - 15 = 15 oz." is an example of a formula written by a pediatrician in 1908, the meaning of which has been lost to posterity (Allen, 1908).

Pediatricians sought to solve a serious public health problem with their formula-writing. **Mothers** appeared to have abandoned their long-time **breastfeeding** habits in favor of artificial feeding. In response, pediatricians wondered: Can we formulate an adequate substitute given the sudden dearth of human milk? This question became so central to pediatricians' professional identity that between 1900 and 1915, members of the American Pediatric Society presented 90 papers on the topic at annual meetings (Wolf, 2006a).

In a brief **history** of **infant feeding** presented to the American Pediatric Society in honor of the organization's 50th anniversary in 1938, Chicago pediatrician Joseph Brennemann recalled the heyday of "scientific" infant feeding, when mathematical formulas were the very foundation of pediatrics. "It became increasingly more complicated and involved as ever . . . so-called 'simpler' methods of calculation appeared until . . . some of the articles [in medical journals explaining how to write formulas] seemed terrifyingly like treatises on mathematics or higher astronomy" (Brennemann, 1938, p. 65).

Despite Brennemann's amusing evaluation of the formula-writing era of American pediatrics, pediatricians' ability to respond to what they quickly termed *the feeding question* helped them to garner professional respect. Before pediatricians took up infant feeding as part of the nationwide campaign in the late 19th-century to lower infant mortality, other physicians persistently denigrated pediatricians as "baby doctors." Parents, who judged doctors by their ability to treat adults, similarly dismissed the need for pediatricians. Thus, despite Joseph Brennemann's entertaining epitaph for the original "formulas," medicalizing infant feeding became pediatricians' entry into both the medical profession and the wider world of mothers and children (Wolf, 2006a).

A Dearth of Human Milk

As the focus of late 19th-century American pediatricians suggests, mothers' infant feeding practices changed dramatically during the last quarter of the 19th century. In the 17th and 18th centuries, mothers of European origin in the American British colonies customarily breastfed their infants through at least their baby's second summer. In an era before refrigerators, pasteurized milk, filtered water, and acceptance of the germ theory of disease, breastfeeding for at least 2 years ensured that human milk was available to rescue an infant or toddler sickened by tainted water or cows' milk or by spoiled adult foods. Thus, through much of the 19th century, most mothers adhered to the custom of breastfeeding for at least 2 years (Salmon, 1994).

By the end of the 19th century, however, change in mothers' traditional breastfeeding habits was manifest. Weaning infants by 3 months of age had become common. Many mothers never breastfed exclusively for any amount of time, supplementing their milk with raw cows' milk or commercially manufactured infant food almost immediately after giving birth. Women offered a uniform explanation for this change: their milk was not up to the task of sustaining their infants. Claims of not-enough or not-good-enough milk were so ubiquitous by 1889 that New England physicians estimated that more than half of American mothers were unable "to properly nurse their offspring" (The Decline of Suckling Power, 1889).

Early weaning and, occasionally, failure to breastfeed at all were seldom mothers' deliberate choices, however. Most women were heartbroken by their inability to adequately breastfeed. When a baby died of diarrhea as a result of artificial feeding, the death was a tragedy beyond measure. In a letter to a popular infant care magazine in 1887, one mother explained the dilemma many women faced: "I cannot refrain from a protest against the injustice done to the mothers of this generation in the way in which they are constantly accused of refusing to nurse their children either from selfishness or laziness, whereas in all of the cases I have known (and they are many) it has invariably been the mother's misfortune and not her fault" (The Mother's Parliament, 1887).

A change in the advice meted out in infant care manuals hints at why so many mothers began to complain of inadequate milk. In the 17th century, women learned to breastfeed according to their infants' cues: "As to the time and hour it needs no limits, for it may be at any time, night or day, when he hath a mind" (Salmon, 1994). In the early 19th century, breastfeeding advice became more explicit, but not overtly so: "The younger the baby, the shorter should be the interval from one feeding time to another" and "allow the baby to continue nursing until it voluntarily ceases" were common recommendations. By the last quarter of the 19th century, however, when mothers began to complain of milk insufficiency, prevailing advice had become strikingly different. Mothers were learning that an infant fed according to a precise schedule "become[s] a creature of habit, and consequently will be less troublesome to care for and will be far more comfortable and happy" (Wolf, 2001, p. 32). By the early 20th century, that sort of advice was universal and unambiguous. The Chicago Department of Health warned mothers that "Spoiling the baby often begins in the first few days. *Doing things by the clock* develops the habit of doing things on time and at the same time makes a baby with good habits" (Bundesen, 1926).

Sweeping Social Change

This change in infant feeding advice reflected sweeping social change. Rapid urbanization and **industrialization** had transformed American life. Until the last quarter of the 19th century, the United States had been a largely rural country, where most citizens lived according to nature's rhythms—the sunrise signaled the start of the day, for example. But with industrialization, life came to be governed by the mechanical clock. With the arrival of the railroad in particular, Americans had to pay attention to artificial, but precise, moments in time. To get their produce to market, farmers had to ensure that their goods were on the railroad platform in advance of the train's arrival. Urban dwellers accustomed to working at home—sewing, or cooking for others, or boarding single men—found themselves increasingly enmeshed in factory work, and so they, too, had to adapt to the mechanical clock to ensure their timely arrival at work. The need to be somewhere at an exact, predetermined time, unrelated to any natural occurrence, transformed not only daily life but also basic cultural values (Wolf, 2001).

The change in attitude toward time affected infant feeding practices particularly and profoundly. Adults, most of whom were having difficulty adjusting to the tyranny of the clock, vowed that their children would learn to adhere to schedules from birth. Even the Women's Christian Temperance Union (WCTU) used their concern about alcohol abuse to jump on the infant-feeding-schedule bandwagon. Mary Wood-Allen, the editor of *New Crusade*, the WCTU's popular national women's magazine, advised that alcoholism, tobacco use, and drug addiction had their origins in "vicious feeding" in infancy. Infants taught self-control via feeding schedules, however, would never succumb to addiction as adults (Wood-Allen, 1895, 1896). The alleged benefits of adopting feeding schedules abounded. Mothers were even told that if they fed babies at precisely the same time each day, they would be able to hold them over the chamber pot at predictable times, eliminating the need for diapers and the onerous task of laundering diapers, as early as 6 weeks of age (Mellin's Food Company, 1907).

Yet a mother's milk supply is based on her baby's demand for her milk. Nipple stimulation is key—the more frequently an infant sucks on their mother, the more milk the mother's body produces. Thus, with even newborns being put to the breast only at specified, widely spaced times, and often kept from the breast altogether at night, women began to complain of insufficient milk. This was not the sole reason for women's reported inability to breastfeed, but it was likely a primary reason.

Other factors prompting the move to artificial food were largely class based. Working-class mothers increasingly worked outside the home. Consequently, they were forced to turn infant care over to older children who had no choice but to bottle-feed their tiny siblings. Wealthy women depended on servants for infant care, and this often precluded breastfeeding. The middle-class marriage, historically a financially based institution focused almost exclusively on economic stability and procreation, was becoming an institution based largely on affection and intimacy. Middle-class men and women alike began to elevate the sexual function of breasts above their physiological function (Wolf, 2001).

The Medicalization of Infant Feeding

Although change in cultural practices and values was the cause of human milk insufficiency, the pediatricians treating sick, artificially fed infants assumed that mothers' complaints of inadequate milk had a physiological basis. Medical theories for lactation failure (or, more accurately, as historians recognize today, *perceived* lactation failure) proliferated. Some physicians argued that "civilization"—a reference to urbanization—had weakened women and destroyed their ability to lactate (Allen, 1889). Others argued it was a matter of heredity. Abt explained in the *Chicago Tribune* in 1904, "Women tend to inherit from their mothers the disability to nurse their offspring, from which it will be seen that the race will eventually suffer from this incapacity, and the nursing function is destined gradually to disappear" (Abt, 1904). By 1910, women's ongoing reports of lactation failure prompted attendees at child welfare conferences to discuss how to handle what appeared to be the next step in human evolution: the inability to lactate (Levenstein, 1983). Still other doctors blamed public education. With girls now attending school longer, some physicians posited that girls' overworked brains were snatching the energy their bodies needed for adequate physical growth during puberty. Difficulty bearing children and failure to lactate upon reaching adulthood were deemed to be two consequences of "overeducating" girls (Clarke, 1873).

With infant feeding now defined as an intractable medical problem, pediatricians joined public health officials to spearhead the Progressive Era crusade to "Save the Babies." This campaign to lower infant mortality focused in large part on infant feeding and called for four simultaneous activities: teaching women that a high infant death was not inevitable but largely preventable, urging women to breastfeed, providing certified milk to the babies whose mothers did not breastfeed, and, because there were not enough dairy farmers willing to adhere to certified milk provisions, pressing for legislation to clean up the dairy industry in order to make clean, unadulterated cows' milk a widely available commodity.

To convey the first two messages, public health workers targeted urban neighborhoods with the highest infant death rates. Visiting nurses traversed streets to talk to new mothers about infant care and feeding. Workers hung heavily illustrated public health posters on the sides of buildings. If the neighborhood housed immigrants, the posters were printed in up to eight different languages. One poster, designed to teach mothers how to prevent infant death, was headlined, "The Preventable Perils Surrounding the Child," and illustrated many of those dangers, including "dirty milk;" the "tuberculous cow;" "foul air;" and childhood diseases such as measles, diphtheria, and scarlet fever (See **Figure 1-1**).

Placards urging mothers to breastfeed were equally ubiquitous. One headlined "Mother's Milk for Mother's Baby, Cow's Milk for Calves," urged "To Lessen Baby Deaths Let Us Have More Mother-Fed Babies. You can't improve on God's plan. For Your Baby's Sake—Nurse It!" and vividly illustrated the hazardous path of cows' milk from careless dairy farmer; to sunny, hot railroad platform; to unrefrigerated railcars; to urban consumer—as opposed to the safe, short, clean route from mother's breast to infant's mouth (Wolf, 2001). (See **Figure 1-2**)

The Milk Wars

By far the longest and most ubiquitous of the efforts to "save the babies," however, was the 40-year crusade to clean up the dairy industry. From roughly the 1880s through the 1920s, public health workers, pediatricians, and citizen-activists living in U.S. municipalities campaigned for tough laws to ensure that all milk sold to the public was pure. Before passage of those laws, cows' milk was the most significant contributor to the high infant death rate. Dairy farmers shipped milk in 8-gallon, uncovered vats that invited adulteration. To increase profits, farmers, shippers, and merchants often added water to the milk. If the milk began to turn gray, as it often did with exposure to dust and dirt, someone along the route would add powdered chalk to the milk to whiten it. Milk was not homogenized in that era, so after the farmer, shipper, or merchant skimmed cream from the top to sell at a premium, plaster would be added to the milk to thicken it and make it appear "whole" (rich with cream) again. After the dubious substance reached stores, merchants placed ladles in the vats so wary customers could sample the milk before placing it into their own vessels. In this way, diphtheria, tuberculosis, typhoid, and scarlet fever, among other illnesses, became milk-borne diseases (Wolf, 2001).

For years, urban newspapers featured the crusade to clean up the urban cows' milk supply, dubbing the crusade the "milk wars." Reporters lamented infants "gone to a premature grave because . . . [their] cry for milk was unwittingly answered by a supply of a weak, unnutritious mixture. . . . Could a proper death certificate be made out many an entry of 'cholera infantum' would be changed to starvation from being fed on watered milk" (Chicago Milk, 1892). Chicago's fight for clean milk was typical of the battle in other cities. Infant diarrhea and its near 100% death rate slowly ebbed in Chicago with each piece of legislation that ended an egregious

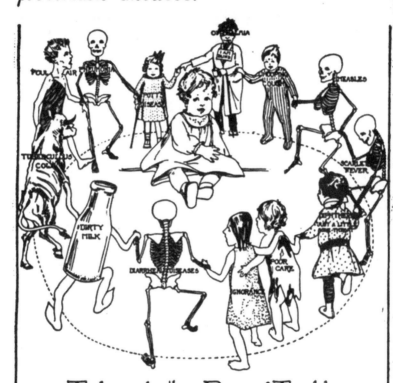

Figure 1-1 "The Preventable Perils Surrounding the Child."

One initiative of the Progressive Era baby-saving campaigns was to teach mothers that infant death was largely preventable rather than, as mothers and even public officials believed at the time, too often inevitable. *Bulletin Chicago School of Sanitary Instruction,* May 18, 1912, p. 80.

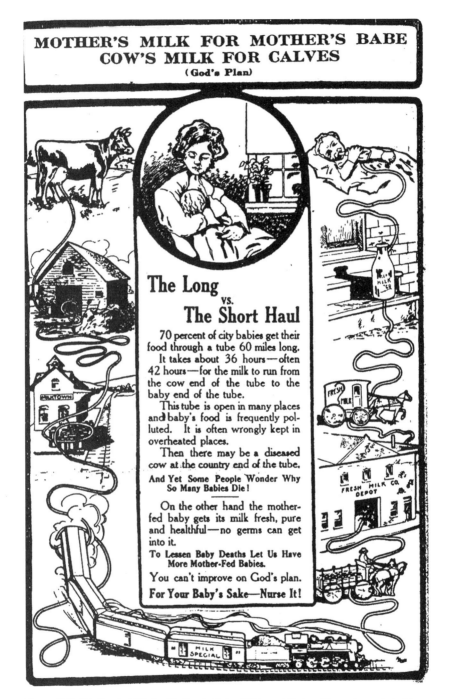

Figure 1-2 "Mother's Milk for Mother's Babe." This public health poster, printed in Chicago in eight different languages, explained in words and drawing why feeding cows' milk to infants was so dangerous.

Bulletin Chicago School of Sanitary Instruction, June 3, 1911 .

dairy industry practice. In 1904, the city ordered that all milk vats be sealed during shipping. In 1912, the city banned the vat shipping method altogether, mandating that milk be sold in individual bottles. In 1916, Chicago's public health officials directed that milk be pasteurized before bottling. By 1920, milk had to be kept cold during shipping. In 1926, Illinois ordered that all dairy cattle be tested for bovine tuberculosis and that any cow testing positive be destroyed (Wolf, 2001). Before passage, the public health rationale for the law was vividly illustrated on a public health poster. (See **Figure 1-3**)

The Paradox of Victory

The paradox of reformers' victories was that the triumphs of the milk wars seemed to solve the problems posed by the use of cows' milk as the primary food for human infants. Thus, in regulating the dairy industry to the benefit of infant and child health, pediatricians and public health officials also unintentionally downgraded the importance of human milk to human health. Forty years of well-publicized pleas for clean cows' milk in order to "save the babies" gave two generations of mothers the distinct impression that cows' milk was an indispensable food for their children. With cows' milk finally an ostensibly safe substance, breastfeeding appeared to be unnecessary.

By the late 1920s, compared to just two decades earlier, artificial feeding seemed to pose little danger. Milk was now bottled and pasteurized, the railroad cars used for shipping were refrigerated, and most homes had "ice boxes" and daily deliveries from the ice man. As one physician explained in the early 1930s, "Except for conferring certain immunity, all other requirements for feeding the baby are more easily met by a formula than by breast feeding." This doctor was not alone in thinking that the benefits of pasteurized cows' milk now outweighed any advantages of what seemed to be mercurial human milk. "Many uncontrollable factors enter into breastfeeding," the doctor complained, while cows' milk could be counted on to "produce consistently normal growth and development" in infants and children (Are Infant Feeding Methods Changing, 1931). By 1972, breastfeeding initiation rates in the United States—with "initiation" defined as breastfeeding once before hospital discharge, an extremely low bar—had plummeted to 22% (Ryan et al., 1991).

With such low breastfeeding initiation rates, several successive generations of women had no opportunity to learn about breastfeeding. There was no information or shared experience to pass from mothers to daughters, grandmothers to granddaughters, between sisters, or among friends. Nor did women have the chance to observe other women breastfeeding. Breastfeeding was no longer on the cultural map. For all practical purposes, it ceased to be an infant-feeding option.

A Resurgence of Breastfeeding

As the breastfeeding initiation rate reached its nadir in 1972, however, an energetic and effective women's health reform movement appeared. This crusade was an offshoot of the broader fight for women's rights that transformed the cultural landscape in the 1970s. Feminist activists in health reform wrested control of women's reproductive health from paternalistic doctors, altering medicine in the United States in

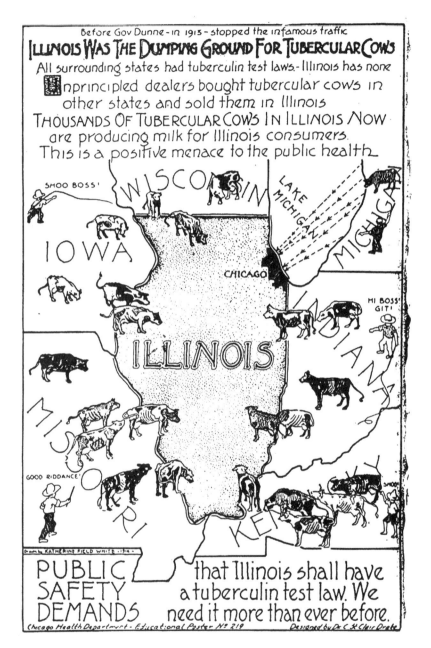

Figure 1-3 "Illinois Was the Dumping Ground."

For years, states surrounding Illinois had laws mandating that dairy cattle be tested for bovine tuberculosis and that any cow testing positive for the disease be destroyed. Because Illinois had no such law, however, rather than destroy a sick cow, dairy farmers in other states simply sold their sick cattle to farmers in Illinois. This public health poster alerts the public to the problem, effectively explaining the public health rationale for a proposed tuberculin test law in Illinois. *Bulletin Chicago School of Sanitary Instruction*, May 2, 1914, p. 78.

many ways that benefitted women and children. Surgeons were forced to alter the protocol for breast cancer diagnosis and treatment (Lerner, 2003). Gynecologists adopted safer and more effective methods of contraception (Watkins, 1998). Researchers began to include women in clinical trials (Merkatz et al., 1993; Merton, 1993). And obstetricians responded to pressure to change longtime, invasive childbirth practices. Stand-alone birth centers, homey birthing rooms in hospitals, meaningful companionship during labor, certified nurse-midwives, abandonment of routine episiotomy, and an end to assorted analgesics during first-stage labor and mandatory general anesthesia during second-stage labor were all offered to pregnant women in response to feminist demands for a more humane, less medicalized approach to childbirth (Wolf, 2009). Along with the interest in "natural" childbirth came a rising breastfeeding rate. By 1982, 62% of mothers initiated breastfeeding—a 182% increase over the initiation rate just 10 years earlier (Ryan et al., 1991)

Yet despite women's renewed interest in breastfeeding just as they began to enter the workforce outside the home in significant numbers, there was no corresponding change in societal infrastructure to support the working mothers who wanted to breastfeed. Breastfeeding did not receive the same attention, from either the media or feminist health reformers, that childbirth did. Although an early edition of the best-selling feminist health manifesto *Our Bodies, Ourselves* contained 62 pages on pregnancy, birth, and postpartum care, the same edition contained barely 2 pages on breastfeeding (Boston Women's Health Book Collective, 1976). Although local and national organizations abounded to lobby for more humane approaches to childbirth (Wolf, 2009), efforts to educate women about the value of breastfeeding and human milk, and to mitigate the factors contributing to women's inability to successfully breastfeed, were largely absent from the agenda of feminist health reformers' (Wolf, 2006b).

Far more influential in the breastfeeding arena than the women's health reform movement was La Leche League (LLL), a voluntary organization that began in a Chicago suburb in 1956 after seven friends who had successfully breastfed began to offer woman-to-woman support and advice to others who wanted to breastfeed. LLL support groups burgeoned around the country. The organization's tome, *The Womanly Art of Breastfeeding*, sold more than a million copies of its 1963 second edition (La Leche League, 1963). Yet the League, too, failed to demand the social supports needed by women to successfully breastfeed in the face of enormous social change. While LLL helped bring breastfeeding to the fore of mothers' consciousness for the first time in decades, the organization also found itself at loggerheads with the budding women's movement (Weiner, 1994; Wolf, 2001).

In 1976, only 31% of women with children under 1 year of age worked outside the home; by the 1990s, 59% did (Blackwelder, 1997). As women moved into the workforce in unprecedented numbers, however, LLL decried the move of mothers away from the full-time care of their children (Weiner, 1994). This twin failure—of feminists active in women's health reform to focus on breastfeeding as a reproductive right, and of breastfeeding advocates, particularly in LLL, to fight for laws, such as nationwide, mandatory paid maternity leave to aid working mothers who wanted to breastfeed—portended scant improvement in breastfeeding rates beyond initiation.

To encourage mothers to breastfeed, and when they did breastfeed to breastfeed for far longer, and to make pediatricians aware of the importance of human milk to human health, the American Academy of Pediatrics (AAP) issued well-publicized breastfeeding guidelines in 1997. The guidelines advised mothers to breastfeed their infants exclusively for 6 months, to continue breastfeeding for at least 1 year as they introduce solid foods, and to breastfeed "thereafter for as long as mutually desired" by mother and baby. The AAP has updated its recommendations since then, most recently in 2012 (AAP, 1997, 2012). Breastfeeding initiation rates kept rising. In 2011, 79% of American mothers initiated breastfeeding (Centers for Disease Control and Prevention [CDC], National Center for Chronic Disease Prevention and Health Promotion, 2014). In 2015, 83.2% did (CDC, 2019).

Despite the improvement in the breastfeeding initiation rate, however, the number is deceptive. While more than 80% of U.S. mothers now initiate breastfeeding, only 25% exclusively breastfeed for 6 months, and only 40% continue to breastfeed for the minimal year (CDC, 2018a, 2018b). In other words, a minority of mothers adhere to the AAP guidelines.

Nevertheless, breastfeeding initiation rates are the only numbers that the media publicizes annually, largely because Ross Products Division of Abbott Laboratories—the manufacturer of Similac—has long conducted an annual survey to determine the breastfeeding initiation rate in the United States (Ryan et al., 2002). Announcing the initiation rate annually to great fanfare is in Abbott Laboratories' interest. As the largest manufacturer of infant formula in the United States, Abbott appears socially responsible by tracking, announcing, and celebrating what looks like progress in increasing the number of breastfed infants each year. Yet in setting itself up as the most visible statistician of U.S. breastfeeding practices, Abbott defines the parameters of data collection—at least the numbers reported by the media. When improved initiation rates become the goal, the public effectively learns that only breastfeeding initiation matters. The implication of that message is that if a baby has been breastfed, no matter how little, supplementation with formula is inconsequential. This message creates a sizeable market for infant formula, even among breastfeeding mothers (Wolf, 2006b).

The Diabolical Formula Industry

The infant **formula industry** has found other diabolical ways to increase market share. As higher breastfeeding initiation rates in wealthy countries began to diminish profits, formula companies devised plans to maintain—even grow—their revenues by marketing their products in developing countries. The Nestlé Company developed a particularly effective strategy. They hired women to dress in white outfits resembling nurses' uniforms and distribute samples of formula for free to new mothers in developing countries. Mothers gratefully accepted the food for their newborns from the saleswomen who, mothers assumed, were medical professionals, only to find their supply of breast milk waning because they had skipped feedings in favor of the free samples. Forced to purchase formula, a product that consumed 50% or more of their weekly income, impoverished mothers watered the food to make it more affordable. In some areas, nonpotable water made formula feeding even more dangerous (Herman, 1980; Muller, 1974).

With babies in developing countries increasingly suffering from starvation and diarrhea, the World Health Organization (WHO) and UNICEF condemned Nestlé's marketing practices as potentially lethal (Herman, 1980). One European pediatrician who had worked in assorted African, Asian, and Latin American countries explained the problem clearly. "Adequate and relatively safe bottle feeding must follow, or at least accompany, but never precede, literacy, education, infection-free water supplies, sanitation and a standard of living which permits the purchase of enough baby foods, equipment and the means of sterilization" (Muller, 1974, p. 8).

The effects of Nestlé's strategy went well beyond the tragedy of increased infant mortality. The number of children affected by formula feeding overtaxed entire national healthcare systems. To counteract Nestlé's schemes (Muller, 1974), countries such as Colombia, Indonesia, Brazil, Thailand, and Mexico began to conduct nationwide breastfeeding campaigns (Hall, 1982), not unlike the campaigns devised by the United States in the late 19th century. But impoverished countries could not muster sufficient funds to counteract the ubiquitous, slick advertising of formula companies.

In 1977, activists in industrialized countries stepped in to help by forming the Infant Formula Action Coalition (INFACT), comprised of national and international religious, labor, and women's organizations. INFACT called for a boycott of all Nestlé products worldwide. The boycott had enormous impact. By 1980, the importance of breastfeeding had become the number-one issue brought before the World Health Assembly (WHA) by an unprecedented number of countries. In 1982, the American Public Health Association endorsed the international boycott of Nestlé products (Hall, 1982; Palmer, 1988).

As the story of deceptive marketing of infant formula in the developing world attests, a mother's decision about how to feed her infant, like most health choices, is not purely voluntary. Although the consequences of formula feeding are not as serious in industrialized countries as in developing countries because potable water is common in industrialized countries and social safety nets often subsidize mothers who need economic help, the United States is currently the only developed country lacking nationwide legislation mandating paid maternity leave for mothers who have infants and work outside the home (Kim, 2015). This makes breastfeeding difficult, even for the mothers living in the United States who prioritize breastfeeding (Rossin, 2011).

Controversies Remain Ongoing

Today, breastfeeding is just as contentious as any other women's reproductive health issue in the United States. The divide over legalized abortion is the best known. But the *Burwell v. Hobby Lobby* U.S. Supreme Court decision spotlighted disagreement over the use of contraception. Natural childbirth in the 1970s was also controversial—proponents characterized birth without medical intervention as empowering; detractors termed it barbaric. For decades, discussion about breastfeeding has been equally hyperbolic. One scholar, a political scientist whose 2011 book questioning the efficacy of breastfeeding received a good deal of publicity, charges that the value of breastfeeding has been exaggerated and that the high costs to mothers who breastfeed have been ignored. In building her case against the value of breastfeeding, she engaged in hyperbole tinged by hysteria, accusing breastfeeding advocates of fear mongering, unethical behavior, and "lobbying for their cause with a single-minded zeal that borders on monomania" (Wolf, 2011). Similarly polarizing rhetoric about breastfeeding, often focusing on "breastfeeding in public" (Wolf, 2008) or characterizing breastfeeding advocates as "fanatics," also appears periodically in popular magazines, receiving widespread, if fleeting, publicity (Rosin, 2009).

Today, much like in the late 19th century when women began to move from breast to bottle, we are once again in the midst of a vast, uncontrolled infant feeding experiment. Women who want to continue to supply human milk to their infants, even after returning to work full time, now commonly pump and store their milk to be fed to their infant later via a bottle by a caretaker. Yet few studies have been done on the effects of this relatively new infant feeding practice, even though researchers predict that pumped milk probably does not provide the same benefits to either infant or mother as feeding directly at the breast (Felice et al., 2017; O'Sullivan et al., 2017).

In the late 19th century, the medical community recognized breastfeeding as a public health imperative that postively impacted children's lives. Reverting to that perspective would be helpful today. Rather than receiving periodic attention primarily as a contentious, polarizing activity, breastfeeding deserves recognition not only as a public health priority but also as a women's and children's rights issue (Ball, 2010; Kent, 2006). Although much has changed since the annual infant mortality rate in the United States was 13%, largely due to artificial feeding, today breastfeeding and human milk continue to contribute immeasurably to infant, child, and adult health even in the sanitized environments of developed countries. In developing countries, breastfeeding remains essential for the maintenance of infants' and children's health. Mothers' ability to fully breastfeed their infants remains a cornerstone of a healthy and happy society; endeavors to maximize women's ability to successfully breastfeed remain ongoing.

Key Points to Remember

1. The economic, social, and cultural change that accompanied industrialization and urbanization contributed to changing infant feeding practices.
2. The switch from mothers breastfeeding their infants to bottle-feeding infants animal milk detrimentally affected infants' and children's health in the 19th century and greatly increased infant mortality.
3. As women returned to breastfeeding in wealthy, industrialized countries in the 1970s, the formula industry began marketing artificial baby milk in developing countries, sickening and killing infants and children in those nations and overwhelming public health systems.
4. Women's right to breastfeed and infants' and children's right to access human milk should be a top public health priority in all cultures and countries; breastfeeding is essential to maintain societal well-being and infants', children's, women's and families' health.

References

Abt, I. A. (1904, April 24). Domestic science conducted by the School of Domestic Arts and Sciences of Chicago Lesson No. 212—Milk Commission. *Chicago Tribune*, 16.

Abt, I. A. (1944). *Baby Doctor*. McGraw-Hill Book Company.

Allen, N. (1889, March). Laws of maternity. *Babyhood, 5*, 111–113.

Allen, T. G. (1908, September). Some observations necessary to successful infant feeding. *Chicago Medical Recorder, 30*, 496–503.

American Academy of Pediatrics. (1997). Breastfeeding and the use of human milk. *Pediatrics, 100,* 1035–1039. https://doi.org/10.1542/peds.2011-3552

American Academy of Pediatrics. (2012). Breastfeeding and the use of human milk. *Pediatrics, 129,* e827–e841. https://doi.org/10.1542/peds.2011-3552

Are infant feeding methods changing? (1931). *Public Health Nursing, 23,* 581–585.

Ball, O. (2010). Breastmilk is a human right. *Breastfeeding Review, 18,* 9–19.

Blackwelder, J. K. (1997). *Now hiring: The feminization of work in the United States, 1900–1995.* Texas A&M University Press.

Boston Women's Health Book Collective. (1976). *Our bodies, ourselves: A book by and for women.* Simon and Schuster.

Brennemann, J. (1938). Periods in the life of the American Pediatric Society: Adolescence, 1900–1915. *Transactions of the American Pediatric Society, 50,* 56–67.

Bundesen, H. N. (1926, April 27). Baby's first month. *Chicago's Health, 20,* 120.

Centers for Disease Control and Prevention. (2018a). *CDC Releases 2018 Breastfeeding Report Card.* https://www.cdc.gov/media/releases/2018/p0820-breastfeeding-report-card.html

Centers for Disease Control and Prevention. (2018b). *Breastfeeding Report Card, United States, 2018.* https://www.cdc.gov/breastfeeding/data/reportcard.htm

Centers for Disease Control and Prevention, National Center for Chronic Disease Prevention and Health Promotion. (2014). *Breastfeeding Report Card United States.* http://www.cdc.gov/breastfeeding/pdf/2014breastfeedingreportcard.pdf

Chicago Milk. (1892, September 30). *Chicago Inter Ocean,* 4.

Clarke, E. H. (1873). *Sex in education; or, a fair chance for girls.* James R. Osgood & Co.

Davis, E. V. (1910, June 18). Breast feeding. *Bulletin Chicago School of Sanitary Instruction,* 2.

Felice, J. P., Geraghty, S. R., Quaglieri, C. W., Yamada, R., Wong, A. J., & Rasmussen, K. M. (2017, July). "Breastfeeding" but not at the breast: Mothers' descriptions of providing pumped milk to their infants via other containers and caregivers. *Maternal & Child Nutrition, 13,* e12425–e12434. https://doi.org/10.1111/mcn.12425

Hall, M. J. (1982, August). The Nestle Boycott: Background and Issues. *Pennsylvania Nurse, 37,* 4.

Herman, N. K. (1980, September/October). Bottle babies: The Nestlé boycott. The bottle baby scandal. *RNAO News.*

Kent, G. (2006). Child feeding and human rights. *International Breastfeeding Journal, 1,* 27. https://doi.org/10.1186/1746-4358-1-27

Kim, S. (2015, May 6). *US is only industrialized nation without paid maternity leave.* ABC News. http://abcnews.go.com/Business/us-industrialized-nation-paid-maternity-leave/story?id=30852419

La Leche League International, (1963). *The womanly art of breastfeeding.* LLLI.

Lerner, B. (2003.) *The breast cancer wars: Hope, fear, and the pursuit of a cure in twentieth-century America.* Oxford University Press.

Levenstein, H. (1983, June). 'Best for babies' or 'Preventable infanticide'? The controversy over artificial feeding of infants in America, 1880–1920. *Journal of American History, 70,* 75–94.

Mellin's Food Company. (1907). *Diet after weaning: A manual for the care and feeding of children between the ages of one and two years.*

Merkatz, R., Temple, R., Sobel, S., Feiden, K. Kessler, D., & Working Group on Women in Clinical Trials. (1993, July 22). Women in clinical trials of new drugs: A change in Food and Drug Administration Policy. *New England Journal of Medicine, 329,* 292–293. https://doi.org/10.1056/NEJM199307223290429

Merton, V. (1993). The exclusion of pregnant, pregnable, and once-pregnable people (aka women) from biomedical research. *American Journal of Law and Medicine, 19,* 369–444.

Muller, M. (1974, March). *The baby killer: A War on Want investigation into the promotion and sale of powdered baby milks in the Third World.* War on Want.

O'Sullivan, E. G., Geraghty, S. R., & Rasmussen, K. M. (2017, July). Human milk expression as a sole or ancillary strategy for infant feeding: A qualitative study. *Maternal & Child Nutrition, 13,* e12332–e12345. https://doi.org/10.1111/mcn.12332

Palmer, G. (1988). *The politics of breastfeeding.* Pandora.

Rosin, H. (2009, April). *The case against breastfeeding.* The Atlantic. https://www.theatlantic.com/magazine/archive/2009/04/the-case-against-breast-feeding/307311/.

Rossin, M. (2011). The effects of maternity leave on children's birth and infant health outcomes in the United States. *Journal of Health Economics, 30,* 221–239. https://doi.org/10.1016/j .jhealeco.2011.01.005

Ryan, A. S., Rush, D., Krieger, F. W., Lewandowski, & G. E. (1991, October). Recent declines in breastfeeding in the United States. *Pediatrics, 88,* 719–727. https://pubmed.ncbi.nlm.nih .gov/1896274/

Ryan, A. S., Wenjun, Z. & Acosta, A. (2002). Breastfeeding continues to increase into the new mil-lennium. *Pediatrics, 110,* 1103–1109. https://doi.org/10.1542/peds.110.6.1103

Salmon, M. (1994, Winter). The cultural significance of breastfeeding and infant care in early mod-ern England and America. *Journal of Social History, 28,* 247–269.

"The decline of suckling power among American women." (1889, March). *Babyhood, 5,* 111–115.

"The mother's parliament." (1887, October). *Babyhood, 3,* 383–388.

Wasserman, M. J. (1972, July–August). Henry L. Coit and the certified milk movement in the devel-opment of modern pediatrics. *Bulletin of the History of Medicine, 42,* 359–390.

Watkins, E. S. (1998.) *On the pill: A social history of oral contraceptives, 1950–1970.* Johns Hopkins University Press.

Weiner, L. Y. (1994). Reconstructing motherhood: The La Leche League in postwar America. *Jour-nal of American History, 80,* 1357–1381.

Wolf, J. B. (2011). *Is breast best? Taking on the breastfeeding experts and the new high stakes of mother-hood.* New York University Press.

Wolf, J. H. (2001). *Don't kill your baby: Public health and the decline of breastfeeding in the 19th and 20th centuries.* Ohio State University Press.

Wolf, J. H. (2006a). The first generation of American pediatricians and their inadvertent legacy to breastfeeding. *Breastfeeding Medicine, 1,* 172–177. https://doi.org/10.1089/bfm.2006.1.172

Wolf, J. H. (2006b). What feminists can do for breastfeeding and what breastfeeding can do for feminists. *Signs: Journal of Women in Culture and Society, 31,* 397–424.

Wolf, J. H. (2008). Got milk? Not in public! *International Breastfeeding Journal.* http://www .internationalbreastfeedingjournal.com/content/3/1/11

Wolf, J. H. (2009). *Deliver me from pain: Anesthesia and birth in America.* Johns Hopkins University Press.

Wood-Allen, M. (1895, September). Baby's firsts. *Mother's Friend,* 13–16.

Wood-Allen, M. (1896, October). Physical nurture. *New Crusade,* 180–181.

CHAPTER 2

Key Concepts of Lactation as Health Promotion

Jolynn Dowling, MSN, APRN, NNP-BC, IBCLC

LEARNING OBJECTIVES

1. Recognize global health promotion strategies to increase initiation and duration of breastfeeding.
2. Describe the health benefits for the breastfeeding parent.
3. Describe the health benefits for the breastfed infant.
4. Apply effective health communication to promote and protect breastfeeding.
5. Differentiate conceptual frameworks for health promotion of breastfeeding.

KEY WORDS

- **Health Promotion:** Social and environmental activities or processes to enhance health and well-being, by addressing and preventing the root causes of illness, not just treatment and cure (World Health Organization [WHO], 2016).
- **Socio-Ecological Model (SEM):** Multilevel framework of health promotion recognizing the interaction of the environment and individual within a social system (Bronfenbrenner, 1977).
- **Exclusive Breastfeeding:** Infant receives only human milk and no other liquids or solids (WHO, 2019).
- **Breastfeeding Dyad:** The infant and the human source of their nutrition. Often this is the biological mother, but this can also be a primary caregiver/ nonbiological parent feeding directly at the breast or through a supplemental feeding system at the breast.
- **Sustainable Food:** Food that has a positive impact on health, climate, economy, and the earth.
- **Health Communication:** Process of communicating health promotion information to influence personal health choices and improve health literacy (Rimal & Lipinski, 2009).
- **Interprofessional Communication:** "Occurs when health providers/students communicate with each other, with people and their families, and with the

community in an open collaborative and responsible manner" (Winnipeg Regional Health Authority, n.d., para 1).

- **Motivational Interviewing:** "A counseling technique designed to meet clients at their point of willingness to change and to support clients in incremental steps toward a goal" (Scherer & Love-Zaranka, 2019, p. 427).
- **Shared Decision Making:** "Form of nondirective counselling where the professional and patient come together as experts, in clinical evidence and lived experience to help the family reach their goals" (Munro et al., 2019, p. 394).
- **Patient Centered Care:** "Providing care that is respectful of, and responsive to, individual patient preferences, needs, and values, and ensuring that patient values guide all clinical decisions" (Institute of Medicine [IOM], 2001, p. 6).
- **Community Coalition Action Theory:** Provides a contextual understanding of inter-organizational collaboration related to community health promotion (Butterfoss & Kegler, 2009).
- **Collective Impact:** "The commitment of a group of important actors from different sectors to a common agenda for solving a specific social problem" (Kania & Kramer, 2011, p. 36).

Overview

The current state of the world's health has been impacted by multiple factors, including climate change, natural disasters, acts of terrorism, and emerging disease. Through this disruption, breastfeeding has remained constant as the best source of nutrition as a *first food*, with the power to make the greatest impact on maternal and infant mortality as well as world economies (Global Breastfeeding Collective, 2017). Sadly, efforts to promote breastfeeding as a public health imperative have remained inadequate. This is a systemic failure from the local, state, provincial, regional, national, and global level. While there has been a shift toward recognizing breastfeeding as the *normal* source of nutrition, unification from multiple sectors toward the goal of supporting the family desiring to provide human milk is needed. These **health promotion** efforts should not only serve the wealthiest of parents but also those who are most vulnerable to the health disparities that exist in our culture today. As health care providers, it is essential that the lens with which breastfeeding is viewed be expanded so that the health of the next generation can be optimized and the human race sustained with improved health outcomes.

This chapter begins by presenting breastfeeding in the context of the socio-ecological framework for health promotion. Breastfeeding and lactation as a global health promotion strategy and investment as well as maternal and infant health benefits are discussed. **Health communication** concepts and additional frameworks for health promotion are included, along with strategies for equitable health promotion. Use of the terms *mother*, *maternal*, *woman*, and *breastfeeding* reflect the current evidence available; however, it is not meant to exclude parents from the lesbian, gay, bisexual, transgender, or nonbinary community who may be breastfeeding or providing human milk to their infant.

Socio-ecological Model to Support Breastfeeding

The **socio-ecological model (SEM)** was first introduced by Bronfenbrenner (1977) as a multilevel framework of health promotion recognizing the interaction of the environment and individual within a social system. This model is widely used within the field of public health and provides a multilevel focus for health promotion. The five levels of influence on health behavior of the SEM include individual, interpersonal (family and peers), community, institutional/organizational, and public policy (Golden & Earp, 2012; United Nations International Children's Emergency Fund [UNICEF], 2018). The construct of the SEM illustrates these levels of influence as nested circles, with the microsystem of the individual at the center and the policy macrosystem as the outer circle. This illustration is provided in **Figure 2-1**.

The SEM guides lactation health promotion through a theoretical understanding of the relationship of multiple factors within these levels of influence. This understanding helps to guide practice decisions as they relate to the breastfeeding dyad, provider, organization, and system. The intrapersonal breastfeeding dyad relationship is at the center of the framework. The factors that influence behavior at this level include breastfeeding motivation and self-efficacy, which directly relates to breastfeeding initiation and duration. The interpersonal relationships with providers influence maternal attitudes and health decisions and include social and educational support. Organizational factors, such as policies to support breastfeeding,

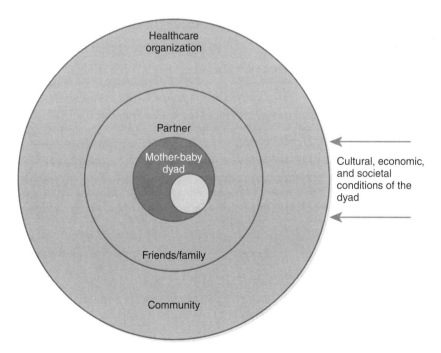

Figure 2-1 Socio-Ecological Model of Health Promotion (Revai, 2017©)
© Tina Revai, 2017.

provide structural and provider support throughout all stages of pregnancy and postpartum. Systems factors influence policy, availability of breastfeeding education and information, continuity of care related to consistent messaging, and breastfeeding support after discharge. Systems factors may also include data tracking mechanisms to determine outcomes of policy and practice on breastfeeding rates (Munn et al., 2016). **Table 2-1** organizes the SEM levels of influence and respective interventions to promote breastfeeding.

Health promotion interventions that impact initiation and duration of breastfeeding for the **breastfeeding dyad** may include prenatal, intrapartum, and postpartum breastfeeding education; one-on-one postnatal support; and postpartum follow-up. Interventions are found to be more effective at improving self-efficacy if delivered both in the inpatient and community setting and using multiple contact points (Brockway et al., 2017; Gupta et al., 2019). Additionally, a comprehensive approach that includes support through legal and policy improvements could positively impact sustainability of breastfeeding interventions across all levels of influence (Gupta et al., 2019).

Breastfeeding Promotion as a Lactation Strategy and Investment

Exclusive breastfeeding during the first 6 months of life has the largest potential to impact infant mortality and pediatric disease, with protection against chronic disease later in life (Global Breastfeeding Collective, 2017). Breastfeeding provides essential species-specific nutrition for a child's growth and development and serves as the first immunization. Even though strategies to improve exclusive breastfeeding have had a significant impact on initiation rates, duration rates up to and beyond 6 months lag behind. Globally, approximately 40% of infants are exclusively breastfed to 6 months, and 69% receive complimentary semi-solid or solid foods at 6 to 8 months along with breastfeeding (Gupta et al., 2019; WHO, 2018).

A global increase in breastfeeding initiation, exclusivity, and duration to the recommended levels could save 823,000 lives per year among children ages 5 years and younger (Victora et al., 2016). Breastfeeding reduces the risk of communicable and chronic disease later in life and also protects women against breast cancer, ovarian cancer, diabetes, cardiovascular disease, and birth-related mortality. Although breastfeeding has significant implications for countries' future prosperity through improving overall population health and decreasing health care costs, countries are not adequately promoting, protecting, and supporting breastfeeding through funding or policies (Global Breastfeeding Collective, 2017).

It is recommended that the initiation of breastfeeding occur within 1 hour of birth, exclusive breastfeeding continue for the first 6 months, and breastfeeding continue with complimentary foods until at least 24 months of age (Gupta et al., 2019; WHO & UNICEF, 2003). The World Health Assembly (WHA) has established a goal of increasing the rate of exclusive breastfeeding in the first 6 months to at least 50% by year 2025 (WHO, 2014). Meeting this goal has the potential to save 520,000 children's lives, generate $300 billion in additional economic gains in lower- and middle-income countries through improved cognitive development and child survival rates, and generate an economic return on investment of $35 for every dollar (Shekar et al., 2017). The United States alone could save $13 billion per

Table 2-1 Socio-Ecological Breastfeeding Health Promotion Interventions

	Individual	Interpersonal	Community	Institutional/Organizational	Systems/Policy
	■ Breastfeeding Dyad	■ Partner ■ Family ■ Peers (other mothers) ■ Co-workers	■ Mother support groups (La Leche League International [LLLI]) ■ Child care providers ■ Local breastfeeding coalitions ■ Special Supplemental Nutrition Program for Women, Infants, and Children (WIC) ■ Worksites ■ Public spaces	■ Hospitals ■ Clinics ■ Health authorities ■ Civic/faith organizations ■ Breastfeeding advocacy and support organizations ■ Universities and medical schools	■ Local/state/federal/provincial governments ■ Professional organizations ■ Health care systems ■ Third-party payers ■ Manufacturers ■ Accrediting/credentialing agencies
INTERVENTIONS	■ Prenatal breastfeeding education ■ Birth plans (natural, C-section; skin-to-skin, visitor limitation, etc.) ■ Nighttime parenting plans ■ Postpartum follow-up at breastfeeding clinic/physician office within 3 days ■ Connection with local breastfeeding resources	■ Education/support for fathers/partners ■ Education for siblings/grandparents ■ Co-worker "sell back" or paid time off (PTO) share to extend family leave for colleagues	■ Breastfeeding friendly child care providers ■ "Breastfeeding Welcome Here" Advocacy and support through LLLI and local coalitions ■ Follow-up with WIC peer counselors ■ Lactation room at employment settings ■ Lactation "tents" at public spaces, such as festivals and fairs ■ Public service announcement (PSA)/billboard marketing to support breastfeeding ■ Signage to support breastfeeding on public transit	■ Baby-friendly Hospital Initiative (BFHI) designated hospitals/health authorities ■ Breastfeeding-friendly physician practice ■ Lactation rooms; mothers' rooms in university buildings; sports arenas, etc. ■ Parish programs to support breastfeeding ■ State/federal/national health authority coalitions	■ Parental leave ■ Employer worksite policy to support breastfeeding employees ■ Policy to support parenting students (high school, university, medical residency programs, etc.) ■ Insurance policy incentive through reduced deductible for breastfeeding parents ■ Insurance provision of breast pumps and lactation counseling with credentialed/licensed providers ■ Policy to support public breastfeeding ■ Breastfeeding-friendly airports ■ Local/state/national funding to support breastfeeding programs ■ Tracking mechanisms

Data from Birch, L. (2015). Public health: Breastfeeding battles. British Journal of Midwifery, 23(6), 438–441. https://doi.org/10.12968/bjom.2015.23.6.438; Global Breastfeeding Collective. (2017). Nurturing the health and wealth of nations: The investment case for breastfeeding. United Nation Children's Fund & World Health Organization. https://www.who.int/nutrition/publications/infantfeeding/global-bf-collective-investmentcase.pdf?ua=1; Munn, A. C., Newman, S. D., Mueller, M., Phillips, S., & Taylor, S. (2016). The impact in the United States of the Baby-Friendly Hospital Initiative on early infant health and breastfeeding outcomes. Breastfeeding Medicine, 11(6), 1–9. https://doi.org/10.1089/bfm.2015.0135; Reis-Reilly, H., Fuller-Sankofa, N., & Tibbs, C. (2018). Breastfeeding in the community: Addressing disparities through policy, systems, and environmental change interventions. Journal of Human Lactation, 34(2), 262–271. Doi: 10.1177/0890334418759055; Rollins, N., Bhandari, N., Hajeebhoy, N., Horton, S., Lutter, C., Martines, J., ... Victora, C. (2016). Why invest, and what it will take to improve breastfeeding practices? The Lancet, 387(10017), 491–504. https://doi.org/10.1016/S0140-6736(15)01044Z; World Health Organization. (2014). Comprehensive implementation plan on maternal, infant and young child nutrition. https://apps.who.int/iris/bitstream/handle/10665/113048/WHO_NMH_NHD_14_1_eng.pdf?ua=1; © Jolynn Dowling 2020.

year if 90% of families met the recommendation to exclusively breastfeed for up to 6 months (American Academy of Pediatrics Section on Breastfeeding, 2012; Bartick & Reinhold, 2010). Strategies to reach the global target include full implementation of the *International Code of Marketing of Breastmilk Substitutes*, improvement of maternity care practices, and improved access to skilled lactation support. Funding for national breastfeeding promotion and program/policy evaluation to achieve the global breastfeeding targets should also be included in the strategic plan (Global Breastfeeding Collective, 2017). An analysis by the World Bank, Results for Development Institute (R4D), and 1,000 Days showed the financial investment needed to help mothers exclusively breastfeed for the first 6 months to be less than $5 per newborn (Walters et al., 2017).

Maternal Health Outcomes

Maternal health is positively impacted by breastfeeding and is enhanced the longer breastfeeding continues. Targeting health promotion strategies to the father or partner increases breastfeeding exclusivity and duration and may enhance maternal self-efficacy (Mahesh et al. 2018). Breastfeeding protects the mother from birth-related complications through the release of the hormone oxytocin to enhance uterine involution and decrease postpartum hemorrhage. Oxytocin release during breastfeeding and a decrease in cortisol decrease the stress response, so when breastfeeding is going well it enhances the bond between the mother and infant and decreases the risk of postpartum depression (Figueiredo et al., 2014; Kendall-Tackett, 2007). Optimal breastfeeding has the potential to impact maternal health and mortality outcomes, with a reduction of an estimated 20,000 maternal deaths from breast cancer each year (Rollins et al., 2016; Victora et al., 2016). Breastfeeding is associated with decreased risk of ovarian cancer and also protects against cardiovascular disease, including hypertension and stroke (Jacobson et al., 2018; Luan et al., 2013; Rameez et al., 2019; Schwarz et al., 2009). Breastfeeding reduces the risk of type 2 diabetes and may protect against obesity helping the mother to return to her prenatal weight faster (Rameez et al., 2019; Schwarz & Nothnagle, 2015).

Infant Health Outcomes

Human milk is a highly complex and unique fluid with marked differences from the milk of other species. It has adapted throughout human existence to meet the nutritional and anti-infective needs of the human infant to ensure optimal growth, development, and survival. These biospecific nutrients are neither interchangeable, nor equivalent, with artificial human milk substitutes. Infant feeding is a process that is always changing. There is consistent evidence showing that any breastfeeding (versus no breastfeeding) protects against infant mortality (Victora et al., 2016). Although the quality and quantity of evidence are increasing related to the health benefits of breastfeeding and human milk to infants, it is important to acknowledge that higher-level research, such as randomized control trials, is not ethical on this population; so much of the evidence is qualitative. Breastfeeding confers multiple health benefits to the infant, which are enhanced with exclusivity and duration. It is considered the normative standard of infant nutrition. However, it is challenging for many countries to fully adopt the *International Code of Marketing of Breastmilk Substitutes*, which is further complicated by advertising and marketing strategies of formula companies (Brady, 2012). Breastfeeding provides lifelong protection against upper and lower respiratory tract infections, otitis media, gastrointestinal disease, sepsis, meningitis, urinary tract infection, leukemia, lymphoma, and neuroblastoma (Lauwers, 2018). Breastfeeding is associated with higher cognition, which is dose dependent, so the longer the infant breastfeeds, the higher the intelligence quotient (IQ) (Horta et al., 2015a). There is a decreased risk of necrotizing enterocolitis, and breastfeeding protects against sudden infant death syndrome. Breastfeeding reduces the risk of both type 1 and type 2 diabetes and positively impacts weight control and feeding self-regulation, including protection against obesity (American Academy of Pediatrics Section on Breastfeeding, 2012; Horta et al., 2015b; Victora et al., 2016).

Sustainable Food Source and Access to Human Milk

Human milk is a renewable food produced by the human body. It is environmentally safe, doesn't require packaging, and does not produce waste. In contrast, human milk substitutes require manufacturing, packaging materials, water, fuel, and cleaning agents for preparation. This increases the ecological footprint and pollutants that are generated in this process (Rollins et al., 2016). In situations of natural or man-made emergency disaster, human milk is available to nourish the child without the need for clean water or supplies for preparation. Human milk is always warm, ready to eat, and available to the infant in an active breastfeeding relationship. If there is an anatomical or medical condition that prohibits the mother from producing an adequate supply of milk for her infant, human milk can be obtained through formal donor milk banks or informal milk sharing. While there has been an increase in commodification of human milk, purchase of human milk through the Internet from an unknown source can present a health risk to the infant and is not recommended (Sriraman et al., & Academy of Breastfeeding Medicine Board of Directors, 2018).

Health Communication

Communication is the core of how humans exchange information. It is societal and involves transmitting and receiving information. Accurate interpretation of the information has become increasingly difficult as technology has advanced and more communication is done without direct human contact. Humans are now communicating without tone of voice, volume, and facial expression to give additional meaning to the information shared. This creates challenges for health communication, health literacy, and change in health behaviors. The U.S. Department of Health and Human Services established health communication as an objective in 2010 and added health information technology to this focus area with the update to *Healthy People 2020* (Office of Disease Prevention and Health Promotion [ODPHP], n.d.). The goal is to improve population health outcomes, the quality of health care, and health equity (ODPHP). While there is the potential to improve health care access, health service delivery, and health care decisions, emerging technology can make it difficult to differentiate between expert and peer health information (Menefee et al., 2016). It can be overwhelming for consumers with limited literacy, skills, and experience using the technology and may negatively impact the use of health prevention services and consequently health status (National Opinion Research Center [NORC] at University of Chicago, 2013). It is important to incorporate multiple methods of health communication, such as social media, printed material, media campaigns, community outreach, and interpersonal communication to positively impact health information delivery and health decisions (Patel et al., 2015).

Although it is the biological norm in some countries, breastfeeding is a very personal health decision and can illicit positive and negative emotional responses depending on the health information that is communicated. There is little mainstream media coverage or marketing of breastfeeding, and that may influence parents to seek health information through the internet. McKeever and McKeever (2017) explored the effects of online health communication and infant feeding practices. Their survey of mothers with young children measuring attitudes toward breastfeeding, perceived behavior control, social norms, and behavioral intention found a direct negative association between the time the mothers spent online and breastfeeding intentions. This negative correlation could be related to mothers seeking health information during breastfeeding challenges or for other reasons. This study reveals that it is important to assess these online communities for accurate health information. Most of the information the mothers accessed online was from parenting groups, mothers' groups, Facebook, and mommy blogs and may have been related more toward the personal experience rather than health-specific or research-oriented health information (McKeever & McKeever, 2017). In a systematic review of information and communication systems to tackle barriers to breastfeeding, Tang et al. (2019) found most health information related to breastfeeding was communicated using Web technologies, text messages, and mobile applications to provide breastfeeding support. They also found that health information did not address all relevant periods of parenting and did not include partners. Although this illustrates the use of technology for health communication related to breastfeeding, most breastfeeding communication, education, and support continue to be delivered primarily through interpersonal communication with the provider, lactation support personnel, or peer support groups. Health care providers must exercise self-awareness of their own biases as they communicate with parents to ensure that it is the parents' goals, and not the health provider's attitude, influencing the plan of care. This has become increasingly apparent with recent testimonies from women of color sharing their personal maternal health care experience.

Interprofessional Communication

Communication with members of different disciplines within the health care team is essential to improve health outcomes. Additionally, this communication must involve the patient or family in order to determine a clear clinical picture. **Interprofessional communication** may also involve different sectors of the community where the patient will be discharged. All disciplines function within a scope of practice that involves specific terminology, or language, and must be understood by others. Some disciplines may communicate more descriptively, while others are more succinct with their communication. This can lead to misunderstanding or different interpretations of a specific clinical situation and ultimately impact the care the patient receives (Fyfe et al., 2016). There has been an increased emphasis on providing interprofessional education within colleges and universities to provide environments where health care students "learn about, from and with each other" (WHO, 2010, p.13). This fosters a safe environment to allow students to become more familiar and establish mutual trust, understanding, and respect that will carry over into the health system to enhance effective collaboration and improve health outcomes (WHO, 2010).

Interprofessional communication between lactation support providers and other health care professionals can be challenging. Physicians are considered the gatekeepers for the availability of patient resources and services (Jabbar, 2011). Although physicians have knowledge of the importance of breastfeeding, their knowledge on more complex lactation issues lags behind (Sigman-Grant & Kim, 2016). International Board Certified Lactation Consultants (IBCLCs) and Lactation Counselors fill this gap with the knowledge and skills to support the breastfeeding dyad and make appropriate referral for diagnosis and treatment (Anstey et al., 2018). However, there is still work to be done for the lactation support provider to be fully recognized and integrated in the health care team as recommended by *The Surgeons Call to Action to Support Breastfeeding* (U.S. Department of Health and Human Services [USDHHS], 2011). The American College of Obstetricians and Gynecologists' (ACOG) Interprofessional Task Force on Collaborative Practice acknowledges that interprofessional communication among health care providers is integral to provide a patient-centered care approach (Jennings et al., 2016). However, barriers to integrated care, lack of provider knowledge, unsupportive work environments, and the influence of the formula industry undermine the interprofessional relationship and care management of lactation support providers (Anstey et al., 2018; Rosin & Zakarija-Grkovic, 2016).

Motivational Interviewing and Shared Decision Making

Motivational interviewing (MI) and **shared decision making (SDM)** are two communication techniques to assist breastfeeding parents to meet their goals. Both require collaboration and communication with the health care provider or counselor. Effective communication using these techniques requires openness, respect, and positive regard for the parents, as well as the intent to meet the parents where they are on the continuum of information and decisions. The culture, values, and relationships of the parents must also be considered. With the description of both of these communication techniques, the word *parent* has been substituted for the word *patient*.

MI assists the parents to increase their desire to change and improve self-efficacy so that they can succeed in meeting their breastfeeding goals. It focuses on behavioral change and is not prescriptive. The parents are the experts. MI involves having the parents set goals, identify personal barriers to the change, and identify potential strategies to overcome barriers. Health care professionals assist the process through active listening and expressing empathy with a nonjudgmental attitude. It is important to avoid arguing with the parents and encourage them to provide answers to their own questions. Support of self-efficacy can be accomplished by affirming and encouraging the parent. With each interaction, the health care provider or counselor can summarize what is discussed, the goals for the parents, and the plan for change (Rollnick et al., 2008). MI shows promise to impact breastfeeding self-efficacy and duration in women who begin to breastfeed within the first hour;

however, further research is needed, especially when implemented in the prenatal period and in women who are not able to breastfeed their infant in the first hour after delivery (Franco-Antonio et al., 2020).

SDM is a communication technique in which the parents and the health care provider come together as experts to reach the desired feeding goals. The conversation shifts from the provider *giving* information to the parents to the *exchange* of information resulting in a shared decision that takes the parents' culture, values, and beliefs, as well as best evidence, into consideration (Munro et al., 2019). Although this shared decision can be made solely between the mother and health care provider, this decision can be influenced by various formal and informal sources of support. It is important to include partners (if they are involved) in these conversations and education, as the attitude and preference of the father has been shown to influence feeding decisions (Wang et al., 2018). The Agency for Healthcare Research and Quality (AHRQ, 2018) developed the SHARE approach to this process. It is a five-step process for shared decision making that includes discussing options in the context of benefit and risk, and then evaluating each option through dialogue of what matters most to the parent. SHARE is an acronym for **S**eek the parents' participation, **H**elp the parents explore and compare treatment options, **A**ssess the parents' values and preferences, **R**each a decision with the parents, and **E**valuate the parents' decision (AHRQ, 2018). Truglio-Londrigan and Slyer (2018) describe that the process of SDM takes advantage of the health care provider's expertise, while allowing the parents to ask questions or express concern. Relationship building, trust, and respect are at the foundation. The relationship is collaborative with sharing of power, as parents who feel trusted and respected are more open to sharing information with their health care provider. Communication is bidirectional, and the tone from the health care provider should convey empathy. There can be challenges for the health care provider to ensure the realities of best evidence and clinical practice, while taking into consideration the parents' preferences. Ultimately the parents will make a decision, with the health care provider following up with the parents on their decision after a period of time (ARHQ, 2018; Truglio-Londrigan & Slyer, 2018). Suggested language for framing conversations using MI and SDM are provided in **Table 2-2**.

Additional Frameworks for Health Promotion

Patient-Centered Care Framework

Patient-centered care is a framework that supports patients to make informed decisions and retain control over their health care choice. The patient is at the center of this framework, and there is partnership between the individual, family, and health care providers. Patient-centered care incorporates SDM to improve communications and health outcomes (British Columbia Ministry of Health, 2015). Although this framework has been implemented in health care systems since the 1990s, there is increasing awareness that changes are necessary to adjust from an acute care focus to implementing the framework across systems to address complex chronic conditions. Recommendations from the Institute of Medicine (2001) include a system to provide patients the care they need, in

Table 2-2 Examples of Motivational Interviewing and Shared Decision Making with Breastfeeding Families

Framing the Conversation	
Motivational Interview	**Shared Decision Making**
Express Empathy: "I appreciate that you made the time for me to visit with you today."	**S**eek the parent's participation: "I would like for you to share with me what you know about breastfeeding."
Develop Discrepancy: "What worries you most about breastfeeding?"	**H**elp parents explore options: "Here are some of the differences between breastfeeding and feeding formula." "Could you tell me some of the health benefits breastfeeding has for you and your baby?"
Avoid Argument: "What would be a first step you could take?"	**A**ssess the parent's values and preferences: "What matters most to you about breastfeeding?"
Support Self-Efficacy: "It is great that despite your uncertainty about breastfeeding, you are willing to try. With a husband who is deployed, and a two-year-old, it can be a lot to manage. I know you can do this too."	**R**each a decision with the parent: "Now that we have had time to discuss breastfeeding, are there any additional questions you have for me to help you make your feeding decision?"
	Evaluate the parents' decision: "Can we talk in two days to see how you are doing with breastfeeding your baby?"

© Jolynn Dowling 2020.

whatever form, utilizing various technologies to ensure continuous healing relationships. This would include responsiveness to individual patient choices, with patients given the opportunity to have a degree of control over the health care decisions that affect them. Additionally, the system should make information available to allow informed choices when selecting health plans, treatments, or facilities to receive care.

This British Columbia Patient-Centered Care Framework (British Columbia Ministry of Health, 2015) describes four core principles as a foundation supporting the relationship between the health care provider and patient. The principles of dignity and respect emphasize the need for active listening to the patient and their families and for honoring their choices and decisions. This would include incorporating their values and beliefs into the plan of care. The principle of information sharing supports the patient and family by providing accurate and timely evidence-based information to assist in decision making. It involves validating what the patient and family have heard and understood so that there is clarity with the informed decisions they make. Through the principle of participation, patients and their families can be involved with their care at whatever level they feel comfortable. Success in implementing this framework depends on a cultural shift from health care providers, organization-wide engagement and support, and a balance in the provider–patient relationship.

Application of this framework for health promotion can be achieved through exploring the patient's past health history and current health status, which takes into consideration the patient's previous health care experiences to develop the health care plan. This approach is thought to decrease the risk of treatment failure and helps to optimize the use of resources for success (Constand et al., 2014).

Community Coalition Action Theory and Collective Impact

It is not enough to support the breastfeeding dyad and family in the inpatient setting through patient-centered care. Continuity of care to sustain breastfeeding after discharge into the community is essential. Since the publication of *The Surgeon General's Call to Action to Support Breastfeeding* (USDHHS, 2011), there has been an increase in community action to support breastfeeding families. This has helped shift the culture to view breastfeeding as the norm. Collaborative relationships through coalition building and collective impact have helped to establish education, programs, and policies to support breastfeeding. This has been accomplished through collective action from the local level to effect change at the local, regional, national, or international level.

Health professionals have embraced coalition building as a method to address complex health issues. **Community Coalition Action Theory (CCAT)** is a theory to increase understanding of how community coalitions work in practice. Coalitions form when different sectors of the community, state, or nation join together to focus on change or create opportunities to impact a mutual goal. These coalitions bring people together to share available resources, focus on a specific community concern, and achieve results that no single agency or person could have achieved alone. Although coalitions are often developed with unselfish motives, difficulties may be encountered when promised resources are not made available, if there is a conflict of interest among members, or when recognition for efforts is not realized. Coalitions may also require a long-term investment of time (Butterfoss & Kegler, 2009, 2012).

Community coalition members may vary, but they usually include professional and grassroots organizations to influence long-term health and welfare practices for their community. Additionally, the most effective coalitions include members that the health issue directly impacts—for example, breastfeeding parents. State and national coalitions facilitate communication and develop strategies over a larger geographical area. These coalitions may serve as a resource for community coalitions and promote breastfeeding through advocacy. The United States Breastfeeding Committee (USBC) is an example of a national coalition with strong advocacy initiatives to promote breastfeeding. Coalition development progresses through formation, maintenance, and institutionalization. As new health promotion initiatives or issues arise, coalitions may reform and begin progressing through the stages again. It is through the institutionalization stage that outcomes to health promotion strategies are realized and sustainability can be achieved (Butterfoss & Kegler, 2012).

Resource allocation for public health and health promotion has decreased, which has impacted sustainability of new and existing programs. Increasingly, funders are supporting initiatives that involve collaboration to address complex health problems. This has made it important for health promotion collaboration across sectors, both public and private. The **Collective Impact (CI)** model by Kania and Kramer (2011) was developed to influence large scale change; however, the evidence to support this model is not as extensive as CCAT. Although this model was initially developed to include only formal organizations, it has evolved in subsequent iterations to include community members. CI has five core tenets: common agenda, shared measurement systems, mutually reinforcing activities, continuous communication, and backbone support organization (Flood et al., 2015). While CI strengths lie in the alignment to CCAT by simplifying the model into five core tenets, criticisms of this model include a top-down approach and omission of grassroots stakeholders as part of the team (Wolfe et al., 2020). CI also does not include social justice and advocacy as a core (Flood et al., 2015). CI aligns to a business model and is not connected with research or scholarly activity to evaluate collaborative development (Wolfe et al., 2020; Wolff et al., 2016).

Collaborating for Equity and Justice

Each of these models has strengths for health promotion; however, a blend of these models has the potential to scale up community programs, health system change, and policy-level change that can transform and promote equity and justice. Wolff et al. (2016) introduced Collaborating for Equity and Justice (CEJ), which includes six principles to facilitate cross-sector collaboration that, when applied to existing models, can improve the potential for lasting systemic change to impact equity and justice for community members. The six principles of CEJ are:

- "Explicitly address issues of social and economic injustice and structural racism.
- Employ a community development approach in which community stakeholders have equal power in determining the collaborative's agenda and resource allocation.
- Employ community organizing as an intentional strategy and as part of the process. Work to build resident leadership and power.
- Focus on policy, systems, and structural change.
- Build on the extensive community-engaged scholarship and research over the last four decades that show what works, acknowledges the complexities, and evaluate appropriately.
- Construct core functions for the collaborative based on equity and justice that provide basic facilitating structures and build member ownership and leadership." (Wolff et al., 2016; p.51).

Wolff et al. (n.d.) have developed a CEJ Toolkit to support implementation of these principles in community collaborations for health promotion that address structural racism.

There is increasing awareness of the impact of health disparities, social determinants of health, and structural racism on maternal and infant health outcomes, including breastfeeding. Incorporating the CEJ principles into the CCAT or CI model may enhance evaluation of the collaborative related to power, equity, and justice.

However, partners must be open to the findings and how they or their organization may be a part of the problem. Leaders should be willing to explore solutions to move forward to achieve health equity (Wolfe et al. 2020; Wolff et al., 2016). More research is needed to validate the impact of the CEJ principles on equity and justice outcomes. Although implementation of the CEJ principles for breastfeeding health promotion has not been documented, integration of these principles into community coalition activities may be worth exploring.

Summary

Local, state, regional, provincial, and national economic, political, and health care system structures influence how families feed their babies. Although breastfeeding has cycled through periods of low rates and high rates of initiation and duration, increasing evidence on the maternal and infant health benefits have influenced parents to have a stronger resolve in their feeding decisions. Health communication and continuity of care that includes the parents as members of the health care team can influence the breastfeeding experience and subsequent health outcomes. As future collaborations are developed to promote and protect breastfeeding, principles of power, equity, and justice must be taken into consideration.

Key Points to Remember

1. The socio-ecological framework for health promotion incorporates multiple levels of influence to support the breastfeeding dyad.
2. Breastfeeding has the potential to have the largest impact on global health and economy if implemented at recommended levels.
3. Breastfeeding research continues to provide new evidence on maternal and infant health outcomes, as well as protection against chronic disease.
4. Interprofessional communication is essential for positive health outcomes.
5. Integration of the lactation support provider into the health care team continues to be a challenge.
6. Motivational interviewing and shared decision making place the parent at the center of health care decisions.
7. Frameworks for health promotion should include the breastfeeding parent as an essential stakeholder for collaborative change.
8. Incorporating Collaborating for Equity and Justice (CEJ) principles into the Community Coalition Action Theory (CCAT) or Collective Impact (CI) model may enhance collaborative outcomes related to power, equity, and justice.

Additional Resources

British Columbia Ministry of Health: Breastfeeding [https://www.healthlinkbc.ca/health-topics /hw91687]

Government of Canada: Breastfeeding [https://www.canada.ca/en/public-health/services/health -promotion/childhood-adolescence/stages-childhood/infancy-birth-two-years/breastfeeding -infant-nutrition.html]

Centers for Disease Control and Prevention: Breastfeeding [https://www.cdc.gov/breastfeeding/index .htm]

Collaborating for Equity and Justice Toolkit [https://www.myctb.org/wst/CEJ/Pages/home.aspx]

UNICEF: Breastfeeding [https://www.unicef.org/nutrition/index_24824.html]

United States Breastfeeding Committee [http://www.usbreastfeeding.org/]

World Health Organization: Breastfeeding [https://www.who.int/health-topics/breastfeeding#tab =tab_1]

References

Agency for Healthcare Research and Quality. (2018, August). *The SHARE approach*. https://www .ahrq.gov/health-literacy/curriculum-tools/shareddecisionmaking/index.html

American Academy of Pediatrics Section on Breastfeeding. (2012). Breastfeeding and the use of human milk. *Pediatrics, 129*(3), e827–e841. https://doi.org/10.1542/peds.2011-3552

Anstey, E., Coulter, M., Jevitt, C., Perrin, K., Dabrow, S., Klasko-Foster, L., & Daley, E. (2018). Lactation consultants: Perceived barriers to providing professional breastfeeding support. *Journal of Human Lactation 34*(1), 51–67. https://doi.org/10.1177/0890334417726305

Bartick, M., & Reinhold, A. (2010). The burden of suboptimal breastfeeding in the United States: A pediatric cost analysis. *Pediatrics, 125*(5), e1048–e1058. https://doi.org/10.1542/peds .2009-1616

Birch, L. (2015). Public health: Breastfeeding battles. *British Journal of Midwifery, 23*(6), 438–441. https://doi.org/10.12968/bjom.2015.23.6.438

Brady J. P. (2012). Marketing breast milk substitutes: Problems and perils throughout the world. *Archives of Disease in Childhood, 97*(6), 529–532. https://doi.org/10.1136/archdischild-2011-301299

British Columbia Ministry of Health. (2015). *The British Columbia patient-centered care framework*. https://www.health.gov.bc.ca/library/publications/year/2015_a/pt-centred-care-framework.pdf

Brockway, M., Benzies, K., & Hayden, K. (2017). Interventions to improve breastfeeding self-efficacy and resultant breastfeeding rates: A systematic review and meta-analysis. *Journal of Human Lactation, 33*(3), 486–499. https://journals.sagepub.com/doi/10.1177/0890334417707957

Bronfenbrenner, U. (1977). Toward an experimental ecology of human development. *American Psychologist, 32*(7), 513–531. https://doi.org/10.1037/0003-066X.32.7.513

Butterfoss, F. D., & Kegler, M. C. (2009). Community coalition action theory. In R. DiClemente, L. Crosby, & M. C. Kegler (Eds.), *Emerging theories in health promotion practice and research* (2nd ed., pp.157–193). Jossey-Bass.

Butterfoss, F. D., & Kegler, M. C. (2012). A coalition model for community action. In M. Minkler (Ed.), *Community organizing and community building for health and welfare* (3rd ed., pp. 309–328). Rutgers University Press.

Constand, M. K., MacDermid, J. C., Bello-Haas, V. D., & Law, M. (2014). Scoping review of patient-centered care approaches in healthcare. *BioMed Central Health Services Research, 14*(271), 1–9. http://www.biomedcentral.com/1472-6963/14/271

Figueiredo, B., Canario, C., & Field, T. (2014). Breastfeeding is negatively affected by prenatal depression and reduces postpartum depression. *Psychological Medicine, 44*, 927–936. https:// doi.org/10.1017/S0033291713001530

Flood, J., Minkler, M., Lavery, S. H., Estrada, J., & Falbe, J. (2015). The collective impact model and its potential for health promotion: Overview and case study of a healthy retail initiative in San Francisco. *Healthy Education and Behavior, 42*(5), 654–668. https://doi .org/10.1177/1090198115577372

Franco-Antonio, C., Calderon-Garcia, J. F., Santano-Mogena, E., Rico-Martin, S., & Cordovilla-Guardia, S. (2020). Effectivness of a brief motivational intervention to increase the breastfeeding duration in the first 6 months postpartum: Randomized controlled trial. *Journal of Advanced Nursing, 76*, 888–902. https://doi.org/10.1111/jan.14274

Fyfe, J. B., Quinn, S., Kiraly, T., & Kernerman, E. (2016). Improving communication and collaboration between lactation consultants and doctors for better breastfeeding outcomes: A review. *Clinical Lactation, 7*(2), 57–61. https://doi.org/10.1891/2158-0782.7.2.57

Global Breastfeeding Collective. (2017). *Nurturing the health and wealth of nations: The investment case for breastfeeding.* United Nation Children's Fund & World Health Organization. https://www.who.int/nutrition/publications/infantfeeding/global-bf-collective-investmentcase.pdf?ua=1

Golden, S., & Earp, J. (2012). Social ecological approaches to individuals and their contexts: Twenty years of *Health Education and Behavior* health promotion interventions. *Health Education & Behavior, 39*(3), 364–372. https://doi.org/10.1177/1090198111418634

Gupta, A., Suri, S., Dadhich, J. P., Trejos, M., & Nalubanga, B. (2019). The World Breastfeeding Trends Initiative: Implementation of the global strategy for infant and young child feeding in 84 countries. *Journal of Public Health Policy, 40,* 35–65. https://doi.org/10.1057/s41271-018-0153-9

Horta, B. L., Loret de Mola, C., & Victora, C. G. (2015a). Breastfeeding and intelligence: A systematic review and meta-analysis. *Acta Paediatrica, 104,* 14–19. https://doi.org/10.1111/apa.13139

Horta, B. L., Loret de Mola, C., & Victora, C. G. (2015b). Long-term consequences of breastfeeding on cholesterol, obesity, systolic blood pressure and type 2 diabetes: A systematic review and meta-analysis. *Acta Paediatrica, 104,* 30–37. https://doi.org/10.1111/apa.13133

Institute of Medicine (IOM) Committee on Quality of Health Care in America. (2001). *Crossing the quality chasm: A new health system for the 21st century.* National Academies Press. Executive Summary. https://www.ncbi.nlm.nih.gov/books/NBK22227

Jabbar, A. (2011). Language, power and implications for interprofessional collaboration: Reflections on a transition from social work to medicine. *Journal of Interprofessional Care, 25*(6), 447–448. https://doi.org/10.3109/13561820.2011.601822

Jacobson, L., Hade, E., Collins, T., Margolis, K., Waring, M., VanHorn, L., . . . Stefanick, M. (2018). Breastfeeding history and risk of stroke among parous postmenopausal women in the women's health initiative. *Journal of the American Heart Association, 7*(17). https://doi.org/10.1161/JAHA.118.008739

Jennings, J., Nielsen, P., Buck, M. L., Collins-Fulea, C., Corry, M., Cutler, C., . . . Ogden, K. (2016). Executive summary: Collaboration in practice: Implementing team-based care: Report of the American College of Obstetricians and Gynecologists' Task Force on Collaborative Practice. *Obstetrics & Gynecology, 127*(3), 612–617. https://doi.org/10.1097/AOG.0000000000001304

Kania, J., & Kramer, M. (2011, Winter). Collective impact. *Stanford Social Innovation Review, 9*(1), 36–41.

Kendall-Tackett, K. (2007). A new paradigm for depression in new mothers: The central role of inflammation and how breastfeeding and anti-inflammatory treatments protect maternal mental health. *International Breastfeeding Journal, 2*(6). https://doi.org/10.1186/1746-4358-2-6

Lauwers, J. (2018). Science of lactation. In Lauwers, J. (Ed.), *Quick reference for the lactation professional* (2nd ed., pp. 57–80). Jones and Bartlett.

Luan, N. N., Wu, Q. J., Gong, T. T., Vogtmann, E., Wang, Y. L., & Lin, B. (2013). Breastfeeding and ovarian cancer risk: A meta-analysis of epidemiologic studies. *The American Journal of Clinical Nutrition, 98*(4), 1020–1031. https://doi.org/10.3945/ajcn.113.062794

Mahesh, P., Gunathunga, M., Arnold, S., Jayasinghe, C., Pathirana, S., Makarim, M., Manawadu, P., & Senanayake, S. (2018). Effectiveness of targeting fathers for breastfeeding promotion: Systematic review and meta-analysis. *BMC Public Health, 18*(11140). https://doi.org/10.1186/s12889-018-6037-x

McKeever, R., & McKeever, B. W. (2017). Moms and media: Exploring the effects of online communication on infant feeding practices. *Health Communication, 32*(9), 1059–1065. https://doi.org/10.1080/10410236.2016.1196638

Menefee, H. K., Thompson, M. J., Guterbock, T. M., Williams, I. C., & Valdez, R. S. (2016). Mechanisms of communicating health information through Facebook: Implications for consumer health information technology design. *Journal of Medical Internet Research, 18*(8), e218. https://www.jmir.org/2016/8/e218

Munn, A. C., Newman, S. D., Mueller, M., Phillips, S., & Taylor, S. (2016). The impact in the United States of the Baby-friendly Hospital Initiative on early infant health and breastfeeding outcomes. *Breastfeeding Medicine, 11*(5), 1–9. https://doi.org/10.1089/bfm.2015.0135

Munro, S., Buckett, C., Sou, J., Bansback, N., & Lau, H. (2019). Shared decision making and breastfeeding: Supporting families' informed choices. *British Columbia Medical Journal, 61*(10). https://www.bcmj.org/sites/default/files/public/BCMJ_Vol61_No10-bc_cdc.pdf

National Opinion Research Center (NORC) at the University of Chicago. (2013). *Understanding the impact of health IT in underserved communities and those with health disparities.* Office of the National Coordinator for Health Information Technology: Department of Health and Human Services. https://www.healthit.gov/sites/default/files/hit_disparities_report_050713.pdf

Office of Disease Prevention and Health Promotion (ODPHP). (n.d.). *Health communication and health information technology.* Retrieved March 10, 2020, from https://www.healthypeople .gov/2020/topics-objectives/topic/health-communication-and-health-information-technology

Patel, V., Barker, W., & Siminerio, E. (2015). *Trends in consumer access and use of electronic health information.* Office of the National Coordinator for Health Information Technology: Department of Health and Human Services. https://dashboard.healthit.gov/evaluations/data-briefs /trends-consumer-access-use-electronic-health-information.php

Rameez, R. M., Sadana, d., Kaur, S., Ahmed, T., Patel, J., Khan, . . . Ahmed, H. M. (2019). Association of maternal lactation with diabetes and hypertension: A systematic review and meta-analysis. *Journal of the American Medical Association Network Open, 2*(10), e1913401. https://doi.org /10.1001/jamanetworkopen.2019.13401

Reis-Reilly, H., Fuller-Sankofa, N., & Tibbs, C. (2018). Breastfeeding in the community: Addressing disparities through policy, systems, and environmental change interventions. *Journal of Human Lactation, 34*(2), 262-271. Doi: 10.1177/0890334418759055

Rimal, R., & Lapinski, M. (2009). Why health communication is important in public health. *Bulletin of the World Health Organization, 87,* 247. https://www.who.int/bulletin/volumes/87/4/08-0567 13/en

Rollins, N., Bhandari, N., Hajeebhoy, N., Horton, S., Lutter, C., Martines, J., . . . Victora, C. (2016). Why invest, and what it will take to improve breastfeeding practices? *The Lancet, 387*(10017), 491–504. https://doi.org/10.1016/S0140-6736(15)010442

Rollnick, S., Miller, W. R., & Butler, C. C. (2008). *Motivational interviewing in health care: Helping patients change behavior.* The Guilford Press.

Rosin, S. I., & Zakarija-Grkovic, I. (2016). Towards integrated care in breastfeeding support: A cross-sectional study of practitioners' perspectives. *International Breastfeeding Journal, 11,* 15. https://doi.org/10.1186/s13006-016-0072-y

Scherer, L. K., & Love-Zaranka, A. (2019). Counseling and communication. In S. H. Campbell, J. Lauwers, R. Mannel, & B. Spencer (Eds.), *Core curriculum for interdisciplinary lactation care* (pp. 427–437). Jones & Bartlett.

Schwarz, E. B., & Nothnagle, M. (2015). The maternal health benefits of breastfeeding. *American Family Physician, 91*(9), 602–604. Retrieved July 3, 2020, from https://www.aafp.org/afp /2015/0501/p602.html

Schwarz, E. B., Ray, R. M., Stuebe, A. M., Ness, R. B., Freiberg, M. S., & Cauley, J. A. (2009). Duration of lactation and risk factors for maternal cardiovascular disease. *Obstetrics & Gynecology, 113*(5), 974–982. https://doi.org/10.1097/01.AOG.0000346884.67796.ca

Shekar, M., Kakietak, J., Eberwein, J., & Walters, D. (2017). *An investment framework for nutrition: Reaching the global targets for stunting, anemia, breastfeeding, and wasting.* Directions in Development. World Bank. http://dx.doi.org/10.1596/978-1-4648-1010-7

Sigman-Grant, M., & Kim, Y. (2016). Breastfeeding knowledge and attitudes of Nevada health care professionals remain virtually unchanged over 10 years. *Journal of Human Lactation, 32*(2), 350-354. https://doi.org/10.1177/0890334415609916

Sriraman, N. K., Evans, A. E., Lawrence, R., Noble, L., & Academy of Breastfeeding Medicine Board of Directors. (2018). Academy of breastfeeding medicine's 2017 position statement on informal breast milk sharing for the term healthy infant. *Breastfeeding Medicine, 13*(1), 2–4. https://www .liebertpub.com/doi/10.1089/bfm.2017.29064.nks

Tang, K., Gerling, K., Chen, W., & Geurts, L. (2019). Information and communication systems to tackle barriers to breastfeeding: Systematic search and review. *Journal of Medical Internet Research, 21*(9), e13947. https://doi.org/10.2196/13947

Truglio-Londrigan, M., & Slyer, J. (2018). Shared decision-making for nursing practice: An integrative review. *The Open Nursing Journal, 12,* 1–14. https://doi.org/10.2174/1874434601812010001

United Nations Children's Fund (UNICEF). (2018). UNICEF 2017 report on communication for development (C4D). https://www.unicef.org/publications/files/UNICEF_2017_Report_on_Communication _for_Development_C4D.pdf

United States Breastfeeding Committee. (2011). *Socio-ecological model.* http://www.usbreastfeeding
.org/p/cm/ld/fid=114

U.S. Department of Health and Human Services (USDHHS). (2011). *The Surgeon General's call to
action to support breastfeeding.* https://www.ncbi.nlm.nih.gov/books/NBK52682/pdf/Bookshelf
_NBK52682.pdf

Victora, C., Bahl, R., Barros, A., Franca, G., Horton, S., Krasevec, J., Murch, S., Sankar, M., . . .
Rollins, N. (2016). Breastfeeding in the 21st century: Epidemiology, mechanisms, and lifelong
effect. *The Lancet, 387*(10017), 475–490. https://doi.org/10.1016/S0140-6736(15)01024-7

Walters, D., Eberwein, J., Sullivan, L., & Shekar, M. (2017). Reaching the global target for breastfeeding. In Shekar, M., Kakietak, J., Eberwein, J., & Walters, D. (Eds.), *An investment framework for nutrition: Reaching the global targets for stunting, anemia, breastfeeding, and wasting*
(pp. 97–116). Directions in Development. World Bank. http://dx.doi.org/10.1596/978-1-4648
-1010-7

Wang, S., Guendelman, S., Harley, K., & Eskenazi, B. (2018). When fathers are perceived to share
in the maternal decision to breastfeed: Outcomes from the infant feeding practices study II. *Maternal and Child Health Journal, 22*, 1676–1684. https://doi.org/10.1007/s10995-018-2566-2

Winnipeg Regional Health Authority. (n.d.). Competency 5: Interprofessional communication.
Collaborate Better Health for All. https://professionals.wrha.mb.ca/files/collaborative-care
-competencies-5.pdf

Wolfe, S. M., Long, P. D., & Brown, K. K. (2020). Using a principles-focused evaluation approach to
evaluate coalitions and collaboratives working toward equity and social justice. In A. W. Price,
K. K. Brown, & S. M. Wolfe (Eds.), *Evaluating Community Coalitions and Collaboratives: New
Directions for Evaluation, 165*, 45–65. https://doi.org/10.1002/ev.20404

Wolff, T., Minkler, M., Wolfe, S. M., Berkowitz, B., Bowen, L., Butterfoss, F. D., . . . Lee, K. S. (2016,
Winter). Collaborating for equity and justice: Moving beyond collective impact. *The Nonprofit
Quarterly.* https://nonprofitquarterly.org/collaborating-equity-justice-moving-beyond-collective
-impact

Wolff, T., Minkler, M., Wolfe, S., Berkowitz, B., Bowen, L, Butterfoss, F.,...Lee, K. (n.d.). Collaborating for Equity and Justice Toolkit. *KU Center for Community Health and Development.* https://
www.myctb.org/wst/CEJ/Pages/home.aspx

World Health Organization. (2010). *Framework for action on interprofessional education and collaborative practice.* https://www.who.int/hrh/resources/framework_action/en

World Health Organization. (2014). *Comprehensive implementation plan on maternal, infant and
young child nutrition.* https://apps.who.int/iris/bitstream/handle/10665/113048/WHO_NMH
_NHD_14.1_eng.pdf?ua=1

World Health Organization. (2016, August). *What is health promotion?* https://www.who.int
/features/qa/health-promotion/en

World Health Organization. (2019). *Exclusive breastfeeding for optimal growth, development and health
of infants.* https://www.who.int/elena/titles/exclusive_breastfeeding/en

World Health Organization. (2020, April). *Infant and young child feeding.* https://www.who.int
/news-room/fact-sheets/detail/infant-and-young-child-feeding

World Health Organization & UNICEF. (2003). *Global strategy for infant and young child feeding.*
World Health Organization. https://apps.who.int/iris/bitstream/handle/10665/42590/924156
2218.pdf?sequence=1

CHAPTER 3

Behavioral Theories Examining Lactation as Health Promotion

Suzanne Hetzel Campbell, PhD, RN, IBCLC, CCSNE

Exclusive breastfeeding is becoming an endangered practice. Breastfeeding has fallen from the foundation of public health to something that is nice but not necessary in the minds of many consumers and health care professionals.

(Walker, 2007)

LEARNING OBJECTIVES

1. Critically analyze behavioral theories that have been used to examine lactation from a health promotion perspective.
2. Identify the assumptions, values, and theories that underpin various conceptualizations of health promotion.
3. Explain why studying lactation as a health promotion behavior should be an integral part of health promotion.
4. Identify the impact of behavioral theories on research examining lactation as health promotion.
5. Compare and contrast behavioral theories usefulness in lactation research.

KEY WORDS

- **Health Belief Model:** A framework for health promotion that motivates individuals to change lifestyle and health behaviors related to their perception of risk of negative health consequences if they do not change their behavior.
- **Social Cognitive Theory:** A learning theory developed by Albert Bandura that incorporates practice, observational learning, modeling, and self-efficacy, which allows enhancement of knowledge, attitudes, and behaviors to positively reinforce one's performance (Bandura, 1986).
- **Self-efficacy:** The confidence individuals have in their ability to enact a behavior or complete a task, a manipulable concept that targeted interventions can affect

and explain changes in behavior. According to social cognitive theory (SCT), self-efficacy as a construct within it explains one's confidence in one's ability and is a product of experience in performing the behavior, vicarious experience (observation), persuasion, and emotional response.

- **Reasoned Action Approach (RAA):** A theory that emerged from the theory of planned behavior and reasoned action, which integrated and redefined initial constructs to create a framework that better predicts human behaviors incorporating attitude; subjective norm; and perceived behavioral control— capacity (e.g., self-efficacy) and autonomy (individual control) (Fishbein & Ajzen, 2011).
- **The Theory of Planned Behavior:** A theory linking one's beliefs and behaviors, taking into consideration the individual's attitude, perception of subjective norms, and perceived behavioral control of the behavior that shapes the individual's behavioral intentions and behaviors (Ajzen, 1985).

Overview

Breastfeeding is a complex health behavior allowing for disease and illness prevention and also acting as health promotion. Models and frameworks for health promotion tend to focus on a risk-based population perspective. This does not work well in the examination of breastfeeding as a health promotion strategy or disease/illness prevention model. It is also why it is so difficult to calculate real-time costs to our planet, parental/infant/child health, and overall long-term effects on the world economy. In this chapter, behavioral theories are outlined with the goal of enhancing understanding about how theories can influence practitioners' ability to arrange, implement, and execute goals as health care professionals with regard to supporting parents in meeting their infant feeding goals. A clear understanding of the theories is necessary to support new parents to set reasonable goals and feel successful in their infant feeding using a strength-based and harm-reduction approach. Understanding parents' goals and helping breastfeeding to work for the family is the only way it will work for the infant. Using an interdisciplinary, social justice, and global lens to understand health promotion theories related to breastfeeding will help to ensure a supportive breastfeeding environment at all levels within society.

Health promotion theories help us to develop organized strategies to enhance efforts and programs within the health care system. There is a strong case for investment in breastfeeding, as a public health issue (Rollins et al., 2016), given the epidemiological studies and knowledge surrounding the role of epigenetics, stem cells, and the origins of health and disease from physical, mental, and intellectual perspectives (Horta et al., 2015; Victora et al., 2015, 2016). Unfortunately, despite increased evidence, we still need to make a case for breastfeeding. For many health care providers, broad public health initiatives can seem overwhelming, so many health care providers take a person-centered approach, think globally, and act locally. Although public health is made up of many different organized systems, these systems consist of teams and individuals who can have significant impact. This chapter examines health promotion theories that have guided research and been used to develop programs to support lactation locally and globally.

The two most prominent health promotion theories used to examine interventions and programs in support of breastfeeding as health behavior include the theories of planned behavior and **self-efficacy**. These theories flow from SCT and the reasoned action approaches, the theory of reasoned action, and **the theory of planned behavior**. Other theories like the **health belief model** and transtheoretical models are often incorporated into programming and intervention development. Components of multiple health promotion theories have been integrated into successful global programs, such as the Baby-friendly Hospital Initiative (World Health Organization [WHO]-United Nations Children Fund [UNICEF], 2009), and these will be explored further in Chapter 6.

Social Cognitive Theory: Self-efficacy and Health Behavior Research

The SCT flows from psychosocial models and behavioral science research and represents one of the dominant health promotion theories used to understand human behavior—initially fearful and avoidant behavior—and to develop interventions targeted to change behavior. Self-efficacy, a component of SCT, is considered a manipulable component in health behavior research (Bandura, 1986; Campbell, 1996). Harnessing SCT's predictive power, Bandura (1986) and others using the theory take into consideration significant changes in human affect, thought, and action, and they considered how individuals learn and the incentives that fuel their desire to change behavior. Health behavior can be difficult to change, and it is affected by individuals' attitudes and beliefs. Bandura (1986) targeted identification of areas where individuals felt less confident about their knowledge, attitude, and skills and provided them with opportunities to master new behavior through enactive attainment, vicarious experience, verbal persuasion, and management of their emotional arousal. Social cognitive theories' broader explanation of human behavior expands definitions of variables, such as learning and incentives. In addition, it draws attention to the cognitive processing of information (e.g., motivations and incentives) that leads to efficacy judgments about one's ability to be successful that, in turn, affect one's behavior (Campbell, 1996).

The important distinction between self-efficacy and other constructs of SCT (e.g., self-esteem and self-concept) is that it is not a personality characteristic or global trait, but rather, it can be perceived to be task and situation specific. Over time, Bandura (1986) further refined the theory to better explain the role of goals; perceived environment and triadic influence; and behavioral, personal, and environmental factors. The importance of fostering self-efficacy in breastfeeding parents has been studied over time and supports Bandura's theory that successful performance and developing favorable perceptions of their outcomes (e.g., healthy thriving infant, bond, and positive experience) identify breastfeeding exclusivity and duration.

Incentive to action and knowledge are other key concepts related to self-efficacy, and incentive to breastfeed has been found to be a very important variable for self-efficacy as it mediates the relationship between knowledge and behavior. Most parents, given the science and present benefits of breastfeeding, have incentive to breastfeed. Although knowledge is necessary to determine behavior, this alone cannot explain parents' success in meeting their infant feeding goals as it is imperative for them to overcome barriers, maintain motivation, and persist at the behavior. When adequate skills are present, SCT postulates that self-efficacy will determine the intensity and persistence of effort to meet those goals, or rather the concentration and strength of effort in the face of barriers (e.g., breast pain, nipple trauma, and infant growth). An individual with a higher judgment of self-efficacy will persist longer and with greater intensity than someone with a low judgment of breast-feeding self-efficacy. If someone loses confidence in their ability to breastfeed, they are more likely to discontinue breastfeeding, especially when faced with multiple obstacles and repeated perceived failures.

An important distinction of this theory for examining breastfeeding as a health behavior is the inclusion of the emotional state of arousal. Because breastfeeding is a physiological and psychological behavior, consideration of this cognitive component of arousal, with its behavioral component of performance fear, is especially important. The stress of pregnancy, birth, and responsibility for a new life can lead to new parents' decreasing self-efficacy, fear of lack of breastfeeding success, requirement of more effort, and performance fear arousal. Without confirmation of normalcy of the process of breastfeeding, infant cues and patterns, and ways to evaluate the "success" of their behavior, new parents can become at risk of discontinuing breastfeeding and not meeting their infant feeding goals. SCT can help us understand the processes occurring and identify specific interventions to support parents and provide incentives (benefits), knowledge (information and vicarious experience), accurate feedback on the behavior (e.g., comfortable latch, milk transfer, infant growth, organizing and implementing new patterns of behavior), and verbal persuasion with positive reinforcement that help new parents manage their emotional arousal and feel efficacious in their "performance" of this new health behavior of breastfeeding. The role of health care providers in educating and supporting new parents using SCT requires understanding of foundational information about lactation and breastfeeding as well as helping parents manage preconceived standards and evaluation of their own ability to succeed and develop breastfeeding self-efficacy.

The following framework was proposed in the development of a Breastfeeding Promotion Nursing Intervention (BPNI) to describe the structural relationships of self-efficacy with other concepts in **social cognitive theory** (Campbell, 1996). This framework supports an internally consistent theory that allows predictions and is logically adequate. There are many intermediary steps between self-efficacy and breastfeeding performance, which weakens the heuristic power of the theory as a whole but lends itself to the testing of specific aspects of the theory within this framework. **Figure 3-1** illustrates this framework (Campbell, 1996).

Campbell (1996) used this model to test the manipulation of self-efficacy in an experimental group by providing information (text and resources, including a step-by-step practice sheet), persuasion (verbal support), role modeling (vicarious experience), demonstration (enactive attainment, practice), guided imagery, and measuring variations in outcome behavior as a way of testing self-efficacy's effect on behavior. These early findings of a Breastfeeding Promotion Nursing Intervention (BPNI) supported a 1-hour prenatal intervention and postpartal follow-up with a visit within 72 hours of birth and phone calls at 2, 3, and 6 weeks postpartum in a sample of highly educated, middle-class, primiparous women who intended to breastfeed, which resulted in high breastfeeding self-efficacy scores at 6 weeks (100% experimental) (Campbell, 1996).

Since the introduction of the Innocenti Declaration and Infant and Young Child Feeding (IYCF) by UNICEF and the WHO, breastfeeding self-efficacy (BSE) theory has been well utilized to examine breastfeeding behavior (Campbell, 1996;

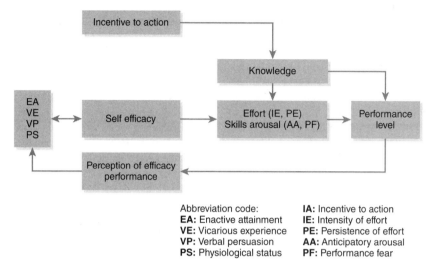

Figure 3-1 Structural relationships: Self-efficacy and related concepts interpreted from Bandura's (1982, 1986) writings by Campbell (1991b, 1991c).

© Suzanne Hetzel Campbell 1991.

McCarter-Spaulding & Gore, 2009; Noel-Weiss et al., 2006; Pollard & Guill, 2009; Tuthill et al., 2016). Several studies found that mothers with a higher level of BSE were more likely to breastfeed their newborns exclusively in the immediate postpartum period (Dennis & Faux, 1999; Loke & Chan, 2013). A systematic review and meta-analysis of the research analyzing interventions to enhance BSE support that BSE is modifiable and can be targeted with a positive effect on rates of breastfeeding in mothers of full-term infants. The interventions having the most effect on BSE include education and support at hospital discharge and at 1 and 2 months postpartum. Similarly, improvements in BSE predicted increases in exclusive breastfeeding rates (Brockway et al., 2017). Finally, a systematic review and meta-analysis found an association between educational programs targeted to enhance BSE and parents' perceptions of insufficient milk supply.

These compilations of the research done on BSE, examining interventions to effect it, and breastfeeding outcomes suggest that BSE as a social change theory can explain breastfeeding behavior.

The next most commonly used theory for breastfeeding health promotion research is the reasoned action approach.

A critical review of the use of these theories (SE, TPB, SCT) to research breastfeeding interventions found that the interventions developed did not use the theories to adequately guide interventions for testing the proposed outcomes, thus results were inconclusive (Bai et al., 2019).

Reasoned Action Approach

The **reasoned action approach** to health promotion (Fishbein & Ajzen, 2011) emerged from two theories: the theory of reasoned action and the theory of planned action. The approach redefines the initial constructs of attitude, subjective norms, perceived behavioral control, and autonomy and combines them to examine changes in behavior. Attitude was expanded and stratified into subdimensions to distinguish the instrumental or cognitive feature from the experiential or affective feature. In lactation, for instance, new parents intend to breastfeed their infants (i.e., the experiential aspect of attitude) because it is identified as the gold standard of infant feeding methods and is recommended for good health (instrumental aspect of attitude). Next, subjective norm was expanded to take into consideration the perception of support from significant others compared to how prevalent the behavior is in one's immediate social environment. Given the above example, the same parents' ability to meet their infant feeding goals will be influenced by their perceptions of how supportive significant others are and whether they believe society and their immediate environment are supportive of the behavior. Finally, in relation to beliefs in this expanded approach, parents' perceived behavioral control—capacity (e.g., self-efficacy) to enact the behavior and their autonomy or perceived individual control—will affect their success at meeting their goals. One of the major criticisms of the theory is that "few interventions led to significant changes in behaviours," so although there might be some guidance in identifying intervention targets, exactly *how* to act on these targets is not clearly identified in the research (Rootman et al., 2017, pp. 71–72). The original authors of the theories suggest integrating this approach with other theoretical models (Fishbein & Cappella, 2006; Fishbein & Yzer, 2003).

The Theory of Reasoned Action

The theory of reasoned action (Fishbein & Ajzen, 1975) posits that behaviors are driven by people's intentions; they have a mental plan for their action and to meet their goals. For parents, this often involves attending parenting and breastfeeding classes; talking to family, friends, and peers about their experiences; and creating a "plan" to meet those goals. These intentions and the motivation they demonstrate toward the behavior are also influenced by their attitudes, which include the value they place on the importance of breastfeeding, directly affecting their ability to meet their infant feeding goals. In addition, the subjective norms they are exposed to—in the form of approval or disapproval from peers, friends, loved ones, society and others related to their breastfeeding—will affect their ultimate behavior and success. This theory was written and tested long before the advent of social media, and new parents' exposure to this subjective norm is in the early stages of being tested, but research suggests that it is a powerful influence on breastfeeding behavior (Nguyen et al., 2016; Tharmaratnam, 2019).

The Theory of Planned Behavior

The theory of planned behavior (TPB) links beliefs to behavior by considering attitudes, norms, and perceived behavioral control to shape an individual's intentions and achievement of the desired behavior. Those who have used the theory of planned behavior (Ajzen, 1985) to examine breastfeeding behavior usually identify the presence of external or internal obstacles, especially those affecting an individual's perceived behavioral control.

This theory has been used to examine breastfeeding intentions and outcomes in a variety of populations (Avery et al., 1998; Bai et al., 2010, 2011; Dodgson et al., 2003; Horodynski et al., 2011; Rempel, 2004; Wambach, 1997; Wambach et al., 2011; Wambach & Koehn, 2004) and even to examine the intention to donate to human milk banks (Grunert, 2018). There is evidence that it is important for health care providers to take into consideration the beliefs held by individuals' social networks and individuals' perceptions of those beliefs and social norms. These social networks, including the general public, can affect parents' decision making, motivation, and success around meeting their infant feeding goals. For example, research has shown that social stigmas around breastfeeding in public have affected parents' motivation and led to extreme reactions (Sheehan et al., 2019). Social stigmas have ranged from breastfeeding parents' being asked to leave such places as restaurants, malls, and swimming pools to the arrest of the breastfeeding parent for indecent exposure. Some reactions have included "sit-ins," where breastfeeding mothers show up in large numbers where a breastfeeding parent may have been asked to leave, or legal battles over parental and child rights leading to local, national, and global policies to support the right of parent–infant dyads to breastfeed anywhere, anytime. The importance of this health promotion theoretical approach is its consideration of the complexity of parents' beliefs, attitudes, and perceptions of social norms in light of their own personal tendencies to conform or not and is influenced by their perception of their status in society. Chapter 10 further explores these complexities in examining inequities in the area of lactation health promotion.

A systematic review of observational studies that examined breastfeeding duration related to the theory of planned behavior (TPB) and breastfeeding self-efficacy (BSE) frameworks found that the most important predictors of breastfeeding duration were maternal intention and breastfeeding self-efficacy. Other variables, including maternal attitudes, subjective norms, and perceived control, provided inconsistent findings with regard to their relationship to breastfeeding duration (Lau et al., 2018). This points to the fact that many more studies need to be done.

The Health Belief Model

The health belief model (HBM) is a social psychological model developed in the 1950s to explain and predict health behavior change (Rosenstock, 1974). As one of the oldest models, it has been widely used, and many of the theories that came after it incorporated some of the underlying constructs. In examining health-promoting behavior, the HBM proposes that beliefs about a potential health issue—including how susceptible individuals believe they are and what the perceived threat of the disease is to them specifically—weighed against their perception of the benefits and barriers to action to resolve or prevent it, and self-efficacy, explain whether or not individuals engage in health promotion behavior. It identifies demographic variables and cues to action as modifying factors affecting individuals' perceived threat, and the model predicts the likelihood of them taking preventive action. There are several limitations in use of the HBM, one being that it does not consider individuals' attitudes, beliefs, or other factors affecting their behavior, such as perceptions and influence of social norms. It also suggests people are intentional in their decision making about healthy lifestyles and behaviors, evaluating their risk of disease, likely severity of illness, and benefits and barriers to taking action (Rootman et al., 2017). Research in areas such as hypertension, coronary artery disease, diabetes, and mental health has found that individuals often underestimate their risk of disease and its severity because of "invisible" symptoms and/or little signs of change when enacting the behavior. The HBM also does not take into consideration identification of personal goals, desires, and the difficulty of maintaining healthy lifestyle changes. The "cues to action" imply that the individual is dependent on health care providers and social or political structures to provide the impetus to change behavior. The major limitation is that, unless all four of the components of the model are present, it is unlikely that interventions will lead to permanent or sustainable behavior change (Rootman et al., 2017).

Research on lactation has used the HBM to analyze individuals' intentions to breastfeed, perceived risks, and breastfeeding duration. Regardless of the long-term health benefits of breastfeeding to mothers and infants (Rollins et al., 2016; Victora et al., 2016), they are difficult motivators in stressful moments when breastfeeding may not be going as expected and parents are feeling sleep deprived and uncertain. In addition, the social pressure to conform to the "breast is best" gold standard of infant feeding can make it a challenge for health professionals to present a balanced case of the benefits of breastfeeding. The HBM has been used to identify the benefits of breastfeeding and perceived barriers in programs like those developed for the Supplemental Nutrition Program for Women, Infant, and Children (WIC) in the United States. In this program, the HBM was not sufficient in isolation to create a program; the program also incorporated Stages of Change (e.g., contemplators answer "breastfeed" to the question "How do you plan to feed your baby?") and social learning theory/SCT incorporating motivators, facilitators, and barriers as well as interventions to enhance BSE (Lindenberger & Bryant, 2000; WIC, 2020). **Figure 3-2**. shows the major constructs for the HBM.

Recognizing the core components of key health promotion theories and how they have been used to develop interventions, programs, and approaches to supporting and sustaining breastfeeding globally will be incorporated throughout other areas of the text. This list is in no way exclusive, and as you can see, theories are continually expanding and changing as they are tested and used over time.

Summary

The efficacy of any of these health promotion studies to fully explain the complex behavior of lactation is still to be seen, yet systematic reviews and meta-analyses of studies provide greater support for approaches based on these theories. A meta-synthesis on the efficacy of the TPB to predict breastfeeding found 10 studies with 2,694 participants using a structural modeling equation method determined that attitude, subjective norms, and perceived behavioral control were significant predictors of breastfeeding intention, which in turn was a strong predictor of breastfeeding behavior (Guo et al., 2016). Having statistical methods to help consolidate

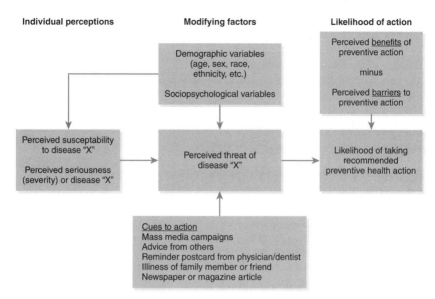

Individual perceptions   **Modifying factors**   **Likelihood of action**

Figure 3-2 Health belief model.

Modified from Janz, N. K., & Becker, M. H. (1984). The Health Belief Model: A Decade Later. *Health Education Quarterly, 11*(1), 1–47. doi:10.1177/109019818401100101

the published evidence will help to further direct us in the testing, shaping, and transforming of our health promotion theoretical models to benefit breastfeeding families globally. Chapter 4 will explore the important role of policy in the promotion and support of breastfeeding families.

Key Points to Remember

1. Many factors affect individuals' decision making related to healthy behavior, and many theoretical models help identify key components for successful programs, policies, and models of care.
2. Working with parents to set their infant feeding goals requires developing trust and rapport to help them identify their attitudes and beliefs in this important area of parenting.
3. In light of the theories examined, directing conversations with new parents to address their concerns (perceived barriers) and balancing messaging of the benefits and risks of breastfeeding are important approaches for health care providers.
4. Discussing perceptions around intentions, motivators, barriers, self-confidence, social support, and setting realistic goals with identified support systems is most likely to lead to success in creating a plan with parents to meet their goals.
5. Several factors represent unique challenges in approaching lactation as a health-related behavior, such as that it cannot be practiced prior to the birth of the parents' first infant; parents represent specific attitudes, beliefs, and subjective norms; and parents are exposed to vicarious experiences of both breastfeeding and bottle feeding, which can affect all the other compounding factors.

Self-Reflection

1. Consider your exposure to breastfeeding. Do you have family members, friends, or colleagues who have breastfed?
2. Analyze your own beliefs about breastfeeding: the benefits, risks, myths, contraindications.
3. Have you had any personal experience with breastfeeding? Might this affect your ability to support parents?

Case Study with Questions Based on the Scenario

Robin and her partner are in their early 30s and are excited about the upcoming birth of their first child. They have heard and read a lot of conflicting information about breastfeeding, and although they just assumed that was how they would feed their infant, now that the due date is coming up they are feeling nervous about it.

1. Outline your approach with this couple from three perspectives:
   a. Using an HBM theoretical health promotion model
   b. Using a TPB model
   c. Using a BSE model
2. What are the advantages and limitations of each model for helping this couple to meet their goals?

Additional Resources

Special Supplemental Nutrition Program for Women, Infants, and Children (WIC) https://www.fns.usda.gov/wic

WIC Breastfeeding Support https://www.fns.usda.gov/wic/wic-breastfeeding-support

Website Resources

Theory of Planned Behavior Diagram
https://people.umass.edu/aizen/tpb.diag.html

References

Ajzen, I. (1985). From intentions to actions: A theory of planned behavior. In J. Kuhl & J. Beckmann (Eds.), *Action-control: From cognition to behavior* (pp. 11–39). Springer.

Avery, M., Duckett, L., Dodgson, J., Savik, K., & Henly, S. J. (1998). Factors associated with very early weaning among primiparas intending to breastfeed. *Maternal and Child Health Journal, 2*(3), 167–179.

Bai, Y., Middlestadt, S. E., Peng, C. Y. J., & Fly, A. D. (2010). Predictors of continuation of exclusive breastfeeding for the first six months of life. *Journal of Human Lactation, 26*(1), 26–34. https://doi.org/10.1177/0890334409350168

Bai, Y., Wunderlich, S. M., & Fly, A. D. (2011). Predicting intentions to continue exclusive breastfeeding for 6 months: A comparison among racial/ethnic groups. *Maternal and Child Health Journal, 15*(8), 1257–1264. https://doi.org/10.1007/s10995-010-0703-7

Bai, Y. K., Lee, S., & Overgaard, K. (2019). Critical review of theory use in breastfeeding interventions. *Journal of Human Lactation, 35*(3), 478–500. https://doi.org/10.1177/0890334419850822

Bandura, A. (1986). *Social foundations of thought and action: A social cognitive theory.* Prentice-Hall, Inc.

Brockway, M., Benzies, K., & Hayden, K. A. (2017). Interventions to improve breastfeeding self-efficacy and resultant breastfeeding rates: A systematic review and meta-analysis. *Journal of Human Lactation, 33*(3), 486–499. https://doi.org/10.1177/0890334417707957

Campbell, S. H. (1996). *Breastfeeding self-efficacy: The effects of a breastfeeding promotion nursing intervention.* (PhD Doctoral Dissertation). University of Rhode Island, Dissertations and Master's Theses (Campus Access). http://digitalcommons.uri.edu/dissertations/AAI9707172 (Paper AAI9707172)

Dennis, C., & Faux, S. (1999). Development and psychometric testing of the Breastfeeding Self-Efficacy Scale. *Research in Nursing & Health, 22*(5), 399–409. https://doi.org/10.1002/(sici)1098-240x(199910)22:5<399::aid-nur6>3.0.co;2-4

Dodgson, J. E., Henly, S. J., Duckett, L., & Tarrant, M. (2003). Theory of planned behavior-based models for breastfeeding duration among Hong Kong mothers. *Nursing Research, 52*(3), 148–158. https://doi.org/10.1097/00006199-200305000-00004

Fishbein, M., & Ajzen, I. (1975). *Belief, attitude, intention and behavior: An introduction to theory of research.* Addison-Wesley.

Fishbein, M., & Ajzen, I. (2011). *Predicting and changing behavior: The reasoned action approach.* Taylor & Francis.

Fishbein, M., & Cappella, J. N. (2006). The role of theory in developing effective health communications. *Journal of Communication, 56*(s1), S1–S17. https://doi.org/10.1111/j.1460-2466.2006.00280.x

Fishbein, M., & Yzer, M. C. (2003). Using theory to design effective health behavior interventions. *Communication Theory, 13*(2), 164–183. https://doi.org/10.1111/j.1468-2885.2003.tb00287.x

Grunert, D. (2018). *Decision making surrounding human milk donation: Attitudes, subjective norms and barriers* (MSN MS). University of British Columbia. https://open.library.ubc.ca/collections/ubctheses/24/items/1.0365593

Guo, J. L., Wang, T. F., Liao, J. Y., & Huang, C. M. (2016). Efficacy of the theory of planned behavior in predicting breastfeeding: Meta-analysis and structural equation modeling. *Applied Nursing Research, 29*, 37–42. https://doi.org/10.1016/j.apnr.2015.03.016

Horodynski, M. A., Olson, B., Baker, S., Brophy-Herb, H., Auld, G., Van Egeren, L., Lindau, J., & Singleterry, L. (2011). Healthy babies through infant-centered feeding protocol: An intervention targeting early childhood obesity in vulnerable populations. *BMC Public Health, 11*, 868–868. https://doi.org/10.1186/1471-2458-11-868

Horta, B. L., Loret de Mola, C., & Victora, C. G. (2015). Long-term consequences of breastfeeding on cholesterol, obesity, systolic blood pressure and type 2 diabetes: A systematic review and meta-analysis. *Acta Paediatrica, 104*, 30–37. https://doi.org/10.1111/apa.13133

Lau, C. Y. K., Lok, K. Y. W., & Tarrant, M. (2018). Breastfeeding duration and the theory of planned behavior and breastfeeding self-efficacy framework: A systematic review of observational studies. *Maternal Child Health Journal, 22*(3), 327–342. https://doi.org/10.1007/s10995-018-2453-x

Lindenberger, J. H., & Bryant, C. A. (2000). Promoting breastfeeding in the WIC program: A social marketing case study. *American Journal of Health Behavior, 24*(1), 53–60. https://doi.org/10.5993/AJHB.24.1.8

Loke, A. Y., & Chan, L. K. (2013). Maternal breastfeeding self-efficacy and the breastfeeding behaviors of newborns in the practice of exclusive breastfeeding. *Journal of Obstetric, Gynecologic & Neonatal Nursing, 42*(6), 672–684. https://doi.org/10.1111/1552-6909.12250

McCarter-Spaulding, D., & Gore, R. (2009). Breastfeeding self-efficacy in women of African descent. *JOGNN: Journal of Obstetric, Gynecologic & Neonatal Nursing, 38*(2), 230–243. https://doi.org/10.1111/j.1552-6909.2009.01011.x

Nguyen, P. H., Kim, S. S., Nguyen, T. T., Hajeebhoy, N., Tran, L. M., Alayon, S., Ruel, M. T., Rawat, R., Frongillo, E. A., & Menon, P. (2016). Exposure to mass media and interpersonal counseling has additive effects on exclusive breastfeeding and its psychosocial determinants among Vietnamese mothers. *Maternal & Child Nutrition, 12*(4), 713–725. https://doi.org/10.1111/mcn.12330

Noel-Weiss, J., Rupp, A., Cragg, B., Bassett, V., & Woodend, A. K. (2006). Randomized controlled trial to determine effects of prenatal breastfeeding workshop on maternal breastfeeding self-efficacy and breastfeeding duration. *JOGNN: Journal of Obstetric, Gynecologic & Neonatal Nursing, 35*(5), 616–624. https://doi.org/10.1111/j.1552-6909.2006.00077.x

Pollard, D., & Guill, M. (2009). The relationship between baseline self-efficacy and breastfeeding duration. *Southern Online Journal of Nursing Research, 9*(4),1-8. https://doi.org/10.19082/3751

Rempel, L. A. (2004). Factors influencing the breastfeeding decisions of long-term breastfeeders. *Journal of Human Lactation, 20*(3), 306–318. https://doi.org/10.1177/0890334404266969

Rollins, N. C., Bhandari, N., Hajeebhoy, N., Horton, S., Lutter, C. K., Martines, J. C., Piwoz, E. G., Richter, L. M., & Victora, C. G. (2016). Why invest, and what it will take to improve breastfeeding practices? *The Lancet, 387*(10017), 491–504. https://doi.org/10.1016/S0140-6736(15)01044-2

Rootman, I., Pederson, A., Frohlich, K., & Dupere, S. (2017). *Health promotion in Canada: Critical perspectives on theory, practice, policy, and research* (4th ed.). Canadian Scholars.

Rosenstock, I. M. (1974). Historical origins of the health belief model. *Health Education Monographs, 2*(4), 328–335. https://doi.org/10.1177/109019817400200403

Sheehan, A., Gribble, K., & Schmied, V. (2019). It's okay to breastfeed in public but. . . . *International Breastfeeding Journal, 14*(1), 24. https://doi.org/10.1186/s13006-019-0216-y

Tharmaratnam, T. (2019). *Mothers' perspectives on smartphone use while breastfeeding* (MSN Master of Science in Nursing). University of British Columbia. https://open.library.ubc.ca/collections/ubctheses/24/items/1.0385536

Tuthill, E. L., McGrath, J. M., Graber, M., Cusson, R. M., & Young, S. L. (2016). Breastfeeding self-efficacy: A critical review of available instruments. *Journal of Human Lactation, 32*(1), 35–45. https://doi.org/10.1177/0890334415599533

Victora, C. G., Horta, B. L., de Mola, C. L., Quevedo, L., Pinheiro, R. T., Gigante, D. P., Gonçalves, H., & Barros, F. C. (2015). Association between breastfeeding and intelligence, educational attainment, and income at 30 years of age: A prospective birth cohort study from Brazil. *The Lancet Global Health, 3*(4), e199–e205. https://doi.org/10.1016/S2214-109X(15)70002-1

Victora, C. G., Bahl, R., Barros, A. J. D., França, G. V. A., Horton, S., Krasevec, J., Murch, S., Sankar, M. J., Walker, N., Rollins, N. C., & The Lancet Breastfeeding Group. (2016). Breastfeeding in the 21st century: Epidemiology, mechanisms, and lifelong effect. *The Lancet, 387*(10017), 475–490. https://doi.org/10.1016/S0140-6736(15)01024-7

Walker, M. (2007). International breastfeeding initiatives and their relevance to the current state of breastfeeding in the United States. *Journal of Midwifery and Women's Health, 52*(6), 549–555. https://doi.org/10.1016/j.jmwh.2007.06.013

Wambach, K. A. (1997). Breastfeeding intention and outcome: A test of the theory of planned behavior. *Research in Nursing & Health, 20*(1), 51–59. https://doi.org/10.100 2/(sici)1098-240x(199702)20:1<51::aid-nur6>3.0.co;2-t

Wambach, K. A., Aaronson, L., Breedlove, G., Domian, E. W., Rojjanasrirat, W., & Yeh, H.-W. (2011). A randomized controlled trial of breastfeeding support and education for adolescent mothers. *Western Journal of Nursing Research, 33*(4), 486–505. https://doi.org/10.1177/0193945910380408

Wambach, K. A., & Koehn, M. (2004). Experiences of infant-feeding decision-making among urban economically disadvantaged pregnant adolescents. *Journal of Advanced Nursing, 48*(4), 361–370. https://doi.org/10.1111/j.1365-2648.2004.03205.x

WHO-UNICEF. (2009). *Baby-friendly Hospital Initiative: Revised, updated and expanded for integrated care.* http://www.who.int/nutrition/publications/infantfeeding/bfhi_trainingcourse/en/

WIC Breastfeeding Support. (2020). https://www.fns.usda.gov/wic/wic-breastfeeding-support

CHAPTER 4

Social Policy and Lactation

Rhoda Taylor, BA, MPH, IBCLC
Jolynn Dowling, MSN, APRN, NNP-BC, IBCLC

LEARNING OBJECTIVES

1. Recognize that the impact of policy at regional levels (state/provincial) can have the largest effect on breastfeeding initiation, promotion, and support.
2. Identify public policy antecedents that lead to health inequities related to lactation.
3. Compare and contrast lactation as an individual or social and economic decision.
4. Describe the role of community coalitions in supporting parents to meet their infant feeding goals.
5. Explore where and how policies can support health system changes.
6. Examine the outcome of deliverables from policies and organizations.
7. Understand the responsibility of healthcare professionals to develop and implement appropriate, effective policies influencing breastfeeding mothers, infants, and their families.

KEY WORDS

- **Policy:** A set of ideas or a plan of what to do in particular situations that has been agreed to officially by a group of people, a business organization, a government, or a political party." (Cambridge University Press, 2020)

Overview

This chapter outlines the importance of **policy** on breastfeeding rates and decision making. It discusses possible policy development tools and methods while empha-sizing the value of healthcare professionals' involvement in policy making both by collaboration in advocacy networks and in direct participation within agencies and government.

The experience and knowledge held within the lactation, nursing, and medical professions are invaluable in policy discussions concerning breastfeeding, but it is incumbent upon those with that knowledge to reach out to share it in a format and manner that can be heard by policy makers (Thomas et al., 2019). This requires healthcare professionals to learn the skills to participate in policy discussions by supporting, encouraging, and participating in advocacy groups at local, regional, state, and national levels; participating in policy development within agencies and government departments; and direct engagement with politicians and political staff.

Historical Perspective of Breastfeeding Policy

Policies impacting breastfeeding emerged in the early 20th century as breastfeeding rates declined, the commercialization of alternative human milk substitutes grew, and public health authorities expanded their involvement in public education regarding infant feeding (Palmer, 2009; Papastavrou et al., 2015; Nathoo & Ostry, 2009). By the 1970s, there was an increasing concern worldwide about the impact of the marketing of alternative infant feeding, in particular commercial human milk substitutes (formula). This resulted in a series of international policies and recommendations that had limited results (Rollins et al., 2016). The recognition that breastfeeding rates, in particular rates of breastfeeding duration, were not easily impacted by those policies—however well intended and written—combined with a greater understanding of breastfeeding's importance for public health and economic outcomes has resulted in a greater appreciation of this as a "wicked" public policy problem (Dowling et al., 2018).

"Wicked" policy problems are those that are complex, multicausal; have a number of possible interventions, some of which will have a significant negative impact if the policies are not successful; and for which there is no clear history of success (Rittel & Webber, 1973). Knowledge of "wicked" problems has grown since the introduction of the concept, and experience with what may also be referred to as complexity problems has allowed a greater understanding of what helps to make policies most likely to succeed (Alford & Head, 2017; Peters, 2017).

When policies were first developed with the intent of increasing breastfeeding initiation and duration, there was an anticipation that the problem of mothers not breastfeeding could be resolved with some relatively simple policy interventions. An example was the hope that regulating and controlling the marketing of human milk substitutes would have the result of breastfeeding rates returning to previously higher levels. This led to the World Health Organization (WHO) and United Nations International Children's Emergency Fund (UNICEF) International Code of Marketing of Breast-milk Substitutes (WHO, 1981); Innocenti Declaration on the Protection, Promotion and Support of Breastfeeding (1990, UNICEF 2005); and the Ten Steps, the initial Baby-friendly Hospital Initiative (WHO-UNICEF, 2009). (See chapter 6, Figure 6-2.) Concurrently the right to breastfeed and to receive quality nutrition for women and children was included in both the Convention on the Elimination of All Forms of Discrimination Against Women (United Nations High Commissioner for Refugees [UNHCR], 1979) and in the Convention on the Rights of the Child UNHCR, 1989). In the ensuing decades, it has become clear that while all of these actions and policy developments have been valuable, achieving breastfeeding rates that meet the recommendation of exclusive breastfeeding to

6 months and some breastfeeding to 2 years and beyond will not happen without further action (Centers for Disease Control and Prevention [CDC], 2011; CDC 2018; Protheroe et al., 2003; Victora et al., 2016; WHO, 2016).

Impact of Breastfeeding Policy

While there is some consensus on the goal, there are significant variations in policies across national and regional governments. The variability of jurisdictions and the regional and national culture of each jurisdiction impacts which level of government policy is most probable and effective (Balogun et al., 2016; EU Directorate Public Health and Risk Assessment, 2008; Heyman et al., 2013) Policies that are able to encompass a wide spectrum of government departments and authority are those most likely to have a cross-spectrum impact. It is this wide sociopolitical impact that is most likely to have success. For example, we know that low-income mothers in high-income nations are the least likely to breastfeed; however, why "is best understood as an outcome of political-economic and socio-cultural relations" (Frank, 2015). In order to change the initiation and duration of breastfeeding, it is imperative that policies be established to meet the needs and environment of the specific population in need of support (MacGillivray, 2016). While not without value, a simple public relations campaign is extremely unlikely to result in the required changes.

Policy focus on the ground has primarily been on the individual choice about whether or not to breastfeed. Promotion of breastfeeding in a wide diversity of marketing campaigns has heightened knowledge and impacted initiation but has not dealt with the many underlying barriers. There is some evidence that these promotion initiatives have had a positive impact on breastfeeding initiation rates, but research is less positive regarding a change in the duration of breastfeeding when measured at 6 or 12 months (Bosi et al., 2015; CDC, 2018; Fallon et al., 2019; Rollins et al., 2016). Changing the duration of exclusive breastfeeding and the duration of breastfeeding requires a wider perspective.

Factors Influencing Breastfeeding Policy

There are political, economic, social, and cultural barriers that exist for those who wish to breastfeed or are breastfeeding (Pérez-Escamilla, 2020; Pérez-Escamilla et al., 2016). These are beyond hospital or public health unit walls. They include what may appear to be simple, such as the ability to feel safe while breastfeeding outside one's home. They may be more complex, such as the provision of paid maternity leave or the right to take pumping breaks and have a place to safely store the pumped milk while at work. Policies regarding funding low-income families may provide a subsidy for human milk substitutes (formula) but not for a breastfeeding mother to access quality food. It may be funding of a fixed amount. Mothers will use a subsidy or provided food to feed older children before herself. To be effective, the number of people in the family must be taken into account. There may also be social barriers, such as cultural beliefs that interfere with breastfeeding duration, particularly duration of exclusive breastfeeding (Agunbiade & Ogunleye, 2012; Joseph & Earland, 2019; Kridli, 2011; Mahesh et al., 2018).

At a population health level, few significantly impactful policy changes are made for a purely health outcome reason. Political and economic factors play a significant and often under-recognized role. It is typically necessary to build a business case for why a policy should or could be implemented. Several studies have looked at the potential cost savings of increased breastfeeding rates and particularly exclusive breastfeeding rates to both healthcare systems and specific healthcare facilities in economically developed nations (Bartick & Reinhold, 2010; Renfrew et al., 2012). These cost savings have been dramatic in jurisdictions with initial low breastfeeding initiation rates (Renfrew et al., 2012; Weimar, 2001).

Policy Development

Final decision makers are often short of time and may not be particularly interested in depth or detail. The most common expectation is for a policy research paper to be written. Once completed, this is summarized into a briefing note. Care must be taken to ensure that the research for the paper is both targeted to the purpose and as broad and unbiased as possible. Frequently this involves research in academic areas that are beyond healthcare provision. Briefing notes are preferably one page and do not normally exceed two pages but may be longer when appendixes are attached. A briefing note asking for a decision typically presents three possible options, one of which is usually the status quo. Most organizations have their own preferred briefing note template, an example of which is provided in **Figure 4-1**. The power of using economic, social and political science research to build a case for a breastfeeding policy cannot be overstated. Significant and cross government policies are rarely instituted simply because it may improve health outcomes. It is necessary to look into the population health impact on society, government finance and the political philosophy of the decision makers currently enacting policy.

Working on policy development requires consideration of a range of perspectives. There is a tendency to step back and blame policy makers for not taking action when no attempt has been made to reach out and either educate or be educated. Criticism is easy, while making substantive change across a society through policy and action is not easy. Recognizing barriers and working in collaboration to form a policy is more likely to be successful. Coalitions and partnerships are most likely to have productive impact.

Establishing the Need for Policy Change

When forming a policy, it is necessary to consider several broad questions. Is the policy intended to impact only a narrow range of services, agencies, service providers, or patients? Is it a policy intended to be widely implemented? Would you like the policy to create action or be a statement? If the intent is for change, how will you build the requirement for action into the policy? What action do you wish, and who will be required to make it? Does the policy require legislation or regulation? How much will the action (if there is one) cost? Who will pay? How will you measure outcomes so it can be known that change is taking place and whether that change is positive?

Start by looking at the wider perspectives of those who will be making the policy and those who will be enacting it. How do your goals align with theirs? It may not be as simple as we all want improved maternal/child health. There may be economic or financial impacts that tip the balance. An example of this is the work of the World Bank (Hansen, 2016; Holla et al., 2013, World Bank, 2015).

Figure 4-1 Briefing Note Sample Template

ORGANIZATION TITLE
TYPE OF BRIEFING NOTE (INFORMATION OR DECISION?)

PREPARED FOR:	- FOR (information or policy or action?)
TITLE:	**5 words or less**
PURPOSE:	One sentence – Why are you sending this note? Is it for a specific meeting or time? If so, include this.
BACKGROUND:	Facts only. Use short paragraphs, ideally with only three sentences each. This is typically only one-third of a page
DISCUSSION:	Use this to summarize the position. Include background and the perspective of the organization to which this is directed. Include the current policies or history as well as any economic or financial impacts. This should be less than one-third of a page.
ADVICE:	A summary or conclusion, including next steps or recommendations for action if appropriate. This can be bullets or short paragraphs. Tailor it to the situation (e.g., a meeting or a presentation). Typically, three options are given for action, with the status quo being one of the options.

Drafters:
Date:

NOTES:

Briefing documents must be no longer than two pages.

Briefing documents including data must include footnotes at the end, and the data must be attached as a third page labeled as an appendix.

Appendixes may make the briefing note longer. Attach pertinent information, including legal and financial references if appropriate.

"The World Bank Group is committed to support the expansion of breastfeeding. . . . We are making the economic case to minister of health, finance, and planning, as well to political leaders" (Hansen, 2016, p. 416).

Does bringing in the Baby-friendly Hospital Initiative (BFHI) increase exclusive breastfeeding rates, or does it reduce hospital stays for premature babies or re-admittance of infants and mothers with a resulting reduction in costs? Is there a need for an increased level in staffing? Do the costs balance out in the long term? In a for-profit system does implementing BFHI increase the number of mothers choosing the hospital as well as improve outcomes? If so, this may increase the willingness of hospital administrators to establish the policy. Policy development is more than making nice statements that sound good. You should expect to bring a fully developed argument that extends beyond the language and needs of health outcomes and provides a reasoned plan to measure the results.

Establishing the Audience for Policy Change

Try to establish the audience with whom you are working and use the language with which they are familiar. If you are dealing predominantly with business people, then using medical terminology exclusively may not bring about the results you desire. Significant research exists for the business case for increasing breastfeeding and family-friendly policies (Hansen, 2016; Holla et al., 2013, Kim et al., 2019). Perhaps you can reach your goals through alternative routes. Across many jurisdictions in North America, significant policy changes have taken place as a result of human-rights agencies declaring that breastfeeding is a human right. Where this has happened, the right to breastfeed in public has become a de facto policy for all public and private agencies across the jurisdiction. This has been one of the most significant population-wide policy changes that we have seen in recent years.

Leveling the Policy Change

Identify the level at which you want the policy effected. Is it at a senior political or regional level or at a local agency or healthcare facility level? This will alter both the policy and the strategy required to have it declared and implemented. For example, there may be a policy to have "Breastfeeding Week" declared by a regional government every year. While this is a wonderful public awareness initiative, it may have no impact on the government's day-to-day operation. A policy at a regional government level requiring each facility to establish an appropriate breastfeeding pumping location would create a change in practice in those facilities. Ensure that you are taking into consideration all aspects of the policy.

Questions to consider: *What are the impact and cost of providing a pumping location? What guidelines are provided to ensure that the space is adequate, private, and safe? Is the space required in all facilities or only specified ones?*

Policy Implementation

A critical part of policy development is developing an understanding of the evolution a policy may take over time. Equal importance must be given to both writing the initial policy and evolving the policy as it moves toward implementation. A frequently missed step is building in a method of measuring outcomes in a frequent and reliable way. For example, in the United States, as well as in Canada, breastfeeding rates are collected but are generalized and not tied back to a small enough regional unit to be able to closely measure outcomes or impacts (CDC, 2016; Public Health Agency of Canada, 2018). This limits the knowledge gained and restricts the ability, at a local level, to understand the impact of policy changes and create amendments, if needed, to improve effectiveness.

The policy structure varies considerably across jurisdictions. Malta is a country consisting of a series of islands in the middle of the Mediterranean Sea. Its government structure does not face the complexity of a larger country. In 2015, the Maltese government brought in a National Breastfeeding Policy and Action Plan intended to be applied at five levels: marketing of human milk substitutes; hospital policy; training; promotion and support of breastfeeding in the community, including the workplace; and setting targets for monitoring. This policy builds upon an initial breastfeeding policy from 2000. The goal of the policy was to reestablish and reinforce a breastfeeding culture. Breastfeeding rates at discharge changed from 45% in 1995 to 66% in 2008, and more slowly they increased to 71% in 2014 (Bosi et al., 2015). This is a significant increase, but Malta continues to have one of the lowest breastfeeding initiation rates in the European Union (see **Table 4-1**). The 2015 policy supports parents prenatally

Table 4-1 Overview of breastfeeding practices in the WHO European Region* (data from 1998 to 2013)

	Breastfeeding within 1 h after birth (%)	EBF under 4 months (0–3.9 months; %)	EBF under 6 months (0–5.9 months; %)	EBF under 6 months (%)	Continued breastfeeding at 1 year (%)	Year of data collection
Albania	42.9	50.2	38.6	–	60.6	2008–2009
Armenia	35.7	47.9	35.0	–	44.2	2010
Austria	78.1	33.0	32.6	10.0	16.0	2006
Azerbaijan	31.9	16.0	11.8	–	26.4	2006
Belarus	53.0	–	19.0	–	27.9	2012
Belgium	–	–	–	11.8	–	2012
Bosnia and Herzegovina	42.3	23.6	18.5	–	12.4	2006/ 2011–2012
Bulgaria	4.6	5.7	2.0	–	–	2010
Croatia	–	–	52.4	–	–	2011
Cyprus	–	–	–	12.4	–	2004
Czech Republic	–	–	–	17.8	–	2011
Denmark	–	–	–	17.2	–	2012
Finland	–	–	–	1.0	–	2011
Georgia	66.3	–	54.8	–	36.5	2009
Germany	–	–	22.4	–	–	2003–2006
Greece	–	–	–	0.7	6.4	2009
Hungary	–	–	–	43.9	–	2007
Iceland	–	–	–	13.0	16.0	2011
Ireland	33.5	–	–	–	–	2008
Israel	–	–	–	11.2	11.8	1998–1999
Italy	–	–	–	5.0	12.0	1999
Kazakhstan	67.8	–	31.8	–	50.8	2010–2011
Kyrgyzstan	83.8	66.2	56.1	–	68.3	2012
Latvia	–	–	–	164	22.4	2011
Luxembourg	66.5	–	–	60	11.8	2008
Malta	–	–	–	35.9	–	2004–2005
Montenegro	25.2	25.8	19.3	–	24.6	2005
Netherlands	–	–	–	18.0	–	2010
Norway	–	–	–	7.0	–	2003
Poland	–	–	3.7	–	40.0	2013
Portugal	–	54.7	–	34.0	–	2003
Republic of Moldova	61.0	–	36.0	–	48.0	2012

(continued)

Table 4-1 Overview of breastfeeding practices in the WHO European Region* (data from 1998 to 2013) (*continued*)

	Breastfeeding within 1 h after birth (%)	EBF under 4 months (0–3.9 months; %)	EBF under 6 months (0–5.9 months; %)	EBF under 6 months (%)	Continued breastfeeding at 1 year (%)	Year of data collection
Romania	12.0	–	15.8	–	–	2004
Serbia	7.6	23.4	13.7	–	18.4	2005–2006/ 2010
Slovakia	–	–	–	49.3	–	2010
Spain	–	–	–	28.5	–	2011–2012
Sweden	–	–	–	14.0	–	2011
Switzerland	–	–	14.0	–	–	2003
Tajikistan	49.6	42.1	34.3	–	1.3	2012
The former Yugoslav Republic of Macedonia	21.0	–	23.0	–	33.8	2011
Turkey	39.0	–	41.6	–	66.7	2008
Turkmenistan	–	15.0	11.0	–	72.0	2009
Ukraine	65.7	–	19.7	–	37.9	2012
UK	–	–	–	1.0	–	2010
Uzbekistan	67.1	36.9	26.4	–	78.3	2006

EBF, exclusive breastfeeding; –, no data.
* No data for Andorra, Estonia, France, Lithuania, Monaco, Russian Federation, San Marino and Slovenia.
Overview of breastfeeding practices in the WHO European Region* (data from 1998 to 2013) Bosi, A.T. B., Eriksen, K. G., Sobko, T, Wijnhoven, T. M. A., & Breda, J. (2015). Breastfeeding Practices and policies in WHO European region member states

by providing prenatal classes. It supports professionals by providing training at many levels. Postnatally, it invests in public health support, including lactation consultants. Crucial sections include goals to develop facilities in workplaces and communities to facilitate the mother's normal social activity. The specificity of the goals is important, but adding a strong monitoring and reporting system is as or more important (Health Promotion and Disease Prevention Directorate, 2015).

The Maltese example is worthwhile, but the complexity of a country, such as the United States with its multiple jurisdictions and governing structures, changes policy development, monitoring, and enforcement. The layering of national, state, and local jurisdictions; social and cultural differences; and the complex corporate healthcare system can make policy development and application challenging. At the same time, existing structures, such as the CDC; U.S. Surgeon General; and effective networking of knowledgeable and experienced organizations, such as the United

Figure 4-2 United States Affordable Care Act (2010)

Health Benefits & Coverage
Breastfeeding Benefits

Most Marketplace plans must provide breastfeeding equipment and counseling for pregnant and nursing women.

You may be able to get help with breastfeeding at no cost.

Health insurance plans **must** provide breastfeeding support, counseling, and equipment for the duration of breastfeeding. These services may be provided before and after birth.

This applies to Marketplace plans and all other health insurance plans, except for grandfathered plans.

Coverage of Breast Pumps

Your health insurance plan **must** cover the cost of a breast pump. It may be either a rental unit or a new one you'll keep. Your plan may have guidelines on whether the covered pump is manual or electric, the length of the rental, and when you'll receive it (before or after birth). But it's up to you and your doctor to decide what's right for you.

Centers for Medicare & Medicaid Services. *Health benefits & coverage: Breastfeeding benefits.* https://www.healthcare.gov/coverage/breast-feeding-benefits

States Breastfeeding Committee (www.usbreastfeeding.org) and Baby-Friendly USA (www.babyfriendlyusa.org), provide a framework for innovation, policy development, and enforcement. This has led to an impressive policy framework but an uneven impact on the initiation and duration of breastfeeding (CDC, 2011, 2016; Gonzalez-Nahm et al., 2019; United States Breastfeeding Committee, 2020).

An example of a policy change that would not have taken place without a significant investment in research and advocacy is the inclusion of professional breastfeeding support in the Affordable Care Act. This is an example of a policy being implemented at a U.S. national level that has had profound local impact. See **Figure 4-2**.

Funding professional breastfeeding support on an individual level is not frequently mandated across a healthcare system. Countries with established local maternal healthcare may provide maternity care visits for a varying length of time pre- and postpartum, but the provision of qualified, professional support by lactation professionals to all breastfeeding mothers is not as common. It is difficult to overestimate the impact of treating professional breastfeeding support reimbursement as a valuable and important investment in healthcare provision. It not only provides personalized support; it also reinforces the importance of breastfeeding as something worthy of time and investment.

Role of the Health Professional

It is important to emphasize the requirement for healthcare professionals to learn the skills to participate in the policy discussions by supporting, encouraging, and participating in advocacy groups at local, regional, state, and national levels as well as through direct engagement with politicians and political staff. The experience and knowledge held within the nursing, medical and allied health professions are invaluable in the discussion, but it is incumbent upon those with the knowledge to reach out to share it in a format and manner that can be heard by policy makers.

Breastfeeding policy has a crucial impact on both the decision to breastfeed and the circumstances that support women to meet their goals for the duration of breastfeeding. It is critical that healthcare professionals learn the skills necessary to engage at all levels to advocate for and develop appropriate, effective policy (Horsley, 2010; Schmied et al., 2011). Working across disciplines and partnering with economists, businesses, and politicians provides the most effective way to create the necessary change. It is useful to learn from effective advocacy groups such as the U.S. Breastfeeding Committee and observing the impact made by a cross-government approach such as has been taken by the Government of Malta. Policy is all too often criticized both for its absence and for its presumed lack of effect. The best way to change this is to take the initiative to learn how to instigate policy change, measure its success or failure, and take the steps to move forward.

Learning Activities

1. Name three international policy initiatives.
2. Research policy initiatives from two countries. Which one is most likely to be effective and why? How would you measure outcomes?
3. Consider possibilities for dealing with decision and policy makers who are not healthcare providers. Which method do you feel would be most effective, and why?
4. Identify the pros and cons of specific policies, such as parental leave, workplace regulations and childcare availability on women's breastfeeding decisions and outcomes, recognizing the importance of the social determinants of health.

Key Points to Remember

1. Policies are key to assisting mothers to decide on and achieve their breastfeeding goals.
2. It is incumbent on all health care professionals to understand the policy-making process and to engage with that process.
3. Policies differ across jurisdictions. Learning from the experience of others assists in the development and implementation of effective policy at all levels of health care.

Case Study

Amy is a 16-year-old female high school student who is 16 weeks pregnant with her first child. She is in her second (sophomore) year and is not married. The father of her baby is neither involved nor supportive of the pregnancy, and he has told Amy he no longer wants anything to do with her or the baby and "doesn't want it." Amy has supportive parents who have attended prenatal classes with her. The classes have provided education on labor and delivery, breastfeeding, car seat safety, and parenting. After attending the prenatal breastfeeding class and learning the infant and maternal health benefits, Amy plans to breastfeed her infant as long as possible—not only for the infant's health but also her own, as she has a family history of breast cancer. Her parents are willing to care for the infant during the day while Amy is at school. Amy will need to express her milk at least three times during the day while she is separated from her infant. When Amy meets with her high school administrators to discuss her lactation needs, she discovers that there is no policy to support students to be excused from class to express their milk. She also discovers that there is no private space where she could express her milk. Her requests for break time from class to express her milk is met with some resistance, and she is asked "Why don't you bottlefeed your baby like everyone else?" Encouraged by her parents, Amy reaches out to the local breastfeeding clinic and lactation providers for support and help to work with the school to develop an action plan and policy to support her in the school environment.

As part of Amy's support team, answer the following questions:

- How can you help Amy meet her breastfeeding goals?
- What is the primary issue/barrier for Amy?
- Based on the primary issue, what would an action plan include?
- What legal and policy precedents are already in place to support Amy in the school setting?
- Is a policy needed?
- What level of policy should be considered?
- Who should be involved in the process? Who are the stakeholders?
- What elements should be considered to draft the policy? What must be included?
- Who will approve the policy?
- What communication, training, or education should be considered for the high school personnel around implementation of the policy?
- How will the policy be monitored and reviewed in order to determine that implementation has met the intended outcome?

References

Agunbiade, O. M., & Ogunleye, O. V. (2012). Constraints to exclusive breastfeeding practice among breastfeeding mothers in Southwest Nigeria: Implications for scaling up. *International Breastfeeding Journal 7*, 5. https://doi.org/10.1186/1746-4358-7-5

Alford, J., & Head, B. W. (2017). Wicked and less wicked problems: A typology and a contingency framework. *Policy and Society, 36*(3), 397–413. https://doi.org/10.1080/14494035.2017.1361634

Balogun, O. O., O'Sullivan, E., McFadden, A., Ota, E., Gavine, A., Garner, C., Renfrew, M. J., & MacGillivray, S. (2016). Interventions for promoting the initiation of breastfeeding. *Cochrane Database of Systematic Reviews, 11*, CD001688. https://doi.org/10.1002/14651858.CD001688.pub3

Bartick, M., & Reinhold, A. (2010). The burden of suboptimal breastfeeding in the United States: A pediatric cost analysis. *Pediatrics, 125*(5), e1048–1056. https://doi.org/10.1542/peds.2009-1616

Bosi, A. T. B., Eriksen, K. G., Sobko, T., Wijnhoven, T. M. A., & Breda, J. (2015). Breastfeeding practices and policies in WHO European region member states. *Public Health and Nutrition 19*(4), 753. https://doi.org/10.1017/S1368980015001767

Cambridge University Press. (2020). Policy. In *Cambridge Dictionary*. Retrieved July 9, 2020, from https://dictionary.cambridge.org/dictionary/english/policy?q=Policy

Centers for Disease Control and Prevention (CDC). (2011). *Five-year progress update on the Surgeon General's call to action to support breastfeeding.* https://www.cdc.gov/breastfeeding/pdf/five-year- progress-update.pdf

Centers for Disease Control and Prevention (CDC). (2016). *Results: Breastfeeding rates.* Retrieved July 9, 2020, from https://www.cdc.gov/breastfeeding/data/nis_data/results.html

Centers for Disease Control and Prevention (CDC). (2018). *Breastfeeding report card.* Retrieved July 9, 2020, from https://www.cdc.gov/breastfeeding/pdf/2018breastfeedingreportcard.pdf

Centers for Medicare & Medicaid Services. (2010). *Health benefits & coverage: Breastfeeding benefits.* Retrieved July 9, 2020, from https://www.healthcare.gov/coverage/breast-feeding-benefits

Dowling, S., Pontin, D., & Boyer, K. (2018). *Social experiences of breastfeeding, building bridges between research, policy and practice.* Policy Press.

EU Directorate Public Health and Risk Assessment. (2008). *Protection, promotion and support of breastfeeding in Europe: A blueprint for action* (revised 2008). https://www.aeped.es/sites/default/files/6-newblueprintprinter.pdf

Fallon, V. M., Harrold, J. A., & Chisholm, A. (2019). The impact of the UK Baby friendly Initiative on maternal and infant health outcomes: A mixed-methods systematic review. *Maternal & Child Nutrition, 15*(3), e12778. https://doi.org/10.1111/mcn.12778

Frank, L. (2015). The breastfeeding paradox, a critique of policy related to infant food security in Canada. *Food, Culture and Security, 18*(1), 107. https://doi.org/10.2752/175174415X14101814953927

Gonzalez-Nahm, S., Grossman, E. R., & Benjamin-Neelon, S. E. (2019). The role of equity in US States' breastfeeding policies. *JAMA Pediatrics, 173*(10), 908–910.

Hansen, K. (2016). Breastfeeding: A smart investment in people and in economics. *Lancet, 387*(10017), 416. https://doi.org/10.1016/S0140-6736(16)00012-X

Health Promotion and Disease Prevention Directorate. (2015). *National breastfeeding policy and action plan 2015–2020.* Malta. https://deputyprimeminister.gov.mt/en/Documents/National-Health-Strategies/BF_EN.pdf

Heyman, J., Raub, A., & Earle, A. (2013). Breastfeeding policy: A globally comparative analysis. *Bulletin World Health Organization, 91*, 398. https://www.who.int/bulletin/volumes/91/6/12-109363.pdf

Holla, R., Iellamo, A., Gupta, A., Smith, J., & Dadhich, J. P. (2013).The need to invest in babies: A global drive for financial investment in children's health and development through universalising interventions for optimal breastfeeding. *The World Breastfeeding Costing Initiative.* IBFAN Asia. https://www.worldbreastfeedingcosting.org/wbci/The-Need-to-Invest-in-Babies.pdf

Horsley, S. E. (2010). *The politics of breastfeeding, an exploration of the effectiveness of UK breastfeeding policy and barriers to breastfeeding.* https://www.academia.edu/22148044/ The_Politics_of_Breastfeeding_An_exploration_of_the_effectiveness_of_UK_Breastfeeding_Policy_and_barriers_to_breastfeeding._The_Politics_of_Breastfeeding

Innocenti Declaration. *On the protection, promotion and support of breastfeeding.* (1990). UNICEF.

Joseph, F. I., & Earland, J. (2019). A qualitative exploration of the sociocultural determinants of exclusive breastfeeding practices among rural mothers, North West Nigeria. *International Breastfeeding Journal, 14*(38). https://doi.org/10.1186/s13006-019-0231-z

Kim, J. H., Shin, J. C., & Donovan, S. M. (2019). Effectiveness of workplace lactation interventions on breastfeeding outcomes in the United States: An updated systematic review. *Journal of Human Lactation, 35*(1), 100–113. https://doi.org/10.1177/0890334418765464

Kridli, S. A. (2011). Health beliefs and practises of Muslim women during Ramadan. *MCN: American Journal of Maternal Child Nursing, 36*(4), 216. https://doi.org/10.1097/NMC.0b013e3182177177

Mahesh, P. K. B., Gunathunga, M. W., Arnold, S. M., Jayasinghe, C., Pathirana, S., Makarim, M. F., Manawadu, P. M., & Senanayake, S. J. (2018). Effectiveness of targeting fathers for breastfeeding promotion: Systematic review and meta-analysis. *BMC Public Health, 18*(1), 1140. doi: 10.1186/s12889-018-6037-x

Nathoo, T., & Ostry, A. (2009). *The one best way? Breastfeeding history, politics, and policy in Canada.* Wilfred Laurier University Press.

Palmer, G. (2009). *The politics of breastfeeding. When breasts are bad for business.* Pinter and Martin.

Papastavrou, M., Genitsaridi, S. M., Komodiki, E., Paliatsou, S., Midw, R., Kontogeorgou A., Iacovidou N. (2015). Breastfeeding in the course of history. *Journal of Pediatric Neonatal Care, 2*(6), 00096. https://doi.org/10.15406/jpnc.2015.02.00096

Pérez-Escamilla, R. (2020). Breastfeeding in the 21st century: How we can make it work. *Social Science & Medicine, 244*(1). https://doi.org/10.1016/j.socscimed.2019.05.036

Pérez-Escamilla, R., Martinez, J. L., & Segura- Pérez, S. (2016). Impact of the Baby-friendly Hospital Initiative on breastfeeding and child health outcomes: A systematic review. *Maternal and Child Nutrition. 12*(3), 402. https://doi.org/10.1111/mcn.12294

Peters, B. G. (2017). What is so wicked about wicked problems? A conceptual analysis and a research program. *Policy and Society, 36*(3), 385–396. https://doi.org/10.1080/14494035.2017.1361633

Protheroe, L., Dyson, L., & Renfrew, M. J. (2003, June). *The effectiveness of public health interventions to promote the initiation of breastfeeding. Evidence briefing.* 1st edition. Retrieved July 9, 2020, from http://citeseerx.ist.psu.edu/viewdoc/download?doi=10.1.1.563.9281&rep=rep1&type=pdf

Public Health Agency of Canada. (2018). *Breastfeeding. Chapter 6. Family-Centered Maternity and Newborn Care: National Guidelines.* Retrieved July 9, 2020, from https://www.canada.ca/content/dam/phac-aspc/documents/services/publications/healthy-living/maternity-newborn-care-guidelines-chapter-6/maternity-newborn-care-guidelines-chapter-6.pdf

Renfrew, M. J., Pokhrel, S., Quigley, M., McCormick, F., Fox-Rushby, J., Dodds, R., . . . Williams, A. (2012). *Preventing disease and saving resources: The potential contribution of increasing breastfeeding rates in the UK.* UNICEF UK. Retrieved July 9, 2020, from https://www.unicef.org.uk/babyfriendly/wp-content/uploads/sites/2/2012/11/Preventing_disease_saving_resources_policy_doc.pdf

Rittel, H. W. J., & Webber, M. M. (1973). Dilemmas in a general theory of planning. *Policy Science, 4*, 155–169. https://doi.org/10.1007/BF01405730

Rollins, N. C., Bhandari, N., Hajeebhoy, N., Horton, S., Lutter, C. K., & Marines, J. C. (2016). Why invest, and what it will take to improve breastfeeding practices? Lancet Breastfeeding Series Group. *Lancet, 387*(10017), 491–504. https://doi.org/10.1016/S0140-6736(15)01044-2

Schmied, V., Gribble, K., Sheehan, A., Taylor, C., & Dykes, R. C. (2011). Ten steps or climbing a mountain: A study of Australian health professionals' perceptions of implementing the baby friendly health initiative to protect, promote and support breastfeeding. *BMC Health Services Research, 11*(1), 208. https://doi.org/10.1186/1472-6963-11-208

Thomas, T., Martsolf, G., & Puskar, K. (2019). How to engage nursing students in health policy: Results of a survey assessing students' competencies, experiences, interests, and values. *Policy, Politics, & Nursing Practice, 21*(1), 12–20. https://doi.org/10.1177/1527154419891129

UNICEF. (2005). *Innocenti Declaration 2005 on infant and young child feeding.* https://www.unicef-irc.org/publications/435/

United Nations High Commissioner for Refugees (UNHCR). (1979). *Convention on the elimination of all forms of discrimination against women.* Retrieved July 9, 2020, from https://www.ohchr.org/en/professionalinterest/pages/cedaw.aspx

United Nations High Commissioner for Refugees (UNHCR). (1989). *Convention on the rights of the child.* Retrieved July 9, 2020, from https://www.ohchr.org/en/professionalinterest/pages/crc.aspx

United States Breastfeeding Committee. (2020). *Federal policies, programs, & initiatives.* http://www.usbreastfeeding.org/p/cm/ld/fid=26

U.S. Department of Health and Human Services. (2011). *Executive summary: The Surgeon General's call to action to support breastfeeding.* https://www.hhs.gov/sites/default/files/breastfeeding-call-to-action-executive-summary.pdf

Victora, C. G., Bahl, R., Barros, A. J. D., França, G. V. A., Horton, S., Krasevec, J., & Rollins, N. C. (2016). Breastfeeding in the 21st century: Epidemiology, mechanisms, and lifelong effect. *The Lancet, 387*(10017), 475. https://doi.org/10.1016/S0140-6736(15)01024-7

Weimer, J. (2001). *The economic benefits of breastfeeding: A review and analysis.* Economic Research Service /USDA. https://www.ers.usda.gov/webdocs/publications/46471/15897_fanrr13_1_.pdf?v=1772.5

Weimer, J. (2001). *The Economic Benefits of Breastfeeding: A Review and Analysis.* U.S. Government Printing Office. Retrieved July 9, 2020, from https://play.google.com/books/reader?id=EHpBBFuP j4EC&hl=en&pg=GBS.PP1

World Bank. (2015). *An investment framework for nutrition: Reaching the global targets for stunting, anemia, breastfeeding and wasting.* https://www.worldbank.org/en/topic/nutrition/publication/an

-investment-framework-for-nutrition-reaching-the-global-targets-for-stunting-anemia-breastfeeding-wasting

World Health Organization (WHO). (1981). *International Code of Marketing of Breast-milk Substitutes*. Geneva, Switzerland. https://www.who.int/nutrition/publications/code_english.pdf

World Health Organization (WHO). (2016, May). *Maternal, infant and young child feeding. Guidance on ending the inappropriate promotion of foods for infants and young children*. Sixty-ninth World Health Assembly. Provisional agenda item 12.1. Geneva, Switzerland. Retrieved July 9, 2020, at http://apps.who.int/gb/ebwha/pdf_files/WHA69/A69_7Add1-en.pdf?ua=1

World Health Organization (WHO) and United Nations Children's Fund (UNICEF). (2018). Implementation Guidance. Protecting, promoting and supporting breastfeeding in facilities providing maternity and newborn services: the revised Baby-friendly Hospital Initiative. *Geneva: World Health Organization*. https://www.who.int/nutrition/publications/infantfeeding/bfhi-implementation-2018.pdf

CHAPTER 5

Relational Practice and Lactation

Tina Revai, MN, RN, IBCLC
Stephanie George, BA, Indigenous Midwife, IBCLC

LEARNING OBJECTIVES

1. Identify key concepts in relational practice theory.
2. Differentiate cultural humility and implicit bias as they affect interactions with parents related to infant feeding.
3. Describe ways to incorporate reflective practice in your day-to-day work.

KEY WORDS

- **Center their story:** A way of providing context and meaning to their experience through careful listening and relational practice, a main goal of the relational framework of breastfeeding
- **Cultural Humility:** A process of self-reflection to understand personal and systemic biases and to develop and maintain respectful interactions and relationships based on mutual trust. Cultural humility involves humbly acknowledging oneself as a learner when it comes to understanding another's experience (First Nations Health Authority, n.d.).
- **Implicit Bias:** Associations outside of conscious awareness that lead to negative evaluation of a person on the basis of irrelevant characteristics, such as race or gender, and are known to contribute to systemic inequities in healthcare service delivery, both broadly in healthcare and specifically in lactation care (Fitzgerald & Hurst, 2017; Thomas, 2018).
- **Listening from the heart:** Listening in a deep way that includes letting go of oneself and one's own agenda.
- **Reflective Practice:** A way of being that involves both an examination of experiences to understand situations for improvement of practice and the deeper process of questioning assumptions and interrogating the power and morality infused in practice to raise one's awareness and critical conscience (Wigginton et al., 2019).
- **Renewed understanding of the situation:** During a lactation consult, integrating the parent's story, goals and information gathered during the history and/or assessment to arrive at a new more holistic understanding of the issue.
- **Trauma-Violence-Informed Care:** A universal approach to care where an understanding of the prevalence and effects of trauma are taken into account and priority is placed on the individual's safety, choice collaboration, connection, and empowerment (BC Provincial Mental Health and Substance Use Planning Council, 2013).

Overview

Health is "a state of complete physical, mental and social well-being and not merely the absence of disease or infirmity" (World Health Organization [WHO], 1946) and is uniquely experienced and meaning laden. Respectful, strength-based, relational lactation support is fundamental not only for self-defined lactation success but also for the parent's emerging identity as part of a significant life transition. Students and practitioners benefit from a framework that guides practice in a way that foregrounds how experience, context, history, and meaning are relationally mediated, as this potentiates the ability to resist and disrupt systemic inequities. We recognize that much of the language around feeding a baby is gendered in a way that may not match how all people identify and that not all people who carry/give birth identify as women, nor that all people who feed their babies with the milk their body produces identify with the word "breasts." A relational approach is to make space for this diversity and to use the preferred language of the person that we are serving. This chapter focuses on why and how a relational approach is foundational to the provider–parent interaction for health promotion of lactation.

Introduction

As with all mammals, breastfeeding is the original first food for humans. As the evolved, traditional food for our species, human milk and breastfeeding play a critical role in survival and well-being. This is of particular importance for us as highly social animals: breastfeeding primes our first relationships, thus laying the groundwork for all future relationships. As social beings, caretaking of the new dyad has been fundamental to our collective survival. This means that we all have a stake in what happens for next generations, and a critical first task after birth is successfully feeding the new infant. Breastfeeding support has been and should be a collective responsibility.

Mapping the history of breastfeeding is a worthwhile project, but beyond the scope of this chapter (see Chapter 1). Briefly, in many Western cultures, the convergence of industrialization and medicalization around the beginning of the 20th century led to the emergence of bottle feeding with human milk substitutes (formula) dominance. Thus, the experiential and embodied knowledge that had been historically passed from aunties, grandmothers, and wise elders through the generations was questioned and moved to the margins (see **Box 5-1**). New, scientific, "convenient" commercial feeding methods were favored.

In some cases, the loss of traditional breastfeeding knowledge and skills spread to non-Western communities as part of political and/or cultural colonization. Thus, a general trend is the shift from a breast to a bottle-feeding culture paralleling colonization and Eurocentric thinking.

In North America, a challenge to this shift began in the middle of the 20th century. Feminism and consumer movements began to question and resist the privileging of medical and scientific ways of knowing, particularly knowledge as it related to feeding and the female body. Groups like La Leche League resisted the dominant messages of that time, leading to a reassertion of the legitimacy of breastfeeding and the establishment of the International Board Certified Lactation Consultant (IBCLC) as a recognized healthcare credential.

Box 5-1 Exploring Your Roots

Explore your own roots. How were you fed as an infant? How did that compare to previous generations in your family? What has been the "story" of how to feed an infant among the people with whom you identify as family? What about messages received through any school or professional training—what have you been taught as the "right way" to feed an infant? Were there differences, and if so, how have you reconciled this in your practice? Why might it be important to map your own story of infant feeding prior to supporting others in their journey?

However, a critique is that the relatively recent reestablishment of breastfeeding culture has left some groups behind. Unless the uniqueness of human experience is acknowledged, breastfeeding success may become too narrowly defined. Breastfeeding support must work to disrupt existing inequities that are often mirrored in breastfeeding rates. This is especially relevant, given the missed opportunity for breastfeeding to ameliorate the harms associated with inequity (Hallowell et al., 2017).

A person-centered, culturally humble approach offers a path to a truly enabling environment that is inclusive of the full range of human experience. Thus, strength-based, person-centered care happens when supporters undertake a responsive, tailored approach while holding a commitment to the determinants of health and the creation of an enabling environment. The framework is meant to guide a practice that seeks to unlock potential for all families by working in partnership and centering their experience.

What Does *Relational* Mean?

Relational means recognizing that for humans all experience becomes meaningful through relationship. A relational view challenges individualism and recognizes all aspects of interconnection. A basic assumption of the framework is that personal experience is contextual and emerges from a unique situatedness in time, place, and history. The relational framework for breastfeeding support seeks to center the unique story, the lived experience, and the goals of each person, while using the best available knowledge to help families attain their goals. An underlying assumption of the framework is that all parents do their best within their capacity and context.

The Relational Framework for Breastfeeding Support

The relational framework honors that relevant, traditional knowledge has been relationally acquired and passed from generation to generation, while holding in balance the importance of scientific contributions to knowledge regarding lactation. Specifically, this framework looks beyond the technical aspects of lactation support and accounts for the primacy of the socio-emotional interconnection in feeding. This includes the bond between parent and child and the task of feeding as foundational to identity and feelings of success as a new parent.

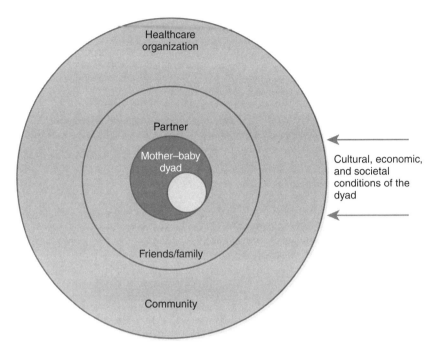

Figure 5-1 Socioecological model of breastfeeding.
© Tina Revai, 2017

Being relational means recognizing that breastfeeding support work is not only a relational process: the "outcome" is relational in nature. As supporters, we are working with a dyad, and the dyad is nested in a family, in community, and within greater society. Although the site for most breastfeeding support takes place at the level of the breastfeeding parent and child, this model asserts that the supporter is obligated to think and act beyond this level to contribute to a truly enabled environment. A visual that may be useful for this is the socio-ecological model (see **Figure 5-1**).

In the relational framework, role and context matter. Most supporters are sought out or brought in because of a challenging situation for the dyad. Rather than jumping to problem solving, a relational approach recognizes strengths and puts the person's experience and meaning in the situation in the foreground.

Case Study

Diane is married 7 years, gravida 3, para 2, living rural, and away from family. She is 30 years old and 8 months pregnant. Her husband is a full-time student and works. Diane is a stay-at-home mother and has access to the family vehicle, depending on her partner's schedule and which she needs to negotiate ahead of time. Diane attends local moms and tots group.

Thinking to the ecological model, what do you know about Diane and her context? What areas might you not yet know about but are curious to know as they relate to her situation?

■   What are the strengths and possible limitations of Diane's current social support?
■   What might you wonder about in terms of her access to material resources?

The first step in the first encounter with a breastfeeding parent is to **center their story**. We are there for a very small part of the journey and, yet, this an important and vulnerable time. This is also a chance to realize that we might be making some assumptions about the situation. Listening in this deep way is letting go of oneself and our own agenda and **listening from the heart**.

Consistent with many well-known therapeutic communication frameworks, focusing on strengths is important to demonstrate positive regard. Many health-care providers are trained in a problem-solving approach. Focusing on strengths may mean thinking a little differently: we frame our work toward self-efficacy, capacity building, and partnering rather than an expert-driven perspective. (See **Figure 5-2**.)

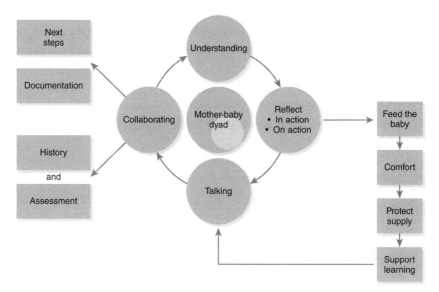

Figure 5-2 Relational framework to guide breastfeeding support.
© Tina Revai, 2017

[Case Study (continued)]

You are the peer supporter in the local mother–tot group. Part of your role and training is to provide general breastfeeding support. You get to know Diane through that group. Diane has a 3-year-old and a 5-year-old. During the times that she's attended, you notice polite friendliness but a distance with other participants in the group. She is very responsive to her children. As part of your process with pregnant participants, you ask her how feeding went with her older children. She shares that milk took a long time to come in with her first baby but that she figured it out. For the second baby it went easier, and she stopped at 6 months because her husband wanted more time with the baby and wanted to bottle-feed the baby. Diane shares that she wants to breastfeed longer this time because she feels she gave up early last time.

The first round of the reflecting stage is focused on foregrounding strengths. Thinking to what we now know about Diane, consider the following:

What are her strengths?

- Compassion, evoking, and honoring autonomy/self-determination
- Attitudes and beliefs of the parent and the parent's partner and family—how they might be influencing the experience
- Material or power constraints that the parent might be experiencing—the opportunities and challenges in this situation
- Listening carefully for real or potential red flags
- Being a reflective practitioner

Specifically, being a reflective practitioner means becoming aware of our own assumptions, judgments, and thinking related to our history and location.

[Case Study (continued)]

Consider the perspective of the peer supporter in this story and how context might affect how he or she sees Diane and her situation:

- The peer supporter breastfed her children until they self-weaned and has a sense of accomplishment about that. How might that be different if the supporter did not have children or did not have their own breastfeeding success?
- As this scenario unfolds, consider how the situation might be different if Diane was approaching the facilitator for support around her breastfeeding.

Consider the following reflective questions:

- How do my personal story, history, and experiences influence my first impressions?
- How might my own narrative/assumptions facilitate or block being fully present for this dyad?
- What is my role in this situation?

Also see **Box 5-2**.

Box 5-2 Implicit Bias

Implicit bias has been well documented as a barrier to equitable care in healthcare both broadly (Fitzgerald & Hurst, 2017) and specific to lactation (Thomas, 2018). We all have implicit bias—it is part of our situated and constituted frame or point of view. This perspective is ever evolving, and we can bring it to consciousness through reflective questions that challenge us to take a critical view of our beliefs and attitudes, which is necessary to unpack unconscious bias. The goal is to align our actions with our ethics.

The first talking step focuses on clarifying and demonstrating positive regard. It can be very powerful to let the parent know what you see as strengths.

[Case Study (continued)]

What are the strengths that you hear in Diane's situation? The following are some we've identified:

- Diane attends group regularly, and we might express this to her (and check our perceptions) by saying "I imagine it can't be easy to get you and your children out of the house with your husband in school, and I am glad you made it here today."
- Diane nursed her two older children. In particular with her first, she "figured it out." This seems to indicate that breastfeeding was a priority for her and that she made it happen.

Many people lack support that centers their experience and is reflected back to them in a strength-based way. This may include the following (also see **Box 5-3**):

- Reflecting any strengths in their story
- Stating what you understand to be the issue and goals
- Using LOVE or OARS to ensure that you understand

By taking an **appreciative approach,** we acknowledge the breastfeeding parent as expert in her own situation. The following are our hopes for the breastfeeding parent:

- They will experience more confidence and feel energized by focusing on what is going well.
- They will see a connection between any actions and their own desired breast-feeding goals.
- They will be more likely to stay motivated.

In the collaborating stage, a basic first step is to **ask permission,** including asking permission to ask more questions. From a parent's perspective, being asked a series of questions can feel invasive and asking permission sets the stage for what will happen and empowers the parent about the process.

Box 5-3 Listening Skills Frameworks

LOVE = Listen, Offer, Validate, Empathize
OARS = Open-ended questions, Affirmations, Reflective listening, Summarizing
   There are many good skills for building frameworks and solid listening skills. Find the one that will work best for you to develop your listening.

[Case Study (continued)]

What might be helpful to know more about as the support person in this situation? Here are some examples:

- It sounds like she worked hard to make breastfeeding work for her previously. Is that how she sees it?
- Given that she has shared wanting to nurse longer with this baby, what are her thoughts on her husband's previous preference for bottle feeding? Is this still the case?
- What, if any, were her supports previously? She has shared that she is away from her family. How is she planning to juggle parenting her older two children, her toddler in particular, and to navigate learning to breastfeed the newborn?

How might you word the questions to get the above information in a way that is affirming and respectful?

History taking may be formal, depending on your setting and role. For example, you may have an intake form with an expectation that it is completed. In this case, think through how you can introduce the process so that the parent is centered. Additionally, you may think that more information is needed and can be obtained by completing a physical assessment of the breasts/chest, the baby, and/or watching the dyad feeding as they usually do. These are intimate processes. Consider how this can be done in a way that is **trauma-violence-informed** (see **Box 5-4**).

[Case Study (continued)]

If your place of work is informal, how would you proceed? Would you encourage the mother to talk about her personal, medical, and lactation history or do something else? Active listening while you are having group discussions can lead to questions you could ask her later in private conversation, such as the following:

- "I heard you say that you think the epidural you had with your first baby made the breastfeeding difficult in the first few days. Have you thought about your plans if you need another epidural? Can I share what I know on this topic?"
- "If your husband wants to bottle-feed the baby again, have you thought about how this might go? May I suggest some ideas that other mothers have shared with me over the years?"

Following Diane's suggestions and desires, you teach her about how medications can affect the baby's first hours and days, the importance of skin to skin, and proper hand expression techniques so she understands the choices she can make to nurse her baby.

Box 5-4 Trauma-Violence-Informed Care

The four core principles of trauma-violence-informed care are awareness of trauma and a universal precaution approach; emphasis on safety and trustworthiness; opportunity for choice, collaboration, and connection; and strengths-based skill building (BC Provincial Mental Health and Substance Use Planning Council, 2013).

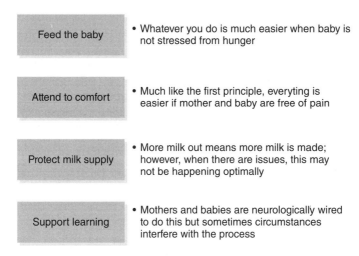

Feed the baby	• Whatever you do is much easier when baby is not stressed from hunger
Attend to comfort	• Much like the first principle, everyting is easier if mother and baby are free of pain
Protect milk supply	• More milk out means more milk is made; however, when there are issues, this may not be happening optimally
Support learning	• Mothers and babies are neurologically wired to do this but sometimes circumstances interfere with the process

Figure 5-3 Feed the baby; attend to comfort; protect the milk supply; support learning.

© Tina Revai, 2017

The framework is cyclical, and after gathering more information we arrive at a **renewed understanding of the situation**. By integrating the parent's story and goals as well as including information gathered during the history and/or assessment, we arrive at a new, more holistic understanding of the issue. Considering this more fulsome view of the situation, we think through to the goal(s) to **generate ideas**, based on our own level of knowledge and experience, guided by the above principles. (See **Figure 5-3**.)

[Case Study (continued)]

■ You get a message to call Diane at the hospital. She tells you she birthed yesterday. She had an epidural for 12 hours. Baby hasn't nursed well yet, but she has kept the baby skin to skin as much as she can. She also said that she has been hand expressing but feeling poorly that she only expressed 5 mL. She is exhausted and overwhelmed.

What would be the first things you would say to Diane? Here are some ideas we have:

■ Remind her of her strengths.
■ Remind her about proper and expected colostrum amounts.
■ Discuss self-attachment by the baby.
■ Discuss hand expression after each feeding session, if she is up to it.
■ Help her to remember supports available to her.
■ Ask if you can do a home visit, or if she can come to see you when she's out of the hospital.

Thus, we move away from the idea of fixing and recenter the parent as expert in their own situation. *What might be gained by resisting the role of the supporter as expert?*

The guiding principles are meant to help the supporter prioritize what to focus on as they make a plan in collaboration with the parent. Consistent with trauma-violence-informed care, we first attend to the immediate needs of the presenting dyad: hunger and pain (if they are experiencing either). It is always useful to check with the parent about our understanding of what they are working toward. Thus, we move away from the idea of fixing and recenter the parent as expert in their own situation. What might be gained by resisting the role of the supporter as expert?

[Case Study (continued)]

Would your first impressions change if the person self-identified as indigenous, or transgender, or Muslim?

If you were at Diane's home for a visit, would you change your opinion of her if she lived in a small apartment, a shelter, or a mansion?

We must decide to relate to Diane where she is and help her to get to where she wants to go. It doesn't matter where a breastfeeding person lives if they have pain while latching. We help her to feed the baby

For an assessment during the first days, we should ask her about her birth. Was she given the option to do skin to skin for a long time? Was it a medicated birth? Did she have private healthcare? Knowing if she felt empowered in her birth experience could give us insight as to how much confidence she has about breastfeeding or if she feels she is failing at nursing like she did right after birth.

We must assist her in her desire to feed the baby and to attain an improved latch that she can do by herself. There are professional organization standards that identify that hands-on care does not take place without consent (Registered Nurses' Association of Ontario [RNAO], 2018). We must help a mom feel like she can breastfeed without hands-on help so she will have faith in herself after the appointment. Use language that the parent understands. Some parents are still traumatized by their birth experiences and may not be able to verbalize. If the baby needs a supplement, we should facilitate an informed-choice discussion between hand expression, donated milk, and human milk substitutes (formula) to assist her with her decision.

If Diane is nursing, we can help her to feed her baby without pain, remembering how she birthed (vaginal, cesarean-section, surrogate, or adoption). We should work with both parents to find out what will work for them: positions, timing, pumping, and so on. We should see Diane nurse where she will most likely be feeding at home. We should help her by breaking down breastfeeding into workable steps or in 12-hour increments, if she is very overwhelmed.

To support Diane's learning after we leave, handouts and videos can work well if we send them to her via email. She can refer to them when we are no longer in front of her.

New parents can have trouble understanding or remembering if we give a long list of rules. At times, a parent needs more than an IBCLC can give. With clear charting and succinctly worded referral letters, we can involve the family doctors, pediatrician, or obstetrician. Including the parent in deciding which specialist (perhaps the family had a bad experience with a previous healthcare practitioner), we can be sure of referring her to someone who will listen and help without judgment.

No matter the mom's economic or family situation, all parents still need to feed the baby; attend to her comfort; protect the milk supply; and support her learning. By working with the parents where they are physically and emotionally, we can help

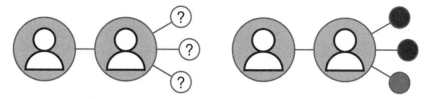

Figure 5-4 Collaboration–communication options.
© Tina Revai, 2017

them to feel our support and be more trusting with our knowledge. A parent with holes in her roof can have their same latch issues as those who own an expensive house. Where they live and what their economic status is doesn't matter. The relational support we give can work with parents in any situation when we remember we are there to learn as well as teach. We are there to learn about the family to discover how best to help them.

Practitioners using this process collaborate with the parent to generate ideas about what might work whenever possible. Our goal is to talk it out and acknowledge that there may be more than one way to approach the issue. Together we want to explore what might fit best. (See **Figure 5-4**.)

Collaborating to settle on a plan is checking that the options chosen are parent focused and realistic?. In general, the more challenging the situation, the more it may be helpful to focus on actions that are easy to do, short term, and concrete. It is usually more empowering to share the rationale for what we are thinking; however, can you think of situations where it might not work to discuss the rationale for your thinking? In our experience, if a parent is upset, keeping the plan clear and short term with another chance to check in soon works best most times. When things are calmer, we can have a more fulsome discussion about the why of any decisions.

Once we've partnered to come up with a **collaborative plan**, we need to decide on next steps. Next steps are appropriate to the plan. It may involve sharing information, with consent, with the primary healthcare provider (HCP) or making a referral elsewhere. The range of options comes from what has been decided and may include the following:

- Involving the primary HCP or a specialist as needed
- Arranging for next contact
  - When/where/how
- Leaving it up to the parents to decide if they have a need for follow up

As part of professional responsibility and accountability, we document according to our role.

This completes the two cycles of the framework at the level of engaging with the parent, but the framework is iterative and **reflection** is encouraged *in action, on action,* and *for action.* Thus, we are invited to engage with the reflective process throughout our practice. The following questions may be a useful guide after we have had an encounter to take our practice deeper:

- How did my personal story, history, and experiences influence my view of the situation?

- Did my narrative/assumptions facilitate or block being fully present for this dyad (family)?
- What did I do well in this interaction?
- What might I do differently next time?
- Do I feel I fulfilled my role and obligations? Did my communications and actions align with my ethics?
- Are there patterns to this situation that reflect the broader context or determinants of health?
- What are the ways I can address this to contribute to a more enabled environment for all breastfeeding and human milk-feeding families?

Summary

The relational framework for breastfeeding support seeks to honor feeding as a critical, meaning-laden task that in many situations contributes to a story about the parent's emergent identity. It is meant to highlight and respect the constituted and situational perspective of each person who comes into the care of a breastfeeding supporter and does not put breastfeeding ahead of the dyad. Enacting this way of being and doing means centering the breastfeeding person and considers problem solving to be collaborative. The support provided is relational as the knowledge and skills are shared from parent to supporter (and vice versa), parent to parent, across generations, and within a cultural and societal landscape. Finally, the outcome is relational as we are working with a dyad, nested in a family, which means that a relational perspective holds commitment to ensuring that all parents are supported in their infant feeding goals and that the environment is an enabling one.

Key Points to Remember

1. The infant feeding journey is critical to the emerging identity of the parent.
2. A relational view of breastfeeding support centers the parent and their goals while understanding that they are uniquely situated in a complex web of relationships.
3. The view of breastfeeding is focused not only on the dyad achieving individualized goals; it also advocates for a truly enabled breastfeeding environment where all experiences of infant feeding are honored and respected.

References

British Columbia (BC) Provincial Mental Health and Substance Use Planning Council (2013, May). *Trauma-informed practice guide.* http://bccewh.bc.ca/wp-content/uploads/2012/05/2013_TIP -Guide.pdf

First Nations Health Authority. (n.d.). *Cultural humility.* https://www.fnha.ca/wellness/cultural-humility

Fitzgerald, C., & Hurst, S. (2017). Implicit bias in healthcare professionals: A systematic review. *BMC Medical Ethics, 18*(1), 19. https://doi.org/10.1186/s12910-017-0179-8

Hallowell, S. G., Froh, E. B., & Spatz, D. L. (2017). Human milk and breastfeeding: An intervention to mitigate toxic stress. *Nursing Outlook, 65*(1), 58–67. https://doi.org/10.1016/j .outlook.2016.07.007

Registered Nurses' Association of Ontario (RNAO) (2018). *Breastfeeding—Promoting and supporting the initiation, exclusivity, and continuation of breastfeeding in newborns, infants, and young children.* https://rnao.ca/bpg/guidelines/breastfeeding-promoting-and-supporting-initiation-exclusivity-and-continuation-breast

Thomas, E. V. (2018). "Why even bother; they are not going to do it?" The structural roots of racism and discrimination in lactation care. *Qualitative Health Research, 28*(7), 1050–1064. https://doi.org/10.1177/1049732318759491

Wigginton, B., Fjeldsoe, B., Mutch, A., & Lawler, S. (2019). Creating reflexive health promotion practitioners: Our process of integrating reflexivity in the development of a health promotion course. *Pedagogy in Health Promotion, 5*(1), 75–78. https://doi.org/10.1177/2373379918766379

World Health Organization. (1946). *Constitution. Definition of health.* Retrieved July 10, 2020, from https://www.who.int/about/who-we-are/constitution

CHAPTER 6

Baby-friendly Initiatives

Suzanne Hetzel Campbell, PhD, RN, IBCLC, CCSNE

"(It is time) to discuss some of the progress and programs that can help return breastfeeding to its rightful place as the initial and most basic act of health protection"

— **Walker, 2007, p. 549.**

LEARNING OBJECTIVES

1. Describe the main components of the Baby-friendly Hospital Initiative.
2. Examine lactation in the global context of health promotion in practice.
3. Identify key components of health care professionals' role in protecting, promoting, and supporting breastfeeding families.
4. Recognize the use of socio-ecological theory and the social determinants of health in supporting families' infant-feeding decisions.
5. Identify ways to translate evidence-based practice into health care professionals' community of practice with a goal of supporting parents.

KEY WORDS

- **Baby-friendly Hospital Initiative:** A global initiative that began in 1991 to protect, promote, and support breastfeeding in facilities that provide maternity and newborn services. (Nyqvist et al., 2013; World Health Organization [WHO], 2018a)
- **The WHO Code (see International Code of Marketing of Breast-milk Substitutes; Gray, 2017):** A short hand reference to the international code developed by the WHO and United Nations International Children's Emergency Fund (UNICEF) and signed by the majority of countries worldwide to minimize marketing of human milk substitutes.
- **Innocenti Declaration on the Protection, Promotion and Support of Breastfeeding (1991; UNICEF, 2005):** A document capturing the renewed commitment on the 15th anniversary of the 1990 Innocenti Declaration, which added five operational

targets as part of the ongoing global strategy on Infant and Young Child Feeding. Endorsed by the Standing Committee on Nutrition on March 17, 2006. The World Health Assembly welcomed the Call to Action made in the declaration on May 27, 2006.

- **International Baby Food Action Network (IBFAN, 2017):** Consists of public interest groups around the world working to safeguard infant and young child health and to reduce morbidity and mortality. It calls for laws to end predatory marketing and ensure food safety and monitoring so that systems are free from commercial influence (https://www.ibfan.org).
- **International Code of Marketing of Breast-milk Substitutes (1981):** A set of recommendations from the WHO member states designed to regulate marketing of human milk substitutes, feeding bottles, and teats; also known as the "WHO Code." The general aim is to shield breastfeeding from commercial promotion that can affect mothers, health workers, and health care systems.
- **Skin-to-Skin contact (S2S):** A practice supported early after delivery and throughout early infancy in which the infant is placed in an upright position with only a diaper on, the parent's chest is without clothing, and the dyad is covered with a blanket for warmth. Especially beneficial in the first few hours after birth for newborn transition and premature infants (Conde-Agudelo & Díaz-Rossello, 2016).
- **The Global Strategy for Infant and Young Child Feeding (WHO, 2003)/Global Strategy for Infant and Young Child Feeding (GSIYCF):** Aims to revitalize efforts to promote, protect, and support appropriate infant and young child feeding.
- **UNICEF:** A United Nations agency that is responsible for humanitarian and developmental aid being provided to children worldwide. With a presence in 192 countries and territories, it is one of the most widespread and recognizable social welfare organizations in the world (https://en.wikipedia.org/wiki/UNICEF).
- **United Nations Convention on the Rights of the Child:** One of the most widely ratified human rights treaties in history. An international agreement on childhood created in 1990 as a commitment to the world's children to protect and transform their lives. The goal is to be sure that children enjoy a full childhood by garnering leaders from government, business, and community to fulfill their commitments to the convention (https://www.unicef.org/crc).

Overview

In this chapter, breastfeeding as a key public health initiative is framed as a responsibility for health care professionals to provide support to families in meeting their infant feeding goals, including exclusive breastfeeding during the first 6 months of life. Key policies are provided to enhance learners' understanding about international policies, such as the **Baby-friendly Hospital Initiative** that can influence practitioners in their ability to support parents. A clear understanding of the global, national, and regional policies is necessary to plan evidence-based support for new parents to meet their infant-feeding goals. The final section outlines successful programs using coalition and community support approaches to health promotion.

Breastfeeding: Health Care Professionals Role

Extensive evidence exists that identifies the role of the health care professional in supporting parents in their transition into parenthood, starting from preconception, through pregnancy, delivery, and postpartum. One of the most important areas of support is related to infant feeding. Given the growing awareness of the health benefits of breastfeeding and its role as a strategy for public health promotion, health system improvements in support of parents to meet their infant feeding goals related to breastfeeding have never been more necessary. Regardless of overall improvements in breastfeeding rates, disparities continue to exist related to racism; socioe-conomic social determinants of health including poverty, income, and food insecurity; and geographic location.

There are key global, national, and local support systems for new parents to support their breastfeeding initiation. These support systems can offer protection and promote their ability to meet their infant-feeding goals. This chapter outlines some of the key global agencies, national and international initiatives, and local coalitions that have successfully implemented health care promotion strategies into socially just programs—beyond single clinical encounters—which take into account that breastfeeding has equity considerations (Campbell et al., 2019; Griswold, 2017).

Global Support of Breastfeeding

International Code of Marketing of Breast-milk Substitutes

A key component of support for breastfeeding began in 1981 when the WHO approved the **International Code of Marketing of Breast-milk Substitutes**, also known as **the WHO Code** (Gray, 2017; WHO, 1981). The goal of this policy was to protect breastfeeding by limiting marketing of human milk substitutes. This WHO Code calls for the prohibition of advertising directly to the consumer (parents), free samples, promotion of formula companies in health care facilities, and health care providers accepting gifts from these companies. In restricting the promotion of human milk substitutes, the WHO Code sets expectations that health care facilities and workers will follow the code. Research has demonstrated that implementation of the WHO Code at a national level, as law, can have an effect on exclusive breastfeeding rates (Michaud-Létourneau et al., 2019; Robinson et al., 2019). This will be covered in more detail in Chapter 9. (See **Figure 6-1**.)

International Baby Food Action Network

The **International Baby Food Action Network (IBFAN)** aims to protect the rights of parents, children, and infants by maintaining vigilance to ensure that the marketing of human milk substitutes and baby foods does not negatively impact their health. IBFAN's seven principles outline the rights of infants and

A Quick Guide to WHO Code Basics (2020)

The International Code of Marketing of Breastmilk Substitutes applies to marketing and promotion; it does not prohibit the sale or use of products. The Code was adopted by the World Health Assembly in 1981 and is updated and clarified by WHA Resolutions every two years.

The Code provides the minimum standard for regulation of marketing practices

What products does the Code cover?

- Formula milks for babies, toddlers and young children up to 36 months, including follow-on and growing-up milks
- Any food or drink marketed for babies under 6 months
- Commercial baby foods or drinks that do not meet global and national standards (marketed for babies, toddlers and young children 6–36 months)
- Bottles, teats or nipples

Who is expected to follow the Code?

- Manufacturers, distributors, and retailers of any of the above items
- Healthcare workers, both professionals and volunteers
- Healthcare facilities – hospitals, clinics, etc.

What must be on the label?

- Labels must be in the local language
- Information must include the hazards associated with artificial feeding
- Labels cannot use idealising language or images, e.g. a happy baby sleeping, or a protective shield suggesting baby is protected by this product

Companies should not create conflicts of interest for health professionals or sponsor health professional and scientific meetings or training, or provide parent education. Health professionals should avoid conflicts of interest.

What is allowed under the code?

✓ Use of formula with safe preparation, for babies who need it

✓ Sale of products with technical information, e.g. "125ml polycarbonate bottle"

✓ Scientific and factual information for healthcare professionals, eg "contains Arachidonic acid (AA)"

✓ Accurate information on safe formula preparation is required on all labels

What is NOT allowed under the code?

✗ Promotion to parents, health professionals, or in health facilities: advertising, free supplies of formula or free samples, gifts, posters

✗ Health claims not substantiated by scientific evidence eg "promotes excellent visual development"

✗ Promotion of unsuitable products for babies (such as sweetened condensed milk)

✗ Donations of formula or feeding equipment in emergencies: instead, cash donations for local agencies to support families

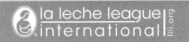

Figure 6-1 WHO Code quick guide.

Reproduced from Gray, H. (2017). A Quick Guide to the WHO Code. Retrieved from https://www.llli.org/quick-guide-international-code-2/

young children toward the highest attainable health, access to adequate nutritious food and water, quality health care services (free of commercial influence), information for parents to make decisions around infant and young child feeding, and the right and support of parents to breastfeed. Global policies and programs have arisen as the last principle supports the individual's right to advocate in international solidarity for change that protects, promotes, and supports basic health (IBFAN, 2017).

United Nations Convention on the Rights of the Child

Another remarkable commitment to children globally is the **United Nations Convention on the Rights of the Child** (https://www.unicef.org/crc). This convention was another worldwide attempt to make leaders accountable for the protection of infants and children by outlining the human rights children have to a healthy and full childhood. Part of this is access to clean water, safe food, and shelter. Additionally, the convention provides a clear way to evaluate leaders in governments, businesses, and communities around the protection of childhood. The rights to breastfeed, have access to the primary caregiver, and be free from the influence of commercialized products, such as human milk substitutes, are covered under this convention. In addition, the convention has been used to further support all aspects of children's safe growth. Sitting within **UNICEF**, this convention outlines areas for support, specifies ways to take action, and shares global stories and successes that encourage communities worldwide.

The Global Strategy for Infant and Young Child Feeding

In 2003, the World Health Organization and UNICEF came together to develop the **Global Strategy for Infant and Young Child Feeding** (WHO, 2003). This global strategy seeks to raise awareness of problems, identify solutions, and provide a framework for interventions to increase government's commitment to an enabling environment for all families. This strategy was introduced in Chapter 2 and is made concrete with examples in Chapter 8 on globalization and Chapter 12 on infant feeding in emergencies.

Following these global initiatives, many countries developed calls to action and frameworks, including the European Blueprint to Action (2004), the U.S. Surgeon General's Call to Action (2011), and launching of 1,000 Days (2010), a nonprofit organization whose goal is to ensure that women and infants have a healthy first 1,000 days. Out of these initiatives arose the Baby-friendly Hospital Initiative (BFHI; WHO-UNICEF, 2009) and the Neo-BFHI (Nyvqvist et al., 2015), with updates on the BFHI came out in 2018. Finally, the Lancet Report 2016, as it has become known, reported on breastfeeding in the 21st century and examined epidemiology and the lifelong effect (Victora et al., 2016) and the returns on investment of breastfeeding practices (Rollins et al., 2016).

Many of these initiatives were introduced in Chapter 2, and you will find them integrated throughout the text. There is a timeline of important events in the evolution of breastfeeding protection, promotion, and support in **Figure 6-2**. In this chapter, we connect the policies to the health care professionals' role and find the synergy with the health promotion theories described in Chapter 3.

Baby-friendly Hospital Initiative

The **Innocenti Declaration** (1991) and the Baby-friendly Hospital Initiative (BFHI; WHO-UNICEF, 2009) are based on evidence-based practice and began in 1991 with the *Ten Steps to Successful Breastfeeding* (Nyqvist et al., 2013), which were revised in 2009 (WHO-UNICEF) and updated again in 2018 (WHO, 2018a). The steps

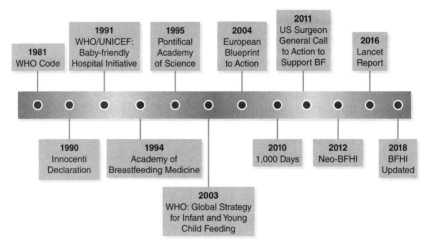

Figure 6-2 Timeline of evolution of breastfeeding initiatives.

© Suzanne Hetzel Campbell

incorporate the same ideals and have added specifics to enhance their usefulness as supported by research and global partners incorporating it for different contexts.

The 2018 updated Ten Steps include the following:

Critical management procedures

1a. Comply fully with the International Code of Marketing of Breast-milk Substitutes and relevant World Health Assembly resolutions.

1b. Have a written infant-feeding policy that is routinely communicated to staff and parents.

1c. Establish ongoing monitoring and data-management systems.

2. Ensure that staff have sufficient knowledge, competence, and skills to support breastfeeding.

Key clinical practices

3. Discuss the importance and management of breastfeeding with pregnant women and their families.

4. Facilitate immediate and uninterrupted **skin-to-skin contact** and support mothers to initiate breastfeeding as soon as possible after birth.

5. Support mothers to initiate and maintain breastfeeding and manage common difficulties.

6. Do not provide breastfed newborns any food or fluids other than breast milk, unless medically indicated.

7. Enable mothers and their infants to remain together and to practice rooming-in 24 hours a day.

8. Support mothers to recognize and respond to their infants' cues for feeding.

9. Counsel mothers on the use and risks of feeding bottles, teats, and pacifiers.

10. Coordinate discharge so that parents and their infants have timely access to ongoing support and care. (WHO, 2018b)

There is substantial evidence that implementing the Ten Steps significantly improves breastfeeding rates. A systematic review of 58 studies on maternity and newborn care published in 2016 demonstrated clearly that adherence to the Ten Steps (see below and **Figure 6-3**) impacts early initiation of breastfeeding

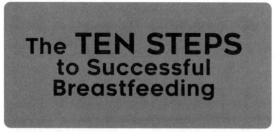
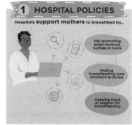
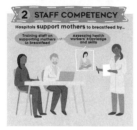
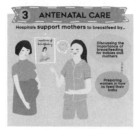
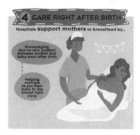
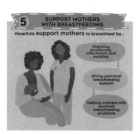
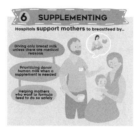
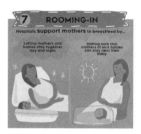
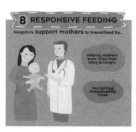
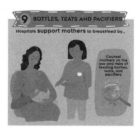
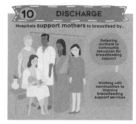
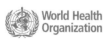

Figure 6-3 The Ten Steps to Successful Breastfeeding InfoGraphic (2018)

Reproduced from World Health Organization, The TEN STEPS to Successful Breastfeeding, Retrieved from https://www.who.int/docs/default-source/nutritionlibrary/bfhi-poster-a2-breastfeeding.pdf?sfvrsn=bcaf8b67_2

immediately after birth, exclusive breastfeeding, and total duration of breastfeeding (Pérez-Escamilla et al., 2016):

1. Have a written breastfeeding policy that is routinely communicated to all health care staff.
2. Train all health care staff in skills necessary to implement this policy.
3. Inform all pregnant women about the benefits and management of breastfeeding.

4. Help mothers initiate breastfeeding within one half-hour of birth.
5. Show mothers how to breastfeed and maintain lactation, even if they should be separated from their infants.
6. Give newborn infants no food or drink other than human milk, unless medically indicated.
7. Practice rooming in—that is, allow mothers and infants to remain together 24 hours a day.
8. Encourage breastfeeding on demand.
9. Give no artificial teats or pacifiers (also called dummies or soothers) to breastfeeding infants.
10. Foster the establishment of breastfeeding support groups and refer mothers to them on discharge from the hospital or clinic. (WHO-UNICEF, 2009)

The infographic of the 2018 Ten Steps outlines 10 key areas of focus, stating the following: "Hospitals support mothers to breastfeed by" and listing key approaches to support under each of the areas:

1. Hospital policies
2. Staff competency
3. Antenatal care
4. Care right after birth
5. Support with breastfeeding
6. Supplementation
7. Rooming-in
8. Responsive feeding
9. Bottles, teats, and pacifiers
10. Discharge

Inherent in these Ten Steps to successful breastfeeding is the need for antenatal information and support and staff competency around hospital policies that support breastfeeding, including encouraging skin-to-skin contact immediately after birth and for as much time as possible in the hospital. Staff competency, both in the hospital and at discharge, infers that health care professionals can check positioning and latch of the infant and evaluate milk transfer, as well as provide practical advice and help parents with common breastfeeding problems. Other key components to support breastfeeding in the hospital include allowing rooming-in of the parent–infant dyad for responsive feeding as indicated by infant cues and, in the case of sick infants, allowing for parents to be in close proximity. Also strict guidelines are required around the use and risks of human milk substitutes, prioritizing the use of human milk whenever possible, and minimizing the use of bottles, teats, or pacifiers. Discharge planning with referrals to community resources and breastfeeding support and continuity of care between delivery and community supports are key for the smooth transition home. Finally, expectations of the Ten Steps are that the health center does not promote infant formula, bottles, or teats and that breastfeeding care is standard practice that is tracked and supported (WHO-UNICEF, 2009; WHO, 2018b). There are implications at many levels for the incorporation of these Ten Steps into hospitals and communities.

When considering the socio-ecological model (SEM) for health promotion, the BFHI supports individuals by considering the breastfeeding dyad and protecting them through skin-to-skin contact, rooming-in for unlimited access to each other, and encouragement to follow infants' cues for hunger. It also considers the interpersonal level by incorporating family members into discharge planning, as well as inclusion of community resource links to community-wide options for support. At the institutional level, when BFHI is in place, policies for staff preparation, hospital guidelines for supplementation and bottle and teat use, and prohibition of marketing of human milk substitutes protect parents from undue pressure. Accrediting hospitals as BFHI has a direct impact on exclusive breastfeeding rates and parents' ability to meet their infant-feeding goals related to breastfeeding.

Within the tenets and recommendations of BFHI, the theory of breastfeeding self-efficacy health promotion strategies are supported. Parents are provided with consistent information to make informed choices, and they are supported during pregnancy, birth, and postpartum by health professionals knowledgeable about breastfeeding, which enhances parents' self-efficacy and ability to meet their goals. Research has connected higher levels of breastfeeding self-efficacy (BSE) to greater likelihood of exclusive breastfeeding, and education targeting BSE has had a positive effect on perceptions of insufficient milk supply (Dennis & Faux, 1999; Galipeau et al., 2017; Loke & Chan, 2013). If the Ten Steps are being followed, BSE should be supported and enhanced for new parents. Similarly, when larger local, community, health authority, and political structures demonstrate support for breastfeeding through their policies and practices, tenets of the theory of planned behavior (TPB) and theory of reasoned action (TRA) are supported, as parents will receive consistent messaging about breastfeeding that will in turn affect the subjective norms, attitudes, and beliefs they are exposed to and will help to support them to meet their goals.

Key Points to Remember

1. The Innocenti Declaration was adopted by policy makers and international agencies in 1990 affirming an infant's right to exclusive breastfeeding for up to 6 months (2001) and thereafter; yet global support and enabling environments for parents to meet their breastfeeding infant-feeding goals are missing. International goals have not been met, and overall fatigue on the part of governments, policy makers, and health care providers should not dissuade us given the health, economic, and global benefits of supporting parents.
2. Adoption of the WHO Code as law is not sufficient to create enabling environments, as the human milk substitute (formula) industry remains an undermining disrupter to parents' and governments' work to improve environments to support breastfeeding. A balance of community support and holding industries and governments accountable is necessary to meet global targets.
3. Creating communities and health care systems that recognize the role of health care professionals in supporting parents to meet their infant-feeding goals and following guidelines from the Baby-friendly Hospital Initiative (BFHI) and the Ten Steps for successful breastfeeding releases the burden on parents.
4. Community Collaboratives and partnerships that include government, community, and health care providers and systems are a powerful way to move forward the international policy in place to support infant and child feeding and access to healthy lives.

Case Study

The following is a case study from 2010–2012 that incorporated all aspects of BFHI on a state level and has been replicated in many other areas since.

Connecticut: Introduction to the Problem

In January 2012, the State of Connecticut had 29 birthing facilities, and 4 of them were BFHI. For context, according to U.S. BFHI (2015) statistics, 245 of 3,250 birthing facilities were designated facilities. The Connecticut Breastfeeding Coalition (CBC) sought to increase BFHI status in the state with a goal to recruit 10 hospitals and increase the number to over 50% of birthing facilities in the state (MacEnroe, 2013).

Baby-Friendly USA (BFUSA) developed what is known as the 4-D Pathway to Baby-Friendly Designation: D1-Discovery, D2-Development, D3-Dissemination, and D4-Designation (2012–2020). This has become the gold standard in the United States to achieving Baby-Friendly Designation and is the tool used to measure a facility's progress toward Baby-Friendly Designation. It is based on the Plan → Do → Study → Act framework used in change management processes for organizations and is often taught as part of leadership theory. It also incorporates components of logic models to assist institutions with developing sustainable plans for incorporation of the Ten Steps and a way to measure for continuous improvement (BFUSA, 2012–2020). The CBC applied for funding and came up with the following plan: (1) Develop and revise materials to assist with implementation in the form of a Tool Kit; (2) Create model action plans rather than work plans; and (3) Design templates for Training, Patient Education, and Data Collection.

One of the major barriers to implementing BFHI is funding staff for training and education. The funding CBC received through the BFUSA's Continuous Quality Improvement (CQI) processes grant allowed dissemination phase fees to be paid for the training of nursing staff. Other ways that barriers around implementation were addressed were the following:

- Provision of mock surveys to allow practice for BFHI review
- Disseminating 20-hour curriculum, 15 education/5 clinical hours at all sites
- Individual consultation for hospitals to address specific issues in their context (up to 40 hours)
- Collaboration and collective problem solving via conference call, workshops, and conveniently scheduled meetings
- Changes to the coalition website to include posting frequently asked questions (FAQs)

The success of the CBC–Connecticut Breastfeeding Initiative (CBI) project was that it addressed specific areas for priority populations, and it provided support in the form of a toolkit in addition to monetary support for education, implementation, application, and continuing education.

Through this project, previously existing hospital-based programs for BFHI were modified into a statewide public health model and a toolkit was created as a replicable model for other states and/or counties (SNAP-Ed Toolkit, 2020). The impact on breastfeeding in the state was significant, as 43% of births occurred at the 10 birthing hospitals that were part of the project, and they focused on underserved, low-income maternity populations (39% of births are public pay at the 10 maternity hospitals). During the project, one hospital achieved Baby-Friendly Designation, and nine hospitals had BFHI steps disseminated by the project's end, including training of 580+ maternity staff with continued education credits secured for all trainees. The coalition was able to leverage other federal funding sources such as the Women, Infant and Children Supplemental Nutrition Program (WIC) Peer Counseling Program to effect other positive changes in the state.

1. Think of other ways coalitions can play a role in effecting institutional changes to promote and support breastfeeding?
2. Can you connect how this CBI project targeted specific aspects of the BFHI?
3. What aspects of the CBI target theoretical components to affect breastfeeding families from the following theories: BSE, TRA, TPB?

Community Support—An Exemplar

Jolynn Dowling, MSN, APRN, NNP-BC, IBCLC

Continuity of care for breastfeeding after discharge is essential for parents to meet long-term breastfeeding goals and extend exclusivity and duration to meet recommendations (Step 10 of BFHI) (McFadden et al., 2017). Community support is key to sustain long-term gains as a result of the BFHI efforts in maternity facilities (Pérez-Escamilla et al., 2016). This continuity of breastfeeding education, care, and support can be provided through a variety of community-based organizations and programs such as hospitals and clinics, mother-to-mother support groups (La Leche League), lactation support providers in private practice, baby cafés, childcare providers, employers, health departments/WIC peer counselors, business, and the general public.

Another source of support to connect breastfeeding parents to community resources is a local breastfeeding coalition. The coalition is comprised of a variety of community partners who have a shared vision to improve breastfeeding outcomes. As such, they bring resources that can be leveraged toward meeting the unique needs of the community. Working together, a network of support can be developed through policy, system, and environmental changes for the promotion and support of breastfeeding (Lilleston et al., 2015).

An example of a promising practice demonstrating this network of support is the Community Supporting Breastfeeding (CSB) program through the Kansas Breastfeeding Coalition (Bandy, 2014). This program recognizes communities that provide breastfeeding support across multiple sectors in the community, as described in the previous paragraph (Bandy, 2014). There is synergy that is needed to sustain long-term community support after funding mechanisms have been depleted. This can be accomplished through engaging key stakeholders and through strategic development to prioritize goals. A part of this process is an evaluation of programs and services to ensure that they are meeting the needs of breastfeeding parents. If the evaluation reveals positive outcomes, then garnering resources for sustainability is enhanced. A variety of tools are available to assist with this evaluation, such as community dashboards, asset maps, and work plan templates (Lilleston et al., 2015). Local community coalitions can find tools and resources through engaging key stakeholders, including state or national coalitions or other agencies that align to promote and protect breastfeeding.

Although breastfeeding parents may be aware of community services through information received during the hospital discharge process, there can be barriers in accessing these services. Recognizing barriers related to transportation, culture, family structure, and social context is essential for the health care provider and community organization in order to meet breastfeeding parents "where they are" so that their breastfeeding goals may be achieved (Lilleston et al., 2015).

Chapter Acknowledgements

USA, Connecticut, WIC Program
- Centers for Disease Control and Prevention
- Connecticut Breastfeeding Coalition (CBC) – Chair, Michele Griswold; CBI Project Consultant, Jennifer Matranga, http://www.breastfeedingct.org
- Connecticut Department of Public Health – Susan Jackman, CBC member
- Connecticut WIC Staff & Patients
- United States Dietetics Association (USDA) – Peer Counselor Program Support – Cathy Carothers
- La Leche League International – Mansfield Center, Connecticut

References

Baby-Friendly USA (BFUSA). (2012–2020). Designation process: Getting started. What are the steps in the 4-D Pathway? https://www.babyfriendlyusa.org/for-facilities/designation-process

Bandy, B. (2014). Communities supporting breastfeeding. *Kansas Health Matters.* https://www.kansashealthmatters.org/promisepractice/index/view?pid=30307

Campbell, S. H., Meek, J., & Revai, T. (2019). Initiatives to protect, promote and support breast-feeding. In S. H. Campbell, J. Lauwers, R. Mannel, & R. Spencer (Eds). *Core curriculum for interdisciplinary lactation care* (pp. 459–475). Jones & Bartlett Learning.

Frenk, J., Chen, L., Bhutta, Z. A., Cohen, J., Crisp, N., Evans, T., Fineberg, H., Garcia, P. Ke, Y. Kelley, P., Kistnasamy, B., Meleis, A., Naylor, D., Pablos-Mendez, A., Reddy, S., Scrimshaw, S., Sepulveda, J., Serwadda, D., & Zurayk, H. (2010). Health professionals for a new century: Transforming education to strengthen health systems in an interdependent world. *Lancet, 376*(9756), 1923–1958. doi:10.1016/s0140-6736(10)61854-5

Conde-Agudelo, A., & Díaz-Rossello, J. L. (2016). Kangaroo mother care to reduce morbidity and mortality in low birthweight infants. *Cochrane Database of Systematic Reviews,* (8). https://doi.org/10.1002/14651858.CD002771.pub4

Dennis, C., & Faux, S. (1999). Development and psychometric testing of the Breastfeeding Self-Efficacy Scale. *Research in Nursing & Health, 22*(5), 399–409. https://doi.org/10.1002/(sici)1098-240x(199910)22:53.0.co;2-4

Galipeau, R., Baillot, A., Trottier, A., & Lemire, L. (2018, April). Effectiveness of interventions on breastfeeding self-efficacy and perceived insufficient milk supply: A systematic review and meta-analysis. *Maternal & Child Nutrition, 14*(3), e12607. https://doi.org/10.1111/mcn.12607

Gray, H. (2017). A quick guide to the International (WHO) Code. *La Leche League International.* https://www.llli.org/quick-guide-international-code-2/

Griswold, M. K. (2017). Reframing the context of the breastfeeding narrative: A critical opportunity for health equity through evidence-based advocacy. *Journal of Human Lactation, 33*(2), 415–418. https://doi.org/10.1177/0890334417698691

Innocenti Declaration. (1991). On the protection, promotion and support of breastfeeding. https://www.unicef-irc.org/publications/435-innocenti-declaration-2005-on-infant-and-young-child-feeding.html UNICEF.

International Baby Food Action Network (IBFAN). (2017). IBFAN statement. http://ibfan.org

Lilleston, P., Nhim, K., & Rutledge, G. (2015). An evaluation of the CDC's community-based breast-feeding supplemental cooperative agreement: Reach, strategies, barriers, facilitators, and lessons learned. *Journal of Human Lactation, 31*(4), 614–622. https://doi.org/10.1177/0890334415597904

Loke, A. Y., & Chan, L. K. (2013). Maternal breastfeeding self-efficacy and the breastfeeding behaviors of newborns in the practice of exclusive breastfeeding. *Journal of Obstetrics, Gynecologic & Neonatal Nursing, 42*(6), 672–684. https://doi.org/10.1111/1552-6909.12250

MacEnroe, T. (2013, May). The Connecticut story. Presentation to Connecticut Coalition for Breast-feeding. https://www.breastfeedingct.org

McFadden, A., Gavine, A., Renfrew, M. J., Buchanan, P., Taylor, J. L., Veitch, E., Rennie, A. M., Crowther, S. A., Neiman, S., & MacGillivray, S. (2017). Support for healthy breastfeeding mothers with healthy term babies (Review). *Cochrane Database of Systematic Reviews, 2:CD001141.* https://doi.org/10.1002/14651858.CD001141.pub5

Michaud-Létourneau, I., Gayard, M., & Pelletier, D. L. (2019). Translating the International Code of Marketing of Breast-milk Substitutes into national measures in nine countries. *Maternal & Child Nutrition, 15*(S2), e12730. https://doi.org/10.1111/mcn.12730

Nyqvist, K. H., Häggkvist, A.-P., Hansen, M. N., Kylberg, E., Frandsen, A. L., Maastrup, R., Ezeonodo, A., Hannula, L., Haiek, L. N., & Baby-friendly Hospital Initiative Expert Group. (2013). Expansion of the Baby-friendly Hospital Initiative Ten Steps to Successful Breastfeeding into neonatal intensive care: Expert group recommendations. *Journal of Human Lactation, 29*(3), 300–309. https://doi.org/10.1177/0890334413489775

Nyqvist, K., Maastrup, R., Hansen, M. N., Haggkvist, A. P., Hannula, L., Ezeonodo, A., Kylberg, E., Frandsen, A., & Haiek, L. N. (2015). The Neo-BFHI: The Baby-friendly Hospital Initiative for Neonatal Wards. https://ilca.org/neo-bfhi/

One thousand (1000) days. (2010). https://thousanddays.org/about/

Pérez-Escamilla, R., Martinez, J., & Segura-Perez, S. (2016). Impact of the Baby-friendly Hospital Initiative on breastfeeding and child health outcomes: A systematic review. *Maternal & Child Nutrition, 12*(3), pp. 402–417. https://doi.org/10.1111/mcn.12294

Robinson, H., Buccini, G., Curry, L., & Pérez-Escamilla, R. (2019). The World Health Organization Code and exclusive breastfeeding in China, India, and Vietnam. *Maternal & Child Nutrition, 15*(1), e12685-n/a. https://doi.org/10.1111/mcn.12685

Rollins, N. C., Bhandari, N., Hajeebhoy, N., Horton, S., Lutter, C. K., Martines, J. C., Piwoz, E. G., Richter, L. M., & Victora, C. G. (2016). Why invest, and what it will take to improve breastfeeding practices? *The Lancet, 387*(10017), 491-504. https://doi.org/10.1016/S0140-6736(15)01044-2

SNAP-Ed Toolkit. (2020). Connecticut Breastfeeding Initiative (CBI). https://snapedtoolkit.org/interventions/programs/connecticut-breastfeeding-initiative-cbi

United Nations Children's Fund (UNICEF). (2005). Innocenti Declaration 2005 on Infant and Young Child Feeding. https://www.unicef-irc.org/publications/435

U.S. Baby-Friendly Hospital Initiative (BFHI). (2015, March 6). https://www.babyfriendlyusa.org/ and https://www.babyfriendlyusa.org/for-parents/find-a-baby-friendly-facility/

Victora, C. G., Bahl, R., Barros, A. J. D., França, G. V. A., Horton, S., Krasevec, J., Murch, S., Sankar, M. J., Walker, N. & Rollins, N. C. (2016). Breastfeeding in the 21st century: Epidemiology, mechanisms, and lifelong effect. *The Lancet, 387*(10017), 475-490. https://doi.org/10.1016/S0140-6736(15)01024-7

Walker, M. (2007). International breastfeeding initiatives and their relevance to the current state of breastfeeding in the United States. *Journal of Midwifery and Women's Health, 52*(6), 549–555. https://doi.org/10.1016/j.jmwh.2007.06.013

World Health Organization (WHO). (1981). International Code of Marketing of Breast-Milk Substitutes. https://www.who.int/nutrition/publications/infantfeeding/WHO_NUT_98.11/en

World Health Organization (WHO). (2003). *Global strategy for infant and young child feeding.* https://www.who.int/nutrition/publications/infantfeeding/9241562218/en/

World Health Organization (WHO)-UNICEF. (2009). Baby-friendly Hospital Initiative: Revised, updated and expanded for integrated care. http://www.who.int/nutrition/publications/infantfeeding/bfhi_trainingcourse/en

World Health Organization (WHO). (2018a). Baby-friendly Hospital Initiative. *Nutrition.* http://www.who.int/nutrition/topics/bfhi/en

World Health Organization (WHO). (2018b). Ten steps to successful breastfeeding. https://www.who.int/activities/promoting-baby-friendly-hospitals/ten-steps-to-successful-breastfeeding

PART 2

Breastfeeding as Developmental Health Promotion

CHAPTER 7

Developmental Processes of Lactation as Health Promotion

Carrie Miller, PhD, RN, CHSE, CNE, IBCLC

LEARNING OBJECTIVES

1. Recognize health promotion during pregnancy as influences of infant-feeding practices.
2. Describe birth practices and the impact of interventions on infant feeding.
3. Describe infant behaviors influencing breastfeeding.
4. Recognize early caregiver practices and behaviors for health promotion of breastfeeding.

KEY WORDS

- **Augmentation:** Used when ongoing labor is determined not to be effective.
- **Birthing Practices:** Based on cultural influences, science, personal references, and health history, birth practices are how a pregnant individual gives birth to another human being.
- **Cesarean Birth:** Surgical removal of a fetus through the abdominal cavity.
- **Electronic Fetal Monitoring:** Use of instruments to monitor the fetal heartbeat and uterine contractions during labor.
- **Endorphins:** Hormones secreted by the body in response to pain, extreme exertion, or high stress.
- **Epidural:** Regional anesthesia that can block pain receptors and numb specific areas in the lower region of the body. Epidural catheters are placed in the epidural space of the spinal column. Epidurals are frequently used during labor.
- **Feeding Cues:** The deliberate body movements and sounds to communicate with caregivers when the infant is ready to feed or is hungry. There are three levels of feeding cues. These include early cues, such as lip smacking and bringing hands to mouth; mid cues: such as more body movements, sucking on hands and rooting; and late signals, such as crying, fussiness, and becoming red in the face.
- **Feeding on Cue:** Parent responsiveness to infant feeding cues.
- **Going Home:** Discharge from a setting that is not home by origination.

- **Hydrotherapy:** The use of warm water to help with pain management.
- **Induction of Labor:** use of medications or natural methods to initiate labor contractions.
- **Infant Behavior:** The cues, actions, and sounds an infant makes to communicate his or her needs to caregivers.
- **Initial Latch:** The first latch after birth.
- **Pitocin:** Synthetic oxytocin. Used to augment labor or reduce risk of postpartum hemorrhage.
- **Placenta:** Essential organ of pregnancy. Attached to the wall of the uterus. The role is to allow for nutrient uptake by and removal of waste from the fetus.
- **Physiological Birth:** Labor is allowed to begin on its own, and there are no routine or medical interventions that alter the course of the labor or birth.
- **Rooming-in:** From birth to discharge (going home), the infant remains in the room with the birthing parent and family members. The infant is only removed from the room for procedures or testing that cannot occur in the parent's birthing suite or hospital room.
- **Skin-to-Skin:** Placing an infant with only a diaper on, or naked, stomach down, between the breasts or on the anterior chest of an awake and alert adult. The premise of skin-to-skin is to promote bonding, help an infant self-regulate, and, if applicable, promote breastfeeding.
- **Uterus:** A pear-shaped organ of the female reproductive system. The uterus is located in the lower pelvis and plays a significant role in reproduction.

Overview

Intuitively, an understanding exists that a fetus is influenced by the environment in which it grows and, subsequently, the journey of birth and the world into which a neonate is born. How a neonate transitions from the **uterus** to the world can be influenced by events that occur during pregnancy, birth, and postpartum. Health promotion activities or processes influence overall well-being (World Health Organization [WHO], 2019) for both parent and infant. Birth practices, including **physiological birth**, **induction of labor**, and surgical birth, can all impact infant-feeding decisions for a birthing parent. A birthing parent's or neonate's interactions in the first moments after birth and into early postpartum all play a role in how a parent bonds, feeds, and nurtures the infant. Despite the intuitive nature of knowing that deliberate actions can influence health outcomes, there appears to be a lack of awareness about how breastfeeding can be impacted. Under optimal conditions, the birthing parent's expectations and the care received facilitate breastfeeding success (Sheeran et al., 2015).

This chapter begins by describing birth practices from physiological and medical management perspectives along with the potential impact of interventions on both the parent and infants. Moreover, the actions and behaviors immediately after birth and in the early postpartum period can potentiate or thwart a parent's sense of confidence and adaptive behaviors as they transition to the role of a parent.

Birthing Considerations

Birthing practices vary across the globe. Giving birth is a personal, intimate, and memorable experience for each person. In considering health promotion, birth can be described as a natural progression from pregnancy to birth without any unnecessary medical interventions. Breastfeeding is part of the birthing experience and responds well to health-promoting attitudes and interventions. Birth requires several interventions to promote the safe passage of a fetus from its birthing parent's body into the world. These include ensuring a safe place to labor and give birth, holistic comfort measures (e.g. **hydrotherapy**), support by trusted companions, and a birth attendant who is educated on the labor processes and mechanisms of birth. Each of these is considered an intervention. These interventions do not impair the anticipated processes of birth. In considering medical interventions, some interventions are lifesaving, such as an emergent **cesarean birth** due to fetal intolerance of labor. However, the question needs to be asked, could the interventions before the emergent birth have contributed to the outcome? Birth settings have the potential to either positively or negatively influence breastfeeding initiation and duration.

Concepts of Physiological Birth

A supportive birth setting can optimize and empower birthing parents during a time of stress and vulnerability. New parents appear to thrive in settings when preferences are considered, honored if possible, and when there is open communication. Due to health care protocols, safety practices, and fear of legal action, many birth settings are strict and policy bound. This creates a division between parents, providers, and caregivers. Furthermore, hospital and birth settings that support the Baby-friendly Hospital Initiative (BFHI) are more likely to respond positively to breastfeeding practices.

Physiological birth, also known as normal birth, is defined as birth with no unnecessary interventions that may disrupt or change the trajectory of the delivery of the infant (Downe, 2008). Birth can proceed in a healthy, physiological fashion. A birthing parent is encouraged or, for lack of a better word, permitted to go into labor spontaneously. Once in labor, the body continues to work through the processes of labor. Giving birth using a physiological approach is not easy to achieve. Westernized culture is steeped in technological advances and expectations of requiring medical assistance to give birth successfully. Interventions may include, but are not limited to, peripheral intravenous catheter placement, **electronic fetal monitoring**, and cesarean birth. Surgical birth occurs due to fetal intolerance to labor, maternal illness or injury, convenience, or maternal request. Over the past decade, cesarean birth has continued to remain steady at approximately one-third of all births across westernized countries (Shee et al., 2019).

Despite established medical policies that meet current standards of best practice, studies suggest the level of interventions and medical management of low-risk birth is not necessary for safe birth outcomes (Shee et al., 2019). In Lamaze Healthy Birth practices, there are six basic premises of giving birth healthily. They are not scripted but, instead, are health-promoting activities that allow the laboring individual to have authority and empowerment. Each birth practice is grounded in scientific evidence and is intended to reduce risk and promote optimal outcomes. Principles surrounding healthy birth practices include the ability to go into labor spontaneously, move around freely and change positions as the laboring person desires and be accompanied by trusted support companions. Moreover, Lamaze birth principles also include avoiding any unnecessary interventions, encouraging laboring parents to listen to their body when it comes time to push, and structuring postpartum settings with both birthing parent and newborn **rooming-in** together. Each of these practices may appear to be grounded in common sense; however, challenges continue to prevail in health care delivery to promote doctrines of physiological birth (Walker, 2017).

When asked, a birthing parent will indicate that the essential aspects of giving birth are curated into four main assumptions. The first and second are to be able to describe their expectations surrounding the birth as well as the level of support with caregivers, partners, and family. The quality of support is vital. Support persons who are caring, attentive, and engaged can reduce stress levels during labor and birth. The third and fourth issues focus on the quality and skills of the caregivers and the birthing parent's ability to be involved in decision making (Downe, 2008).

When considering the quality of care by caregivers during the birth process, the *Theory of Caring* by Kristen Swanson (1991) describes how caregivers can provide caring attitudes for parents and newborns early in their breastfeeding experience (Miller & Wojnar, 2019). Swanson (1991) defines *caring* as "a nurturing way of relating to a valued other toward whom one feels a personal sense of commitment and responsibility" (p. 165). Caring is a fundamental component of a caregiver's contribution to a client's biopsychosocial and spiritual well-being. Swanson Theory of Caring is enacted by five nonlinear processes: (1) Maintaining belief, (2) Knowing, (3) Being with, (4) Doing for, and (5) Enabling. Swanson (1991) defines the caring constructs, beginning with "Maintaining belief," as a philosophical attitude toward persons in general and their abilities to achieve personal goals. "Knowing" encourages the caregiver to avoid assumptions or make decisions based on personal beliefs and bias and rather to center on the birthing parent's and infant's needs. "Being with" represents the emotional and physical presence of the caregiver and expression of understanding and respect. "Doing for" depicts caring acts out of the specific therapeutic actions necessary to optimize care outcomes. This may include providing comfort and physical care because the birthing parent is unable to do it for themselves. The final process, "Enabling," refers to guiding the breastfeeding individual and infant through infant-feeding transitions. When acts of caring are omitted in communications with clients, negative consequences may take place. The usefulness of Swanson's Theory of Caring is demonstrated in research, education, and clinical practice globally (Miller & Wojnar, 2019; Wojnar, 2014).

Birth Partnership

During pregnancy and prenatal care, a partnership has the potential to develop. These partnerships between a pregnant client and health care provider can illuminate a healthier pregnancy and birthing experience. Presently, the birth plan remains a popular option to help guide communication regarding birth environments and practice. Birth plans, although resolute with the intent to advocate for informed consent and a voice in birth settings, have created barriers and obstacles for both providers and clients (DeBaets, 2017). Web-based birth plans are one-way communication and can be created with little or no guidance. Birth plans can create adversarial caregiver/client relationships when wishes or prescribed intents are not met (DeBaets, 2017). According to DeBaets (2017), ongoing conversations during pregnancy, before birth, and after birth are more helpful. Ongoing dialogue will enable a clear understanding of clients' preferences, concerns, and questions. The pregnant parent can share values, beliefs, and concerns. These can then be used to create a person-centered approach to care delivery. These actions facilitate a trusting relationship when there is a need to make unexpected or desired decisions.

Caregivers during the birth process need to be educated about breastfeeding practices and policies. These initial steps during early breastfeeding experiences will impact the breastfeeding relationship and duration. Many new parents lack role models and the self-confidence to breastfeed without support. A knowledgeable caregiver for the **initial latch** and during the first days after birth can influence the success of the breastfeeding relationship.

Hospital Practices

Before the 1970s, all medical care was delivered based on authority or opinion. Whoever had the highest rank, or status, established the patterns and decisions of care. After decades of discussion, legislative action, and scientific research change began to take form. Health care consumers demanded change, and health care providers advocated for evidence-based practice policies (Smith & Kroeger, 2010). Despite calls for action to empower the lay public and careful analysis of the impact of interventions, technological advances in care delivery continued to increase, including interventions such as inducing labor for noncompelling reasons. When a laboring person is induced into labor, the contractions are more likely to be closer together and stronger. The laboring person does not have time to adjust to labor and produces fewer **endorphins**. The lack of sufficient endorphins and lack of time to slowly adapt to the laboring process cause a majority of laboring parents to request **epidural** anesthesia. The act of receiving an induction and epidural anesthesia increases the risk of cesarean birth. In situations where labor began spontaneously, labors that slow down may be subject to **augmentation**. When augmentation occurs, **Pitocin** (oxytocin) is given to increase the intensity of contractions, thus increasing pain, as well as decreasing mobility due to continuous fetal monitoring and, potentially, increasing fetal intolerance to labor.

The risk of complications due to medical interventions may impact the breastfeeding relationship. For example, if labor has been induced for a nonmedical reason and the fetus is not tolerating the labor, cesarean birth is warranted. As a result of the fetal intolerance, the newborn may be taken to the special care nursery for monitoring. This will result in separation from the birthing parent. Due to the surgical nature of cesarean birth, the parent is unable to hold the newborn until after medical stabilization from surgery. Cesarean birth is major abdominal surgery with care issues concerning pain, mobility, and genitourinary and gastrointestinal issues that must be addressed. Studies consistently suggest that infants born via cesarean section are less likely to exclusively breastfeed and are weaned earlier than infants born vaginally (Zhang et al., 2019).

Interventions

When considering health care standards, what may seem essential may not be based on evidence but rather on tradition or fear of legal action. Presently, westernized culture and medical practice influence the birthing process to include scientific or evidence-based interventions intended to support labor clients and the fetus.

The use of medications, anesthesia, and unnecessary procedures can affect early breastfeeding and breastfeeding duration. The American Academy of Pediatrics encourages the avoidance of routine procedures during and after birth until the first breastfeeding has taken place (Eidelman, 2012). Promoting physiological birth enhances the opportunity to have fewer interventions. In 2013, the Listening to Mothers survey was conducted with 2,400 mothers. Findings revealed that the majority of respondents had interventions during labor. Despite recommendations to move freely about during labor, three out of five women did not get out of bed after admission to the birth setting (Declercq et al., 2014). Also, nine out of ten gave birth on their backs or in a semi-reclined position. Mobility during labor and pushing reduces the incidence of episiotomy, abnormal fetal heart rates, and vacuum-assisted deliveries (Declercq et al., 2014).

Furthermore, interventions during labor, such as electronic fetal monitoring, are standard practice. Pragmatically, health care providers know that the fetal heart rate during labor can help determine well-being. Assessing fetal health is critical in the labor process. In the use of electronic fetal monitoring, the caregiver can choose to monitor the fetus intermittently or continuously. In physiological birth, a birthing parent is encouraged to move freely, and intermittent fetal monitoring can be used strategically and within protocols. This allows periods for freedom of movement and opportunities for the laboring parent to be unrestricted in movement or environment. If a cause for concern is noted when assessing fetal well-being, surveillance frequency can be changed to accommodate the needs of the fetus. The use of continuous fetal monitoring can influence the mobility of the laboring patient and increases the risk of further interventions (Heelan, 2013).

Electronic fetal monitoring, created in the 1950s, was intended to reduce the incidence of cerebral palsy (Chez et al., 2000). Using technology to monitor the fetus's heart rate during labor can provide critical information for caregivers on the well-being of a fetus.

The intent is to assess well-being during labor contractions. During labor, when the uterus contracts, there is reduced oxygen to the uterine muscle and the **placenta** (Neilson, 2015). In the majority of situations, the fetus can tolerate labor contractions without any distress. Studies suggest when the continuous fetal monitor is utilized, there is a higher risk of instrumental and cesarean birth (Ayres-de-Campos et al., 2015). Incidentally, the rates of cerebral palsy and birth injuries did not decrease with the use of electronic fetal monitoring over the past 40 years (Chez et al., 2000).

Another common intervention within the hospital birth setting is regional anesthesia, typically known as an an epidural. In most situations, the epidural uses two medications to promote pain relief for the laboring patient. These include a numbing medication and a narcotic. The epidural is placed in the laboring parent's spinal region and is closely monitored by nursing and medical caregivers. The medication used can influence the laboring process, impact mobility, reduce endogenous oxytocin, affect breastfeeding initiation, and reduce the efficacy of the infant's suckle (French et al., 2016; Jonas et al., 2009). Studies have attempted to prove or disprove the impact of epidural medications and breastfeeding outcomes (French et al., 2016). Despite numerous studies suggesting epidurals impede breastfeeding outcomes and studies that dispute these findings, the research clearly states that birth and breastfeeding outcomes are directly linked to factors that may have been influenced by the use of regional anesthesia for pain management in labor, including **infant behavior**, duration of labor, need for instrumental delivery, and cesarean birth (French et al., 2016).

Infant Considerations

Golden Hour

The "golden hour" is identified as a time for a medically stable newborn to be placed between its birthing parents' breasts for 1 to 2 hours. During this time, the neonate remains skin-to-skin with the parent in a quiet, dimmed space. The intent is to allow the neonate to begin the transition to extrauterine life, have the first feeding, and promote optimal neonatal and maternal outcomes (Crenshaw, 2014). Caregivers have a responsibility to support the physiological need of **skin-to-skin** through education, advocacy, and implementation (Crenshaw, 2014). During this time, assessments and care can be delivered as needed; however, the intent is to be an observer of changes and advocate to reduce disruptions unless medically necessary. Tasks such as weight, length, bathing, wrapping, and dressing the newborn can wait until long after the first feeding has taken place. The physiological adaptation that occurs for the newborn and birthing parent is critical.

In the Baby-friendly Hospital Initiative, step four suggests that infants need to be placed skin-to-skin with their mothers in the first hours after birth. During skin-to-skin contact, the breastfeeding reflexes awaken and newborns exhibit a series of behaviors that result in the newborn locating and latching onto the nipple (Widström et al., 2010). These acts during the first hours after birth can have a profound impact on the breastfeeding experience (Bramson et al., 2010; Marín Gabriel et al., 2010; Moore et al., 2012). Promoting physiological birth and careful consideration to interventions can facilitate a higher likelihood of skin-to-skin contact and the initial latch in the immediate postpartum period. Throughout this sensitive period, the newborn is imprinting on parents, similar to what is seen with other animal species. The newborn's cardiac, respiratory, and temperature regulation systems function more effectively during skin-to-skin activities. Infants on the maternal chest can initiate the initial latch and what is known as the breast crawl. Many scientists believe the breast crawl is a natural way for a baby to behave immediately after birth and is essential for optimal self-regulation (Heidarzadeh et al., 2016). The act of the breast crawl appears to be an instinctive behavior during the immediate postpartum period for a full-term infant. The breast crawl is structured with the newborn placed on the maternal abdomen and given 60 minutes to independently reach and latch onto the nipple (Heidarzadeh et al., 2016). As this is occurring, the newborn is covered by a warm blanket and the birthing parent is awake.

In addition to breastfeeding, the newborn is able to imprint and bond with parents. The bonding is strongest during the first 1 to 2 hours of life (Lauwers & Swisher, 2016). After the first 1.5 to 2 hours, routine procedures by caregivers can take place. Bonding is described as close contact between parent and newborn (Kennell & Klaus, 1982). The optimal time for bonding to be established is immediately after birth, and it begins with the first contact between parent and newborn (Brody, 1981). During this time, attachment behaviors are noted through sucking, crying, eye contact, and feeding behaviors (Brody, 1981). In response, the birthing parent will touch, hold, cuddle, and nurse the newborn.

Moreover, the hormonal function of oxytocin increases dramatically during skin-to-skin contact. The increased oxytocin facilitates the uterus to contract and activate the milk ejection reflex (MER). The MER promotes the release of colostrum and human milk. Additional benefits of oxytocin are that it reduces physiological stress and reduces the risk of postpartum hemorrhage (Buckley, 2014). In addition to maternal effects of skin-to-skin contact and the first feeding, studies suggest that paternal roles also have hormonal responses, including a rise of oxytocin, prolactin, and testosterone (Swain et al., 2014). These increasing levels are associated with caregiving attitudes (Rilling, 2013).

Postpartum Practices to Promote Breastfeeding

Through health-promoting partnerships, communication, and policies, the postpartum setting can support the breastfeeding experience. A healing environment, nonjudgmental attitude, and treatment of parents as capable can contribute to breastfeeding success. Active listening and being available will also enable parents to relax and share their ideas, perceptions, and expectations. Although breastfeeding is instinctual, these are learned skills that must be obtained for breastfeeding to continue and be successful. These include parents learning their newborns' behaviors, **feeding cues**, biological needs, and care needs. A sequence of events occurs during skin-to-skin contact. The sequence of events, such as head bopping, bringing hands to the mouth, sucking motions, and nuzzling the breast and nipple, facilitate teaching parents about feeding cues and expected newborn behaviors right after birth (Widström et al., 2019). In BFHI Step 7, Rooming-in, studies suggest that when newborns and birth parents are together, breastfeeding practices can be established and ongoing. Parents learn to care for their newborns, including feeding, diapering, burping, and holding. In addition, newborns feed more frequently with less crying, thus conserving energy (Lauwers & Swisher, 2016). Caregiving staff can offer lactation support and education as needed. Avoiding disruption and providing positive communication all contribute to setting down a solid foundation for lactation.

Summary

Throughout human existence, newborns and parents depend on each other for the intricate dance of life. Newborns come into the world with instincts and foundational skills that must be nurtured and recognized. If provided with the optimal environment, newborns are capable and will be able to navigate to the breast, latch, and suckle. Each of these movements aligns with future feedings and the breastfeeding experience. In promoting lactation and the overall health of the parent and newborn dyad, consideration must be given to both the birthing parent and newborn during pregnancy and birth. In pregnancy, open communication and teamwork guide a birthing parent to consider options and realize that care delivery may need to change when urgent issues occur. During the birth process, protecting physiological birth and avoidance of nonessential, routine medical interventions can optimize birth outcomes and recovery. For newborns, an awareness of expected behaviors along with ensuring that newborns are provided with ample time to acquaint themselves with the breast and bond with parents set the tone for further interactions and the breastfeeding relationship.

Key Points to Remember

1. Breastfeeding-friendly practices and policies can optimize health outcomes for birthing parents and newborns.
2. Through partnerships with parents, breastfeeding can be supported.
3. Careful consideration of birth interventions is essential to optimize breastfeeding outcomes.

Student Questions for Consideration

1. Consider birth experiences you have experienced or witnessed. What interventions do you recall that are considered supportive of physiological birth? What interventions are not supportive of physiological birth?
2. Identify routine procedures seen in maternity care that can impede breastfeeding.
3. Research care practices in a local hospital birth center and in a midwifery-run birthing center. What differences and similarities do you notice?
4. Do the hospitals, birthing centers, and communities in your geographical area practice Baby-friendly Hospital Initiative practices? Can you identify them?

Real-life Stories—Brief Anecdotes from Relative Sources

- Typical case scenario of uncomplicated birth-vaginal-breastfeeding well
  - Lynne woke up with the sensation of a contraction in the middle of her back that seemed to radiate to the front part of her very pregnant belly. She was 40 weeks pregnant and eager to meet her baby. Her pregnancy was healthy. Her midwife was very helpful in explaining all the changes her body was going through. She had breast changes early in her pregnancy and started to leak colostrum about six weeks ago. She was very hopeful to have a physiological birth. She called her midwife and began the drive to the Birth Center. As she arrived at the Birth Center, the contractions were starting to strengthen, and she was feeling confident in her body. After two hours of walking around the Birth Center, she decided to get some fresh air. The midwife assessed Lynne's labor and said she had several hours before her body would be ready to push. Lynne decided to go for a walk outside around the Birth Center. She was able to move freely and to relax between contractions by resting her arms on her partner's shoulders. After about an hour of walking, Lynne was feeling pressure in her pelvis and some back pain, so she headed into the Birth Center. The midwife assessed Lynne's labor and was quite surprised to tell Lynne her body was ready to push the baby if Lynne had the urge to push her baby out. After about a half-hour, Lynne felt the urge to push her baby out and did so with about six pushes. A baby boy was born and placed on Lynne's chest between her breasts. The birth attendant covered both the baby and Erin with a warm blanket and allowed for privacy… observing the baby and Lynne for any concerns or complications. About 15 minutes after the placenta was expelled, the baby began to wiggle toward Lynne's nipple. It took about 20 minutes, but the baby was able to latch independently and suckle for

about 15 minutes. Both mom and baby rested while the birth attendant cared for both of them. Postpartum recovery was uncomplicated, and both Lynne and her baby thrived. Lynne breastfed her baby for two years.

- Typical case scenario of a complicated birth, long labor, sleep baby, and overcoming breastfeeding difficulties.

  - Kim was anxious to leave for the hospital. Her scheduled cesarean birth was taking place in less than two hours, and she did not want to be late. The older children were rustling in their beds at the early dawn, knowing their mum was heading out early this morning. Kim's husband was packing up the car and having the first cup of coffee for the day. There was a lot of activity in the house. Kim was 39 weeks pregnant. The option of surgical birth was chosen because the hospital she was having her baby in did not allow for the attempt of vaginal birth after a cesarean, also known as VBAC. She had her two older children vaginally, but the twins she gave birth to three years ago were by cesarean birth. With everything packed and ready to go, Kim and her husband headed to the hospital. Kim planned to breastfeed her baby. She had breastfed all of her prior children.

    After they checked in to the admitting desk, they were escorted to the birthing suite. After the intravenous catheter was placed and Kim was changed into a hospital gown, she walked to the Operating room suite. In the suite, the fetal monitor was used to assess fetal heartbeat, an epidural was placed, and a tube was placed in her bladder to keep her bladder empty during the surgery. The nursing team washed her belly with an anti-infective solution and put a warm blanket across her thighs and across her shoulders to keep her warm. The surgeons came, gowned, and gloved up. A surgical drape was placed on Kim's belly, and surgery began. Within a few minutes, the surgical drape was lowered just a bit, and Kim was able to see her baby's face and hear a soft cry. Her baby was placed on her chest. During this time, the surgeons changed their gloves and continued with surgery while the nursing staff attended to Kim and her new baby.

    About 15 minutes later, the baby was taken to the warmer to be evaluated and wrapped in warm blankets. The surgeons completed the surgery, and both mom and baby were escorted to the recovery room. In the recovery room, the baby was placed on Kim's chest, avoiding the abdomen for skin-to-skin time. As the baby began to root around searching for the nipple, the nursing staff was there to assist in supporting the baby with the first latch. Baby latched and nursed for several minutes, then became sleepy. During the postpartum stay, the baby struggled to latch and seemed fussy most of the time. The baby was not feeding well. There was difficulty in placing the baby skin-to-skin because of the abdominal incision and recovery pain. The nursing staff asked the lactation nurse to assist in helping Kim with feeding her baby. The lactation nurse visited with Kim and helped her with different positions for breastfeeding and skin-to-skin. The lactation team visited with her with the next three feedings to make sure latching was more comfortable for Kim. The help from the nursing staff and lactation team made a difference, and the baby was breastfeeding well at discharge.

Questions:
1. What is different between each of the case studies?
2. What is similar in both case studies?
3. Is it possible to promote physiological birth aspects for cesarean birth?

Additional Resources

BirthsTools.org—Tools for Optimizing the Outcomes of Labor Safety. https://www.birthtools.org /What-Is-Physiologic-Birth

International Childbirth Education Association—Physiologic Birth. https://icea.org/wp-content /uploads/2016/01/Physiologic_Birth_PP.pdf

References

Ayres-de-Campos, D., Spong, C. Y., & Chandraharan, for the FIGO Intrapartum Fetal Monitoring Expert Consensus Panel. (2015). FIGO consensus guidelines on intrapartum fetal monitoring: Cardiotocography. *International Journal of Gynecology & Obstetrics, 131*(1), 13–24. https://doi .org/10.1016/j.ijgo.2015.06.020

Bramson, L., Lee, J. W., Moore, E., Montgomery, S., Neish, C., Bahjri, K., & Melcher, C. L. (2010). Effect of early skin-to-skin mother-infant contact during the first 3 hours following birth on exclusive breastfeeding during the maternity hospital stay. *Journal of Human Lactation, 26*(2), 130–137. https://doi.org/10.1177/0890334409355779

Brody, S. (1981). The concepts of attachment and bonding. *Journal of the American Psychoanalytic Association, 29*(4), 815–829. https://doi.org/10.1177/000306518102900403

Buckley, S. J. (2014). *The hormonal physiology of childbearing.* Childbirth Connection.

Chez, B., Harvey, M., & Harvey, C. (2000). Intrapartum fetal monitoring: Past, present, and future. *Perinatal Neonatal Nursing, 14*(3), 1–18. https://doi.org/10.1097/00005237-200012000-00002

Crenshaw, J. T. (2014). Healthy birth practice #6: Keep mother and baby together—It's best for mother, baby, and breastfeeding. *The Journal of Perinatal Education, 23*(4), 211–217. https://doi .org/10.1891/1058-1243.23.4.211

DeBaets, A. M. (2017). From birth plan to birth partnership: Enhancing communication in childbirth. *American Journal of Obstetrics and Gynecology, 216*(1), 31.e1–31.e4. https://doi .org/10.1016/j.ajog.2016.09.087

Declercq, E. R., Sakala, C., Corry, M. P., Applebaum, S., & Herrlich, A. (2014). Major survey findings of listening to Mothers[SM] III: New mothers speak out. *The Journal of Perinatal Education, 23*(1), 17–24. https://doi.org/10.1891/1058-1243.23.1.17

Downe, S. (2008). *Normal childbirth: Evidence and debate,* 2nd ed. Elsevier.

Eidelman, A. I. (2012). Breastfeeding and the use of human milk: An analysis of the American Academy of Pediatrics 2012 Breastfeeding Policy Statement. *Breastfeeding Medicine, 7*(5), 323–324. https://doi.org/10.1089/bfm.2012.0067

French, C. A., Cong, X., & Chung, K. S. (2016). Labor epidural analgesia and breastfeeding: A systematic review. *Journal of Human Lactation, 32*(3), 507–520. https://doi.org/10.1177 /0890334415623779

Heelan, L. (2013). Fetal monitoring: Creating a culture of safety with informed consent. *The Journal of Perinatal Nursing, 22*(3), 156–165. https://doi.org/10.1891/1058-1234.22.3.156

Heidarzadeh, M., Hakimi, S., Habibelahi, A., Mohammadi, M., & Shahrak, S. P. (2016). Comparison of breast crawl between infants delivered by vaginal delivery and cesarean section. *Breastfeeding Medicine, 11*(6), 305–308. https://doi.org/10.1089/bfm.2015.0168

Jonas, W., Johansson, L. M., Nissen, E., Ejdebäck, M., Ransjö-Arvidson, A. B., & Uvnäs-Moberg, K. (2009). Effects of intrapartum oxytocin administration and epidural analgesia on the concentration of plasma oxytocin and prolactin, in response to suckling during the second day postpartum. *Breastfeeding Medicine, 4*(2), 71–82. https://doi.org/10.1089/bfm.2008.0002

Kennell, J. H., & Klaus, M. H. (1982). *Parent-infant bonding.* Mosby.

Lauwers, J., & Swisher, A. (2016). *Counseling the Nursing Mother* (6th ed). Jones and Bartlett.

Marín Gabriel, M., Llana Martín, I., López Escobar, A., Fernàndez Villalba, E., Romero Blanco, I., & Touza Pol, P. (2010). Randomized controlled trial of early skin-to-skin contact: Effects on the mother and the newborn. *Acta Paediatrica, 99*(11), 1630–1634. http://dx.doi .org/10.1111/j.1651-2227.2009.01597.x

Miller, C. W., & Wojnar, D. (2019). Breastfeeding support guided by Swanson's Theory of Caring. *MCN: The American Journal of Maternal/Child Nursing, 44*(6), 351–356. https://doi.org/10.1097 /NMC.0000000000000570

Moore, E. R., Anderson, G. C., Bergman, N., & Dowswell, T. (2012). Early skin-to-skin contact for mothers and their healthy newborn infants. *Cochrane Database of Systematic Reviews 5,* CD003519. http://dx.doi.org/10.1002/14651858.CD003519.pub3

Neilson, J. P. (2015). Fetal electrocardiogram (ECG) for fetal monitoring during labour. *Cochrane database of systematic reviews, 12.* https://doi.org/10.1002/14651858.CD000116.pub5

Rilling, J. K. (2013). The neural and hormonal bases of human parental care. *Neuropsychologia, 51*(4), 731–747. https://doi.org/10.1016/j.neuropsychologia.2012.12.017

Shee, A. W., Nagle, C., Corboy, D., Versace, V. L., Robertson, C., Frawley, N., McKenzie, A., & Lodge, J. (2019). Implementing an intervention to promote normal labour and birth: A study of clinicians' perceptions. *Midwifery, 70,* 46–53. https://doi.org/10.1016/j.midw.2018.12.005

Sheeran, L., Buchanan, K., Welch, A., & Jones, L. (2015). Women's experiences of learning to breastfeed. *Breastfeeding Review, 23*(3), 15–22. http://hdl.cqu.edu.au/10018/1041581

Smith, L. J., & Kroeger, M. (2010). *Impact of birthing practices on breastfeeding.* Jones & Bartlett.

Swain, J. E., Kim, P., Spicer, J., Ho, S. S., Dayton, C. J., Elmadih, A., & Abel, K. M. (2014). Approaching the biology of human parental attachment: Brain imaging, oxytocin and coordinated assessments of mothers and fathers. *Brain research, 1580,* 78–101. https://doi .org/10.1016/j.brainres.2014.03.007

Swanson, K. M. (1991). Empirical develop of a middle range theory of caring. *Nursing Research, 40* (3), 161–165. https://doi.org/10.1097/00006199-199105000-00008

Walker, M. (2017). *Breastfeeding management for the clinician* (4th ed). Jones and Bartlett.

Widström, A. M., Brimdyr, K., Svensson, K., Cadwell, K., & Nissen, E. (2019). Skin-to-skin contact the first hour after birth, underlying implications and clinical practice. *Acta Paediatrica, 108*(7), 1192–1204. https://doi.org/10.1111/apa.14754

Wojnar, D. (2014). Kristen M. Swanson: Theory of Caring. In M. Alligood (Ed.), *Nursing theorists and their work.* Elsevier.

World Health Organization. (2019). *Guidelines: Protecting, promoting, and supporting breastfeeding.* https://www.who.int/publications/i/item/9789241550086

Zhang, F., Cheng, J., Yan, S., Wu, H., & Bai, T. (2019). Early feeding behaviors and breastfeeding outcomes after cesarean section. *Breastfeeding Medicine, 14*(5), 325–333. https://doi.org /10.1089/bfm.2018.0150

CHAPTER 8

Globalization and Lactation as Health Promotion: Brazil

Nicole de Oliveira Bernardes, PhD, PT
Suzanne Hetzel Campbell, PhD, RN, IBCLC, CCSNE

LEARNING OBJECTIVES

1. Define the concept of globalization within the context of infant feeding and maternal–infant health promotion.
2. Reflect on ways that globalization may affect health promotion.
3. Compare and contrast facilitators and barriers to the promotion and support of lactation as health promotion from the context of a globalized society.
4. Describe an international perspective on lactation and infant feeding.
5. Analyze multiprofessional and interdisciplinary international experiences supporting and promoting breastfeeding.

KEY WORDS

- **Globalization:** A term used to describe the increasing connectedness and interdependence of world cultures and economies.
- **PAHO/WHO:** Pan American Health Organization/World Health Organization.
- **WHO/UNICEF Baby-friendly Hospital Initiative (BFHI):** World Health Organization/United Nations International Children's Emergency Fund Baby-friendly Hospital Initiative.
- **Global Strategy Infant and Young Child Feeding (GSIYCF):** Aims to revitalize efforts to promote, protect, and support appropriate infant and young child feeding.

Overview

Given the strong evidence of the importance of supporting and protecting breastfeeding as a precious health, economic, and global resource, this chapter will further explore lactation as a global health promotion strategy with an example from Brazil.

Introduction

We live in a world greatly influenced by the processes of **globalization** that are affecting the health outcomes in both positive and negative ways (Labonte, 2007; Lee, 2004). For this chapter we use the term *globalization* within the context of an international health approach related to infant feeding. The comparisons between well-resourced and less well-resourced countries on diseases or health issues—such as comparing maternal and infant morbidity and mortality—could constitute an "international approach" to the situation. In this chapter, a global approach moves beyond a comparison of countries' health and disease states to more critically examine and recognize that both the social determinants of health and the subsequent consequences on an individual's health and well-being are linked to the process of globalization itself (Labonte, 2007; Labonté, 2011). Due to the strong cumulative evidence demonstrating that breastfeeding is one of the highest health promotive impact interventions benefiting children, women, and society (Victora et al., 2016), situating lactation in a global context of health promotion and practice is fitting for this chapter. This topic has great significance for public health, where promoting health is linked to the goals of prolonging life and preventing disease through the organized efforts of society. Our perspective is that everyone is responsible for supporting new parents in their infant-feeding decisions and meeting their goals, and health care professionals are well suited to have great influence, locally and globally. This chapter further explores lactation as a global health promotion strategy with a specific example from Brazil.

The Effect of Globalization on Breastfeeding

Nevertheless, how does globalization affect breastfeeding? On the surface, globalization may appear to have a small effect. However, when examining the impacts of globalization, such as free trade that is not necessarily fair and a system that values profits above people, the effects become more pronounced and more profound. This requires vigilance to avoid compromise of the needs of parents and children and to protect the dyad from the commercialization of human milk substitutes, which has become the norm, not the exception (Henry, 2005). On the other hand, global communication has the potential to educate people regarding breastfeeding and its importance, benefits, and also about the health risks of human milk substitutes for infants (Henry, 2005).

Transforming breastfeeding into a normative behavior in a globalized world is a considerable challenge (Lutter & Lombardi, 2014). Two global events—the World Health Assembly and the Second International Conference on Nutrition—had important roles in shaping the infant and young child nutrition agenda, and breastfeeding was a huge component of both. They identified targets to advance globally in this area through 2025, with a goal to "increase the breastfeeding rates in the first six months up to at least 50%" (Lutter & Lombardi, 2014, p.1). Even with this global movement toward exclusive breastfeeding, several factors can affect parents' ability to adhere to these guidelines, including cultural behavior, lack of support within hospital and health services, lack of maternity protection and programs for breastfeeding in the workplace, and not controlling the marketing of human milk substitutes (Lutter & Lombardi, 2014).

These issues are social barriers and are directly related to diminishing breast-feeding rates all around the world. Another worldwide social barrier is women's pressure not to breastfeed in public. This pressure can be explicit or subtle on breastfeeding parents. To overcome this obstacle, there needs to be social support that allows women to be comfortable breastfeeding their babies anytime and any-place necessary (Henry, 2005; Lutter & Lombardi, 2014).

Questions to Consider

1. *How comfortable are you in the presence of a breastfeeding parent?*
2. *Compare your comfort level at home, in your place of work, in public space. Is there a difference? Why or why not?*

Brazilian Perspective

In 1975, the average breastfeeding duration in Brazil was increased to greater than eight months, with an eight-fold increase in exclusive breastfeeding (EBF) in infants less than 6 months old. Some of the ways the changes occurred were related to mass-media breastfeeding-promotion campaigns that increased the awareness of the public and government officials by providing evidence-based information on the health benefits and cost savings of breastfeeding. All primary health care units supported breastfeed-ing, and all health care staff were educated on the benefits of breastfeeding and risks of artificial breast milk substitutes. Public pressure and attitudes were affected by annual celebrity contests and posters advocating breastfeeding. Parent/peer breastfeeding support groups provided the important support of new parents in meeting their infant feeding goals. This successful national program for breastfeeding promotion presents important lessons to be learned and is related to the social marketing framework used to scale up breastfeeding support as a public health concern (See Chapters 9 and 10). An example of this program, the **Baby-friendly Hospital Initiative (BFHI)**, leans on the strength of product availability, namely human milk, and offers attractive oppor-tunities to support maternal–child health, such as mother-to-mother support groups, and its availability at key locations including the health facilities and communities. Given strong support from the government, civil societies, international agencies [WHO/UNICEF; **PAHO/WHO**; & **Global Strategy Infant and Young Child Feeding (GSIYCF)**], and academic and philanthropic organizations, breastfeeding was pro-moted through mass media, leading to enhanced attitudes affecting a positive public opinion and behavior change. In addition, coordination between civil society, policy

---

Box 8-1 Related Research

Posters designed to promote public acceptance of breastfeeding were placed in doctors' offices and restaurants. Although 50% of those surveyed (n = 117) admitted to discomfort with a mother breastfeeding in public, being shown the posters significantly improved their level of comfort toward seeing breastfeeding in public (Vieth et al., 2015).

makers, professional societies, and medical/nursing schools, as well as government and nongovernment organizations, relied on strong intersectoral communication and decentralization of health promotion messages (Pérez-Escamilla et al., 2012). In other words, all the burden of "exclusive breastfeeding for six months" was not left on mothers' shoulders, and support of the community and broader society (including the government) was made evident. There was a long initial lag time in Brazil between 1975 and the results of the early 1990s through 2000s, whereas other countries with fewer initial barriers may find scaling up happens more quickly.

In 2003, the Brazilian federal government developed the National Program of Humanization (NPH) in health to guarantee free, universal, integral, and equal access to health care for all Brazilian citizens. Following the NPH, in 2009, a regional experiment began that supported the humanization of childbirth, and in 2011, the Stork Network was launched. The Stork Network is a care network that aims to ensure during prenatal, childbirth, and childcare periods that women and children have the right to humanized care in all health services of the Brazilian Unified Health System (SUS). From then on, Brazil faced a national movement to promote and support the humanization of childbirth and to promote vaginal births, as Brazil was ranked first in elective cesarean sections in the world (Caderno Humaniza SUS, 2014).

Still, in 2011, there was a large national women's movement, supported by public health policies, to promote humanized attention to the parent–infant dyad supporting breastfeeding on demand, exclusive breastfeeding for at least 6 months and continued until 2 years or more of the child's life. This movement gained strength as part of a Brazilian and feminist struggle for the right to breastfeed where, when, and how the parent/baby wanted. Also, it became part of the #metoo world phenomenon, which led to more than 12 million people across the world sharing their experiences of sexual abuse on social media. Thus, the "shaming of breastfeeding moms" was exposed as a sexual harassment claim against breastfeeding parents (Aleitamento Materno Solidário, 2014; Hhoo, 2017; Karmaluk, 2011; Segatto, 2016; Yong, 2017).

With the organization and gathering of thousands of women throughout Brazil, sporadic marches began in 2011 and are still occurring today, including parents, families, and women (the famous "Mamaços"). These marches included tens of thousands of people and focused on supporting breastfeeding on demand without embarrassment. Families went to the streets to protest against the sexualization of breasts that led to the taboo of breastfeeding in public (Aleitamento Materno Solidário, 2014; Hhoo, 2017; Karmaluk, 2011; Segatto, 2016; Yong, 2017).

From this national movement, light was shed on an organic problem in Brazilian society, and with the pressure of women, families, and organized society, state and federal laws were created to guarantee women's freedom and safety breastfeeding anywhere, including in public. In addition, it was made illegal to negatively react to women or demonstrate prejudice or violence against breastfeeding parents; thus these actions were criminalized under the law (Agência Senado, 2019; Watts, 2015).

When parents, supported by public policies and laws, breastfeed freely without any social restrictions, they send a powerful message to their family, to the community, and to society that breastfeeding is natural, enjoyable, and helps to affirm that this is a normative behavior for all women. Barriers to breastfeeding in public must be removed to promote breastfeeding, once again, as a norm, recognized, accepted, and valued as the ideal and physiological way to feed a child (Lutter & Lombardi, 2014). The support offered to breastfeeding families is the key to the success of continuous breastfeeding. This adequate groundwork includes support that is offered by trained health professionals/peers/volunteers or a mix (McFadden et al., 2017).

Teamwork and individual improvement in multiple skills in the interdisciplinary context, as well as cooperation between professionals, are fundamental to the fluidity of the health services provided to breastfeeding families. Today, teams are gaining ground in health service organizations thanks to the efficient way of organizing and harnessing human skills. A more global and collective view of work is necessary for a better use of the unique skills and qualities of professionals working in maternal and child health. Identifying the needs of healthcare professionals to better support parents in the promotion of breastfeeding requires examining the policies in place and the actions of administrators in supporting those policies. Chapter 6 outlines the Baby-friendly Hospital Initiative and the policies required in the Ten Steps. This chapter provides further background and acknowledges that verifying administrative, governmental, community, and industry support is paramount to the success of breastfeeding. Nurses, midwives, physical therapists, physicians, nutritionists, speech therapists, social workers, pharmacists, and many other healthcare professionals are working with breastfeeding families; these broad teams are intended to be prepared to help lactating families and to promote breastfeeding through their practices and in their workplaces.

The multiprofessional healthcare team plays a key role related to the duration and exclusivity of lactation by providing women with information and personal support during pre/postnatal care, delivery (intrapartum), immunization appointments, and parent–infant clinical consultations. It is essential that members of the health team welcome parents and infants and are available to listen and explore questions, fears, or barriers to breastfeeding. Conversations to discuss alternative solutions and an exchange of experiences, feelings, and ideas should be encouraged. This support can increase mothers' breastfeeding self-efficacy and may affect the breastfeeding initiation and exclusivity rates; it is more effective when it is expected, scheduled, and face to face (Brockway et al., 2017; McFadden et al., 2017). Thus, a well-prepared health professional team is important in providing a positive influence to promote breastfeeding for the parent–infant dyad (Almeida et al., 2015; Beinner & Beinner, 2004; Martins & Montrone, 2009; McFadden et al., 2017).

Brazilian Experience: A Physical Therapist Professional Supporting Breastfeeding Parents

My first professional contact with breastfeeding parents and babies was during my undergraduate course in physical therapy in 1998, while doing a women's health internship in a maternity hospital. I stayed there for 6 months, three mornings a week, helping postpartum parents with their physical complaints, questions, and managing their pain. One of the most prevalent complaints was their difficulties with breastfeeding. I helped them position the baby, and themselves during lactation, as the major issues centered on nipple trauma with pain and engorgement. I was enchanted by that place and all the help we could give to the new parents and their babies. The year before, I had 1 year of a theoretical course in obstetrics and gynecology as applied to physical therapy. In that moment, I was ultimately in love with the "women's health specialty" and have built my career in this area ever since. But what is the role of a physical therapist in women's health?

In Brazil, the specialty started around the 1980s, and in 1985, the course on gynecology and obstetrics applied to physical therapy was included by the Ministry of Education as part of the regular curriculum of physical therapy undergraduate courses. The course enables the student to work with obstetrics, gynecology, urology, mastology, lymphology, and sexuality. The obstetric topic includes pregnant women's prenatal care related to the pelvic floor muscles, postural assessment and treatment of back pain, edema, muscle and joint pain and instability, muscle preparation for delivery, exercise prescription guidelines for pregnant women, and breastfeeding lectures and simulations. We also support women during labor and delivery, using nonpharmacological analgesic methods, posture positioning, massages, stretching, breathing, and relaxation. At this stage, we can use therapeutic resources, such as high-frequency electrotherapy, hydrotherapy, and heat and cold (depending on the indication) to help control pain during labor and delivery.

During the postpartum period, the physical therapist assists women after the first 6 to 8 hours following delivery with physical and muscular recovery. We work with passive strengthening of abdominal muscles, abdominal pain and flatus, back pain and positioning, breathing, and pelvic floor muscles (pain, exercise, stitch healing), and we give some verbal information related to immediate, late, and remote postpartum. Besides this, we support them while breastfeeding in order to reduce postpartum edema and stimulate them to walk and self-care.

The breastfeeding support is one of the most important topics during our postpartum evaluation. As part of the multiprofessional team, we help with proper latching and positioning, nipple pain, sore breasts and nipples, breast engorgement, breast lumps, feeding issues or concerns, problems with baby latching or sucking, helping a baby who won't latch, and teaching and practicing hand expression of colostrum and breast milk. After the physical therapist's evaluation and treatment, women receive a referral from us to make an appointment in our clinic during remote postpartum to initiate a global rehabilitation, with a focus on pelvic floor and sexuality function/dysfunction.

On discharge day, as part of the Baby-friendly Hospital Initiative (BFHI) guide, one of the maternity health professionals meets with all parents/families. They provide some guidance on breastfeeding and postpartum and newborn care, and they also provide information about human milk donation, immunization, and newborn and parents' civil rights. They also provide a list of public health breastfeeding support in case they have any problems or concerns.

An Interprofessional and Interdisciplinary Obstetric Clinical Case

This clinical case was designed and simulated by a group of professors from five different health courses in a private university in Brazil. The medical, nurse, physical therapy, biomedicine, and psychology departments were involved in this interprofessional and interdisciplinary obstetric clinical case. The students enrolled in this simulation class were in the second year of their programs, and they had two meetings during the interprofessional project. The first meeting consisted of three steps:

Step 1: Simulation of a prenatal medical appointment (a medical professor and an actor). All the five-course students stayed in a separate room, inside the simulation lab behind a two-way mirror, observing the appointment and documenting any pertinent information. Medical and nursing students also complete the perinatal record, and after a brief discussion all students received the written case.

Step 2: During the debriefing phase, vulnerabilities were discussed, as were key clinical issues and elaborate learning questions (LQs) that guided the theoretical research.

Step 3: This step consisted of two phases. Initially, the student wrote their thoughts about the case based on at least two scientific references to respond to LQ. Then, the students met together to elaborate on their points of view or elements that constituted the therapeutic project (TP). They also prepared a presentation for the second meeting. During the second meeting, the students presented their work to the professor and finished the TP.

Summary

This chapter offered an overview of the globalization of infant feeding and lactation as a health promotion resource. We presented the concept of globalization within the context of infant feeding and maternal–infant health promotion, and discussed how health promotion may be affected by it. Moreover, we examined the facilitators and barriers to the promotion and support of lactation from the context of a globalized society. From an international perspective, we described lactation and infant feeding in Brazil, and we analyzed multi-professional and interdisciplinary international experiences supporting and promoting breastfeeding. For clinical purposes, we concluded the chapter with a multi-professional and interdisciplinary obstetric clinical case.

Key Points to Remember

1. Support for new parents in their infant-feeding decisions requires everyone's input.
2. Lessons learned from Brazil support broad political, health system, and social measures to support parents in breastfeeding their infants and children anytime, anywhere.
3. Interprofessional teams have the opportunity to provide a safety net of support to new parents.

Case Study

Medical appointment on May 3.

Silvia was born in Betim, Minas Gerais, Brazil. She lives in the Teresopolis neighborhood and attended a public basic health unit (PBHU). She is 19 years old, white, and completed high school. She got married 2 years ago to 20-year-old

Arcangelo, who was convicted and imprisoned for the second time due to illicit drug trafficking. They have a healthy 1½-year-old son. Silvia is employed cleaning houses. She and her son Francisco have lived with her parents ever since her husband was arrested. Her parents never accepted this marriage but welcomed her and her son into their home. Her mother has diabetes and hypertension and a family history without other pathologies. Francisco was delivered vaginally with the usual prenatal care at a district maternity hospital. According to Silvia, forceps were used during Francisco's birth. An episiotomy was performed with subsequent prolongation of the incision. The procedure was performed under local anesthesia, but she felt immense pain and screamed a lot. "The doctor was very rude and said to me, 'At the time you wanted it and thought it was good, so now just hold on.'" According to Silvia, the stitches of the episiotomy loosened 2 days later, and she was left to heal on her own. She did some sitz baths with herbal tea, as taught to her, in an attempt to relieve the pain. She had postpartum depression, cried a lot for no reason, and didn't care about the new infant. Her mother took care of Francisco because Silvia stated, "I wanted him to die. . . . This all lasted about a month, and I still don't understand why I felt these things, and I have many regrets about it. The health team at my PBHU and my family helped me a lot at that time." Silvia is very afraid of her second birth and having depression again. She was not encouraged to breastfeed Francisco, her first son, during the first hour of his life. He was taken to the nursery for two nights, before their discharge. When she left the hospital, she was bottle-feeding human milk substitutes (formula), and soon her own milk was gone. She didn't breastfeed her first son. She reports that she has been experiencing urinary incontinence since Francisco's birth, that got worse during this pregnancy, as well as dyspareunia. She is also experiencing a lot of pain in the lower back that does not improve with medication, and she is feeling very sick, with a few weekly vomiting episodes. Silvia is a smoker and uses 15 cigarettes a day. She was also using cannabis but stopped after she learned she was pregnant. She denies other previous pathologies. She denies having a previous abortion. She was unsure of her last menstrual period but thought it was about mid-November. This pregnancy wasn't planned as she always used the emergency contraceptive method after intercourse when visiting her husband in prison, as he refused to use a condom. She didn't take the pregnancy shots, and she didn't show her immunization card. She had a prenatal appointment 2 months ago and didn't return for the next one. The health agent went to her home to inform her about this new prenatal appointment, and so she came into the office today. She denied having received the "pregnant woman's book" in the previous consultation and did not perform all the exams requested because, at PBHU, they weren't conducting the exams, and she had no money to pay them all. Silvia's blood type is A, Rh positive, hemoglobin/hematocrit and urine are normal, Toxoplasmosis IgG + and IgM +, rapid test of HIV (negative), hepatitis B (negative), and syphilis (positive).

On physical examination: Normal Stained, hydrated mucosa with no changes in thyroid and lymph nodes. Blood pressure PA 100/80 mmHg, pulse 60 bpm, temperature 36.0 C/96,8 F, weight 67 kg 147,7 lb, height 1.61 m/5,3 ft, without edema. Cardiac and pulmonary auscultation without changes. Breasts without nodules or pathological secretions. Pain in lumbosacral spine compression, Giordano negative. Free abdomen. Performed Leopold maneuvers. Uterine fundus 29 cm from the pubic symphysis. Right fetal back, 130 bpm fetal cardio beats—cephalopelvic (not breech or transverse) presentation. Specular examination observed abundant white, milky discharge with reddish mucosa. Cytological examination performed. Inspection and vaginal touch: perineum with large right middle lateral scar, perineal rupture and cystocele of the first degree, thick neck, softened, closed, anterior, distance between sciatic spines greater than 10 cm and not touching the promontory.

Box 8-2 Interdisciplinary Interaction

- Start with a case study in a simulation scenario.
- Conduct rounds of conversation to discuss vulnerabilities and key problems.
- Discuss some of the learning questions to guide the theoretical investigation.
- Assignment for self-study: Initially, students do their own research on the case. Students write their considerations based on at least two references in order to answer the LQ. In the second assignment, students meet to share the study they researched, raise issues and point out elements that will constitute the therapeutic project (TP), and prepare a presentation for the next class meeting.
- Students will present the result of their work, which will be shared and discussed with their professors.

Case Study Questions

1. How would you communicate with this mother about her upcoming labor and delivery and choices for infant feeding?
2. What approach would you take to learn her goals for infant feeding after the birth of the baby?
3. What other key supports can you identify that will be strengths for her given this present pregnancy and imminent delivery?

Additional Resources

Globalization
https://www.mja.com.au/journal/2004/180/4/globalisation-what-it-and-how-does-it-affect-health
Interprofessional Health Support https://www.ncbi.nlm.nih.gov/pmc/articles/PMC3662612/pdf
/1478-4491-11-19.pdf

References

Agência Senado. (2019). *Senado aprova multa para quem impedir amamentação em local público.* [Senate approves fine for those who prevent breastfeeding in a public place.] https://www12 .senado.leg.br/noticias/materias/2019/03/12/senado-aprova-penalizacao-para-quem-impedir -amamentacao-em-local-publico

Aleitamento Materno Solidário. (2014). *"Hora do Mamaço" – A História do Movimento.* Hora do Mamaço. [The History of a Movement: 'Mamaço's Hour'] https://horadomamaco.wordpress.com /2014/07/18/hora-do-mamaco-a-historia-do-movimento

Almeida, J. M. De, Luz, S. D. A. B., & Ued, F. D. V. (2015). Support of breastfeeding by health professionals: Integrative review of the literature. *Revista Paulista de Pediatria, 33*(3), 356–363. https://doi.org/10.1016/j.rpped.2014.10.002

Beinner, M. A., & Beinner, R. P. C. (2004). The profile of professionals in health and education fields at work in their communities. *Ciência & Saúde Coletiva [Science and Public Health], 9*(1), 77–83. https://doi.org/10.1590/s1413-81232004000100008

Brockway, M., Benzies, K., & Hayden, K. A. (2017). Interventions to improve breastfeeding self-efficacy and resultant breastfeeding rates: A systematic review and meta-analysis. *Journal of Human Lactation, 33*(3), 486–499. https://doi.org/10.1177/0890334417707957

Caderno Humaniza SUS. (2014). *Humanização do parto e do nascimento. [Humanization of childbirth and birth.]* Brasília, DF, Brazil: Ministério da Saúde [Ministry of Health].

Henry, F. J. (2005). *Breastfeeding and Globalization: Implications for the Caribbean.* Presented at the National Launch of Breastfeeding Week 2003 in Jamaica under the theme "Breastfeeding in a Globalized World for Peace and Justice." https://www.unscn.org/web/archives_resources/html /resource_000272.html

Hhoo, I. (2017, October 23). Shaming breastfeeding mamas is form of sexual harassment, says mom Diana Channing. *Huffington Post.* https://www.huffingtonpost.ca/entry/shaming -breastfeeding-mamas-is-form-of-sexual-harassment-says-mom-diana-channing_ca _5cd51122e4b07bc729747597

Karmaluk, C. (2011). *Grande Mamaço Nacional Ato pró-amamentação.* [Great National Mothers Pro-Breastfeeding Act.] Grande Mamaço Nacional. https://grandemamaconacional.wordpress. com

Labonte, R. (2007). Global perspectives on health promotion effectiveness. In D. McQueen & C. Jones (Eds.), *Globalization and health promotion: The evidence challenge* (pp. 181–200). Springer. https://doi.org/10.1007/978-0-387-70974-1_12

Labonté, R. (2011). Toward a post-Charter health promotion. *Health Promotion International,* 26(suppl_2), ii183–ii186. https://doi.org/10.1093/heapro/dar062

Lee, K. (2004). Globalisation: What is it and how does it affect health? *Medical Journal of Australia,* 180(4), 156–158. https://doi.org/10.5694/j.1326-5377.2004.tb05855.x

Lutter, C., & Lombardi, C. (2014). Breastfeeding: A contemporary issue in a globalized world. In *World Alliance for Breastfeeding Action (WABA), PAHO/WHO and SPRING.* PAHO. https://www .paho.org/hq/dmdocuments/2014/WBW-2014-PolicyBrief-Eng.pdf

Martins, R., & Montrone, A. (2009). Implementação da Iniciativa Unidade Básica Amiga da Amamen- tação: Educação continuada e prática profissional. [Implementation of the Breastfeeding-friendly Basic Unit Initiative: Continued education and professional practice.] *Revista Eletrônica de Enfermagem,* [Electronic Journal of Nursing], 11(3), 545–553. https://revistas.ufg.br/fen /article/view/47099 http://www.fen.ufg.br/revista/v11n3/v11n3a11.htmhttps://revistas.ufg.br /fen/article/view/47099

McFadden, A., Gavine, A., Renfrew, M. J., Wade, A., Buchanan, P., Taylor, J. L., . . . Macgillivray, S. (2017, February 28). Support for healthy breastfeeding mothers with healthy term babies. *Cochrane Database of Systematic Reviews,* pp. 1–289. https://doi.org/10.1002/14651858 .CD001141.pub5

Pan American World Health Organization/World Health Organization (PAHO/WHO). (2014). https://www.paho.org/en

Pérez-Escamilla, R., Curry, L., Minhas, D., Taylor, L., & Bradley, E. (2012). Scaling Up of Breast- feeding Promotion Programs in Low- and Middle-Income Countries: the "Breastfeeding Gear" Model. *Advances in Nutrition,* 3(6), 790–800. doi.10.3945/an.112.002873 https://pubmed.ncbi .nlm.nih.gov/23153733/

Segatto, C. (2016, March). *Brasil vira referência em aleitamento materno. Palmas para os "mamaços."* *[Brazil becomes a reference in breastfeeding. Let's hear it for (the mothers)]* Epoca. https://epoca .globo.com/colunas-e-blogs/cristiane-segatto/noticia/2016/03/brasil-vira-referencia-em -aleitamento-materno-palmas-para-os-mamacos.html

Watts, J. (2015, March 19). São Paulo breastfeeding law would fine those who try to stop nursing mothers. *The Guardian.* https://www.theguardian.com/world/2015/mar/19/brazil -law-breastfeeding-mothers-fine-sao-paulo

Victora, C. G., Bahl, R., Barros, A. J. D., França, G. V. A., Horton, S., Krasevec, J., Murch, S., Sankar, M. J., Walker, N., Rollins, N. C., & Lancet Breastfeeding Series Group. (2016). Breastfeeding in the 21st century: Epidemiology, mechanisms, and lifelong effect. *The Lancet,* 387(10017), 475–490. https://doi.org/10.1016/S0140-6736(15)01024-7

Vieth, A., Woodrow, J., Murphy-Goodridge, J., O'Neil, C., & Roebothan, B. (2015). The ability of posters to enhance the comfort level with breastfeeding in a public venue in ru- ral Newfoundland and Labrador. *Journal of Human Lactation,* 32(1), 174–181. https://doi .org/10.1177/0890334415593944

Yong, S. (2017, October 20). Woman calls out breastfeeding shaming as form of sexual harassment. *Independent.* https://www.independent.co.uk/life-style/breastfeeding-shaming-sexual-harassment -women-public-instagram-diana-channing-a8011321.html

International Perspectives: Best Practices for Supporting Breastfeeding Across the Continuum

Suzanne Hetzel Campbell, PhD, RN, IBCLC, CCSNE

"According to the Global Breastfeeding Collective (2017) 'countries are not adequately protecting, promoting, and supporting breastfeeding through funding or policies. As a result, a majority of children in the world are not breastfed as recommended'"

– **(WHO, 2017**, p. 1**)**.

LEARNING OBJECTIVES

1. Describe international examples of successful breastfeeding programs.
2. Identify key areas for scaling up related to public policy, research, and practice.
3. Describe some specific models of success with a health promotion focus.
4. Outline barriers and innovative strategies.
5. Envision application to individual contexts and situations.

KEY WORDS

- **AIDED:** A framework including 22 enabling factors and 15 barriers to breastfeeding promotion that served as the building blocks for the breastfeeding gear model (BFGM) (Pérez-Escamilla et al., 2012).
- **Breastfeeding Gear Model (BFGM):** A model that identifies the key areas, or "gears," that need to be coordinated for synchronization of efforts to enhance (scale up) breastfeeding health promotion programs globally (Pérez-Escamilla et al., 2012).
- **Neo-BFHI:** A core document created to provide three guiding principles and Ten Steps to protect, promote, and support breastfeeding in neonatal intensive care units and for parents of premature infants. The Nordic and Quebec working groups prepared this document based on the Baby-friendly Hospital Initiative (BFHI; Hedberg-Nyqvist et al., 2015; WHO, 2018).
- **Scaling Up Public Health Initiatives:** Specific interventions to increase the quality of and improve specific programs and initiatives, taking into consideration the

political, social, economic, and legislative actions necessary and the context to support public health initiatives.
* **World Alliance for Breastfeeding Action (WABA, 2020):** A global network of individuals and organizations dedicated to the protection, promotion, and support of breastfeeding worldwide (https://waba.org.my).

Overview

Although each family chooses how to feed their infant, this decision will be influenced by many social, political, environmental, and economic factors. One factor is the effect of media, especially related to the decision to breastfeed. Strong marketing and advertisements for human milk substitutes (formula), reflected by the lack of regulation of the formula companies, affect a parent's decision and success. A parent's workplace and access to a support team also influence breastfeeding success. The breastfeeding experience is vulnerable when there is a lack of parental leave, a suitable place for breastfeeding/pumping in the parent's workplace, and a lack of adequate support from the health care team involved with the family (Global Breastfeeding Collective [GBC], 2017). This chapter presents international initiatives that have made progress over the years in supporting parents to breastfeed while focusing on barriers and facilitators to provide support.

World Alliance for Breastfeeding Action

Previous chapters describe international initiatives to protect, promote, and support breastfeeding, and the **World Alliance for Breastfeeding Action** (WABA) is a driving force. WABA is:

> a global network of individuals and organisations dedicated to the protection, promotion and support of breastfeeding worldwide based on the Innocenti Declarations, the Ten Links for Nurturing the Future and the WHO/UNICEF Global Strategy for Infant and Young Child Feeding. WABA is in consultative status with UNICEF and an NGO in Special Consultative Status with the Economic and Social Council of the United Nations (ECOSOC). (WABA, 2020, p.1)

Partners in these efforts with WABA include the Academy of Breastfeeding Medicine (ABM), International Baby Food Action Network (IBFAN), International Lactation Consultant Association (ILCA), La Leche League International (LLLI), United Nations International Children's Emergency Fund (UNICEF), World Health Organization (WHO), and several other international organisations (WABA, 2020).

WABA has a dynamic influence in networking breastfeeding organizations across the globe and provides important links across these groups for advocacy, education, and support. The organization has consolidated global data such that it can provide details about the effects of scaling up breastfeeding in the prevention of 20,000 maternal deaths, 823,000 child deaths, and $302 billion in economic losses annually (WABA, 2020). How can we as a society ignore the overwhelming impact of breastfeeding on our citizens, families, and planet? If we believe that breastfeeding provides a universal solution, laying the foundation for good health and survival of women and children, as WABA (2020) asserts, then supporting parents in exclusive breastfeeding (EBF) will provide an equitable start in life for all infants.

The Sustainable Development Goals (SDGs) (United Nations [UN], 2020) are another measurement of global health, and there are 17 goals identified for achievement by 2030. The WABA website connects breastfeeding to the achievement of all 17 SDGs, providing an example for each goal (WABA, 2020).

Student Activity

1. *Choose one of the SDGs for 2030, and identify how breastfeeding can have an effect on meeting that goal.*
2. *Develop a plan. Choose one area of focus: local, regional, national, international that will address that SDG. How might the plan change given modifications in the area?*
3. *Create intervention targets related to health promotion theories and provide rationale.*

In Chapter 8, we examined how social marketing and strong government, civil society, international agency, academic and philanthropic organizations came together with mass media to provide strong intersectoral communication that decentralized and altered public opinion and behavior change related to breastfeeding in Brazil (Rea, 2003). The lessons learned in framing this national program as a social marketing framework are that social marketing can be useful as a conceptual framework and is consistent with the scaling up **AIDED** model suggested by Pérez-Escamilla et al. (2012). The next section gives an overview of the health impact pyramid and the AIDED framework.

Health Impact Pyramid

Health promotion research often considers the Health Impact Pyramid (Frieden, 2010) as a framework around which to plan public health action. This model, utilized to create the AIDED framework for breastfeeding, considers a pyramid or triangle with interventions beginning at the base and continuing to the tip of the pyramid. Those interventions at the base have the least individual effort required, and they have the greatest potential for population impact because they represent the socioeconomic determinants. The next level on the pyramid examines ways for interventions to change the context so that individuals default to healthy decision making. An example is the breastfeeding lounges instituted in airports that make it easy for parents to find privacy and minimize distraction in a busy public area. In breastfeeding, we have long focused on the next two levels of the pyramid: clinical interventions and ongoing clinical care, including health education and counseling. These levels depend on limited contact, and although they may provide long-term protection, they require much more effort on the part of individuals (Frieden, 2010) (See **Figure 9-1**).

Student Activity

In considering the levels of the Health Impact Pyramid, where would you classify some of the interventions of the BFHI (WHO, 2018) discussed in Chapter 6? Can you think of other examples that represent socioeconomic factors? Is breastfeeding itself a long-lasting protective intervention for parents, infants, and families? Why or why not?

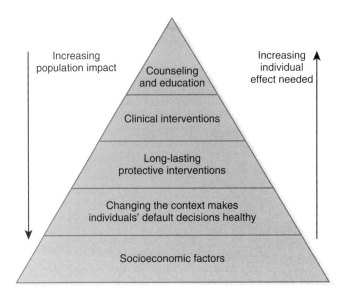

Figure 9-1 Health Impact Pyramid.

Reproduced from Thomas, R., & Frieden, T. R. (2010). A framework for public health action: The health impact pyramid. *American Journal of Public Health, 100*(4), 590–595. doi:10.2105/AJPH.2009.185652. http://www.ncbi.nlm.nih.gov/pmc/articles/PMC2836340/

The AIDED Framework

Given that breastfeeding is one of the most important and cost-effective interventions in protecting and advancing maternal–infant health, examining factors that facilitate its promotion and barriers are necessary to provide sufficient support to families. Pérez-Escamilla et al. (2012) did a systematic review of key barriers and facilitators of low- and middle-income countries scaling up breastfeeding programs. The AIDED Framework was the result of that systematic review and has now been applied as a logical process with the following steps:

1. **Assess** the landscape and the baseline needs of the country.
2. **Innovate** in a way that fits user receptivity.
3. **Develop** support.
4. **Engage** specific user groups.
5. **Devolve efforts** to spread the innovation. (Pérez-Escamilla et al., 2012)

In total, the team identified 22 enabling factors and 15 barriers that were mapped and used to build the parsimonious **Breastfeeding Gear Model (BFGM)**.

Analogous to a well-oiled engine, the BFGM indicates the need for several key "gears" to be working in synchrony and coordination. Evidence-based advocacy is needed to generate the necessary political will to enact legislation and policies to protect, promote, and support BF at the hospital and community levels. This political-policy axis in turn drives the resources needed to support workforce development, program delivery, and promotion. Research and evaluation are needed to sustain the decentralized program coordination "gear" required for goal setting and system feedback. The BFGM helps explain the different levels of performance in national BF outcomes in Mexico and Brazil. Empirical research is recommended to further test the usefulness of the AIDED framework and BFGM for global scaling up of BF programs. (Pérez-Escamilla et al., 2012, p. 790)

Consolidated information and support for becoming breastfeeding friendly and scaling up are available on the Family Larsson-Rosenquist Foundation website (2020).

Key components of the work are essential to foster enabling relationships, environments, and networks among partners for supporting and facilitating one another to spread innovation. The international consensus meetings were critical early events in order to foster the political will, legislation, and workforce development, yet continued investments into the infrastructure are necessary to manage the social determinants of health and make long-term commitments to scaling up the promotion and support for breastfeeding families. This book outlines some of the ways that investing in intersectoral partnerships and politically sensitizing consumers and policymakers related to cost/savings analyses help to mobilize civil society for further engagement.

If we unpack the AIDED framework from an international perspective, we can see how each section of the model correlates with specific health promotion interventions, as well as where the role of health care professionals in collaboration with community and government partners can have the greatest effect.

Assess the Landscape

When evaluating the landscape for breastfeeding support, assessment of the health system, broader community, and sociocultural contexts must occur at the country, state, province, or county level, depending on those managing it. Ideally, assessment begins at the national level by examining specifics such as parental leave policies and return-to-work accommodations for breastfeeding parents. The physical infrastructure for the delivery of breastfeeding support at the facility and community levels must be in place. Initially, this means that health professional support for the acuity level of lactating patients, where the parents are delivering, ideally includes a full-time International Board Certified Lactation Consultant (IBCLC) position (Mannel, 2011; Mannel et al., 2019; Mannel & Mannel, 2006). Although the hope is that every health care provider has foundational knowledge in breastfeeding, and many perinatal nurses may be IBCLCs or have advanced lactation consultation education, without a full-time position, busy perinatal nurses get clinical assignments as staff and cannot act in their position to provide lactation support to higher-acuity patients at risk of difficulties. In addition, it is important to assess the implementation of BFHI (WHO, 2018) in maternity wards, which accommodates key behaviors that facilitate breastfeeding getting off to a good start such as rooming-in, supplementation policies, and encouragement of skin-to-skin between parent and infant. Examples of Community-Level Promotion (Step 10 of BFHI) are outlined in Chapter 6. However, a lack of community-level infrastructure for lactation management support continues to be a major barrier to EBF promotion globally. The WABA (2020) cost-savings information and effect of breastfeeding on the SDG for 2030 (UN, 2020) can influence all levels to commit to identifying key facilitators and barriers to meeting the Ten Steps of breastfeeding. Using the 4-D Pathway, described in Chapter 6, at this stage of assessment and determining the site's readiness for implementation of the Ten Steps is key. Encouraging use of toolkits and curriculum to create policies, educate the public and health care providers, and make a commitment to pursuing BFHI status will scale up services at these sites. Coalitions work well in assessing the landscape because they bring a multitude of providers together to examine where differences have the greatest potential for success. The role of champions cannot be underestimated, and much work is required to allow the networking necessary for changes to the landscape. The next step of the AIDED framework is "I" for "Innovate."

Innovate to Fit User Receptivity

In considering the cultural implications of breastfeeding and societal practices, some key areas identified to support sustainable large-scale breastfeeding promotion include these:

- Maternity leave
- Workplace legislation
- Enforcement of the WHO International Code of Marketing of Breast Milk Substitutes (UNICEF, 2005)
- Training of administrators, health professionals, and paraprofessionals
- Improvements in medical/nursing allied health professional academic curricula

Some other ways worldwide support continues is through coming together to disseminate comprehensive and locally appropriate information on breastfeeding and sharing this information with a broad audience (e.g., websites, open access articles, shared toolkits). Health care professionals need support to improve counseling related to breastfeeding. A key barrier is a lack of communication skills among health care providers and peer counselors/community workers and use of culturally appropriate information, as well as dispelling myths such as perceived insufficient milk supply (see Chapter 14) (Bazzano et al., 2015; Pérez-Escamilla et al., 2012). This text has incorporated concepts of trauma-informed care, relational practice, and forms of communication to take a strengths-based approach to parents related to infant feeding, support them in decisions that best meet the needs of their family, and encourage them when things do not go exactly as planned. Global studies on various cultures and traditions related to breastfeeding can provide important information to identify user receptivity and how best to innovate the message.

World Survey on Timing of Breastfeeding

An interesting study by Morse et al. (1990) did a world survey of the timing of breastfeeding in the postpartum period and found that out of 120 countries, 50 believed that colostrum was "dirty" or "old milk" and withheld feedings for 48 hours. Today we realize the effect this could have on the mother's milk production, the valuable stimulation of her body to make milk, and the infant's risk of dehydration. As an anthropologist, Morse was more concerned about health care providers interpreting this behavior to mean that the mother did not want to breastfeed, and therein lies the danger. It is a reminder to check with new parents about their understanding and help them begin to learn to interpret infant cues of early hunger, satiation, and normal fussiness. Physiologically, an early introduction of supplements, cereals, and solid foods may influence continued breastfeeding and affect the mother's supply. This is the danger in pacifier (or "dummy") use—if we manage the infant's physiological need to suck with a pacifier, the breast is not being stimulated to produce more milk, which the infant needs to survive.

Cultural Implications of Breastfeeding: Understanding User Receptivity

Some cultures fear inadequate milk supplies and value plump babies as healthy babies, which leads to breastfeeding and providing human milk substitutes (formula). This can be seen as reported in Central Karnataka in India (Banapurmath et al., 1996; Sreedhara & Banapurmath, 2014) and the United States with specific populations (Cartagena et al., 2014; Sloand et al., 2018). Helpful to new parents is an explanation of the "supply and demand" process of breastfeeding and how infants' control of how much they eat by feeding to satiation helps encourage healthy weight promotion and avoid obesity (see Chapter 11 for details).

In Native American populations, cultural beliefs may vary between rural and urban settings while support for breastfeeding can come from a variety of individuals, including mothers, grandmothers, sisters, and sisters-in-law (Eckhardt et al., 2014). Examining the beliefs that women hold around infant feeding can also demonstrate similarities and differences in opinion.

An example of an intervention to affect breastfeeding promotion that incorporated cultural beliefs was accomplished with positive results on a Navajo reservation. The qualitative portion of the study included interviews of 250 women who shared beliefs about the importance of breastfeeding as symbolic and holy, being handed down as the "proper way of feeding an infant," and role-modeling of sharing of food. Breastfeeding is considered to be the original symbol of earliest relationships between people, passing on maternal attributes, promoting growth and development, love and security, and self-discipline (Wright et al., 1997). With this information in hand, participants in the project created an intervention that incorporated both social marketing and community participation and included the health care system, the community, and the individual. This three-pronged approach, based on understanding the belief system of the individuals and community, and incorporating them into the process, led to behavioral change. It serves as a wonderful example of health promotion that provides evidence to support how understanding the users' receptivity and including them in the development of innovative promotion plans resulted in parents meeting their infant feeding goals to breastfeed exclusively.

Developing Support

Global Breastfeeding Promotion Efforts Support

It is evidence-based international consensus meetings and declarations that led to global infant-feeding recommendations issued by UNICEF (2005) and the WHO (2018), which in turn resulted in actionable programs like the Baby-friendly Hospital

Initiative (WHO, 2018, WHO-UNICEF, 2009) (also see Chapter 6). This included international advocacy groups (e.g., IBFAN, WABA), local advocacy groups, and coalition building with various stakeholders, including public opinion leaders. The example from Brazil of a social marketing conceptual framework to guide scaling up of national breastfeeding promotion programs suggested that:

- when the **product** (human milk) and
- **process** (breastfeeding)
- are **available** to meet a need, such as parent-child health improvement;
- and when they can be offered in an **affordable** and **accessible** way:
  - such as through the **BFHI**,
  - mother-to-mother **support groups** and
  - **peer counseling** options;
- and it is situated at **locations easily accessible** such as health facilities and community centers;
- then **scaling up** of the public health intervention "support for breastfeeding" is more likely to be **diffused** through the society and uptake of the **behavior is facilitated**. (Pérez-Escamilla et al., 2012).

Engage User Groups: Global Uptake of BFHI

We have opportunities to continue to support the progress made by international, national, and local groups around BFHI (WHO, 2018, WHO-UNICEF, 2009), and now is the time to capitalize on the momentum that COVID-19, #BlackLivesMatter, and the present global crisis has provided to us. In synchronizing efforts, we can support families and put in place structures that eliminate systemic racism and inequities so that all families have the support they need for the best start in life.

Canada

Successes in Canada include the launching of the Baby-Friendly Initiative (BFI): protecting, promoting, and supporting breastfeeding in 2012 (Pound et al., 2012) and reaffirmed in 2020. The initiative has raised awareness for BFI approaches across Canada, based on the BFHI and *Ten Steps for Successful Breastfeeding* (WHO, 2018). A call for the provision of national support and provincial and territorial ministries of health to mandate strategies for the implementation of the BFI across all health care facilities has resulted in coordinated efforts across Canada. The positive influences of national public health care goals along with community-based EBF promotion/support—such as World Breastfeeding Week events, parental leave policies, and attention to health care professionals' education so that they can provide substantial support—is becoming evident.

Specifically, in British Columbia, BC Women's Provincial Milk Bank (BC Women's Hospital + Health Centre, 2020), which has been operating continuously since 1974 and is a founding member of the Human Milk Banking Association of North America (HMBANA, 2020), held media campaigns for milk depots that led to an increase in depots and human milk collections. This means a wider distribution of human milk available for premature infants and infants who are unwell or whose parents are having issues around establishing their own milk supply. The province convened a "Breastfeeding Think Tank" in 2015 and has appointed a provincial Breastfeeding Coordinator who leads the BC Baby-Friendly Network (2020) with representatives from across the province to coordinate efforts, policy making, and education. Two of the challenges are public health support for lactation consultant care and availability of specialists when parents need assistance. Another stronghold in the province to support breastfeeding is the British Columbia Lactation Consultants Association (BCLCA, 2020). Recognizing the gaps to breastfeeding support made more evident than ever by the COVID-19 pandemic crisis, the BCLCA started a petition and created a position paper (BCLCA, 2020) to share with the Ministry of Health. Do other countries struggle with implementing BFHI/**Neo-BFHI**? Let us examine a few other countries' stories, knowing that there are far more than could be included in this text.

India, Vietnam, and China: Comparative Study of WHO Code Compliance

One of the key factors to promoting EBF is in regulating the marketing of human milk substitutes (formula), referred to in the early documentation as 'breast-milk' substitutes (WHO, 1981). A study compared the relationships between code enforcement, legislation, and infant formula (human milk substitutes) sales with EBF in India, Vietnam, and China (Robinson et al., 2019). Findings indicated that "implementation of the Code is a necessary but insufficient step alone to improve breastfeeding outcomes (Robinson et al., 2019, p. 1). The results supported the need for maternity leave, BFHI, and available counseling for improvement of breastfeeding behaviors. A key finding is the need to transition from donor-led breastfeeding programs to large-scale government-owned programs.

Student Reflection

1. *Review the cost-analysis presented by Rollins et al. (2016) or presented on the WABA (2020) website. Calculate the cost per infant born annually to provide point-of-care prenatal education, at delivery support, and follow-up postpartum visits, considering a variety of health professionals and pregnancy care packages in most countries. Is it worth the investment? (Extra credit: Calculate what formula companies spend on marketing human milk substitutes (formula) per infant born annually.)*
2. *How are some of the key targets for BFHI/Neo-BFHI interventions derived from behavioral theories. Where do they fit on the Health Impact Pyramid?*

Global Implementation of Neo-BFHI

Setting the Stage for the Case Study

Up to this point in this text, it may appear our focus has been on providing a general overview of breastfeeding support for full-term infants healthy deliveries. In reality, our most vulnerable infants—those born prematurely, small-for-gestational-age, or substance dependent—demonstrate the most dramatic health benefits from human milk, skin-to-skin contact, and following the Ten Steps to successful breastfeeding (Bharwani et al., 2016; Blomqvist, et al., 2013; Conde-Agudelo & Díaz-Rossello, 2016; MacMillan et al., 2018; Quigley & McGuire, 2014). The case study provided next describes a research project led by Dr. Carmen Scochi at the University of São Paulo, Ribeirão Preto, Brazil, and generously funded by a Bill and Melinda Gates Foundation grant to examine the introduction of the Neo-BFHI program in the neonatal intensive care units (NICUs) of 5 of 10 research locations in Brazil (5 experimental/5 control). This study involved experts from the Nordic and Quebec Neo-BFHI Working Groups, expert research teams in five locations in Brazil, and experts from the University of British Columbia in Vancouver, BC, Canada. Using the Neo-BFHI core principles (Hedberg-Nyqvist et al., 2015), the team worked closely with the five experimental sites to identify barriers and facilitators for the implementation and knowledge translation in each context and reviewed policies, practices, and educational support for staff and research teams. Brazil has one of the highest premature infant birth rates in the world, which prompted the funding from the Gates Foundation to carry out this research (de Oliveira et al., 2016). The research team visited all five locations over a five-week period and provided support to the teams at each site with a review of implementation steps, understanding the context of the site, and providing support at the point of care (Scochi et al., 2014–2016).

Findings from the Neo-BFHI Study in Brazil

Brazilian health professionals in the neonatal units perceived the following barriers to Neo-BFHI implementation:

- Limited infrastructure to support 24-hour parental presence, overcrowded units, and insufficient staff
- Lack of protocols
- Lack of education for clinical staff on preterm breastfeeding and resistance to change
- Inadequate interdisciplinary communication
- Cultural and socioeconomical challenges of families (i.e., social determinants of health)

In contrast, the perceived facilitators identified in the five Neo-BFHI sites included the following:

- BFHI implemented at all sites
- National law permitting parental access to infants (24/7)
- Multidisciplinary teams to assist with families' needs
- Training in BFHI policies
- Support of human milk bank staff (Sochi et al., 2014; Souza et al., n.d.).

Another study in Brazil showed some changes in the hospital on breastfeeding and EBF rates; however, no changes in duration of breastfeeding over 6 months were identified, suggesting the need for health sector and community support to be enhanced (Coutinho et al., 2005). Another country that showed the effects of incorporating the Neo-BFHI to be easier in hospitals with BFHI accreditation was Spain, similar to the Brazilian results reported above (Alonso-Diaz et al., 2016).

Canada

Canada identified the following barriers and facilitators in expanding BFHI in the NICU:

- Barriers included infant health status, parent/infant separation, workloads/patterns of staff, gaps in staff knowledge/skills, and lack of continuity in breastfeeding support.
- Facilitators included breastfeeding education and champions, as well as interprofessional collaboration. BFHI was recognized as a facilitator of family-centered care, and recommendations included promoting it as such, developing champions in the NICU, and increasing access to lactation consultants for parents and staff (Benoit & Semenic, 2014).

Australia

A study examining staff experiences of implementing the Neo-BFHI in Australia in four metropolitan maternity hospitals included focus groups of 47 nursing and midwifery staff, as well as a pediatrician, to identify their perceptions of the process. Although staff held a positive attitude that BFHI could be achieved, they found differences in the four NICUs, that mothers and infants lived in very separate worlds given the NICU environment, and that implementing the BFHI involved a lot of hard work. Some barriers were similar to what we have seen in other countries: lack of resources, wanting a quick fix and not really understanding how the BFHI translated to the NICU, and staff shortages and workloads challenging the staff's ability to bring mothers and infants together. Conclusions were that motivated staff with educational support and clearly identified guidelines were essential to support implementation of the BFHI in NICUs (Taylor et al., 2011). A recurring theme for Neo-BFHI implementation is that high staff workloads act as a barrier to promoting breastfeeding, which matches the findings of a meta-analysis by Renfrew and others (2009).

Changing the culture of the NICU, providing 24-hour rooming-in for parents, unlimited skin-to-skin contact when possible, and parental involvement have comprised a foundational concept for implementation of Neo-BFHI. This is perhaps why it is more successful in Nordic countries (Bloomqvist et al., 2013; Hedberg-Nyqvist et al., 2015; Hedberg-Nyqvist et al., 2019). A NICU in the United Kingdom found that parents benefited when the culture and philosophy of the NICU changed by applying BFI standards and making parents partners in care (Read & Rattenbury, 2018). Seeing parents as partners may be a radical perspective for health care providers in the NICU, but implementation of Neo-BFHI relies on it for the health of parents, infants, and families.

Other Countries' Experience Implementing BFHI

Change within health systems is challenging. Research demonstrates that it takes approximately 17 years for evidence-based-practice (EBP) to reach the bedside (Morris et al., 2011). Countries throughout the world experience facilitators and barriers to implementation of BFHI/Neo-BFHI.

Austria found that a complex interplay of factors is required to become a Baby-friendly hospital, especially during implementation. In hospitals seeking BFHI-certification, distinct and intensive investments in planning and preparation before putting the steps into practice worked well. Best outcomes occurred when staff, mothers, and families were provided the extensive information they required and families also benefited from continuous participation of health professionals. Other approaches allowed room for debate, not attempting to implement all the steps at once, and staggering step implementation according to the context. Adjusting activities or expanding them during the operation of the BFHI certification led to more sustainable implementation (Wieczorek et al., 2015).

Spain identified barriers and challenges to implementation of BFHI through a national survey and developed a new national strategy to promote BFHI with promising results. In the development of the strategy, those involved acknowledged key areas of focus. Initially, health professionals' fear of change and the need to counteract noncompliance with the WHO Code was identified and strategies were developed. Perhaps most important, they recognized the strength present in generous volunteers whose enthusiasm empowered increasing numbers of mothers to recognize their right to attain their breastfeeding goals (Alonso-Diaz et al., 2016; Flores-Antón et al., 2012; Hernández-Aguilar et al., 2014). From there they were able to put steps in place for advancing EBF nationally. The last stage of the AIDED Framework involves decentralizing and transferring the efforts for BFHI implementation.

Devolve the Efforts: Local Support Systems that Work

Similar to the benefits of breastfeeding for premature infants, infants born to families lacking basic social determinants of health, have been found to show minimal discrepancies in growth and ability when breastfed. This is why the U.S. Department of Agriculture (USDA) incorporated the Loving Support Makes Breastfeeding Work campaign, a social marketing program, into the Supplemental Nutrition Program for Women, Infants, and Children (WIC), a program that supports families at the lower end of the income scale. They began by analyzing WIC participants' reasons for not pursuing breastfeeding. Some of the key motivations included embarrassment, work and/or school making it difficult, negative perceptions of breastfeeding, and the fact that they had used a human milk substitute (formula) with a previous child. Those who began breastfeeding disclosed that reasons for using human milk substitutes included work and/or school, perceptions of insufficient milk, sense that the baby did not like the breast, or the infant's condition (e.g., jaundice, low weight gain) (Pérez-Escamilla, 2012). Some of the lessons learned from the WIC campaign include the importance of messaging which targets the societal influences that affect women's decisions. As mentioned throughout this text, those can include family and friends, employers, health care professionals, policy makers, legislators, and human milk substitute (formula) industries. With increasing effects and outreach of social media to new parents, health care professionals need to be vigilant in providing parents with accurate information (Pérez-Escamilla, 2012).

Setting the Stage for Case Study

A major social marketing campaign success was the USDA's Loving Support Makes Breastfeeding Work campaign, of which I was a part in 1997. The United States was spending billions of dollars on human milk substitutes (formula) for WIC. Those working in these programs and at state departments of health realized that women in the WIC program wanted to breastfeed (over 50% at the time), yet there was no support in place at WIC clinics for breastfeeding. Over the past 30 years, the initiation and duration rates of breastfeeding in the WIC population have markedly improved, and the resultant peer counselor program has become a great success as well. One of the key enablers was drawing on women's support for one another, as was identifying the WIC site as the accessible location where change could take place (Chapman et al., 2004; Gill et al., 2004; Lindenberger & Bryant, 2000).

Case Study

In the mid 1990s, as a La Leche League leader, I was approached by a visionary nutritionist who asked me if I might lead a monthly support group at our local WIC center on the day when women came in for their check-ins. This was the beginning of a long relationship for me with WIC in Connecticut and then nationally. Collaboration over time led to positive outcomes, including state funding for WIC staff scaling up. As a consultant, I visited all 19 sites to work with staff contextually on incorporating some of the BFHI at their locations, assessing knowledge, practices, and brainstorming around barriers and facilitators. With input from Connecticut State Department of Health administrators and WIC leaders, I led twice-yearly workshops and provided on-site presentations with the full complement of staff from the 19 sites attending as part of their paid work time. This had an effect in all locations for more baby-friendly practices (e.g., comfortable and private rooms to nurse or pump in; posters of breastfeeding women; removal of all human milk substitute advertising [formula for distribution hidden away]), and it built confidence in the staff of their capability to support parents in their infant-feeding decision making, especially when they decided to breastfeed. A state coalition, the Connecticut Breastfeeding Coalition (described in Chapter 6) and the work of that group led to BFHI scaling up in the state. This work was made possible by support from the Connecticut State Department of Public Health and federal grant funding, yet the leaders, volunteers, and WIC staff are to be congratulated for their vision and perseverance. A national peer counselor program was created with success that can be modeled across other areas (Bronner et al., 2001; Chapman et al., 2005, 2010).

Case Study Questions

1. Identify how a health system, community, and individual intervention approach to health promotion might work in your local area to promote, support, and protect breastfeeding.
2. Who are some of the key stakeholders you would want to involve?
3. What are the first steps to rolling it out?
4. What types of social marketing would you use to launch your intervention/program?

Summary

This chapter has focused on international key strategies that have been incorporated in many countries to advance implementation of BFHI (WHO, 2018) and Neo-BFHI (Hedberg-Nyqvist et al., 2015). Ensuring continuity of care for new parents to support breastfeeding can be achieved through professionally mediated sessions and/or through peer support programs and was identified to be of paramount importance. In order for continuity of care to occur, education and training in BFHI policies and foundational lactation knowledge are necessary for all health care providers in the health system and the community. Another effective strategy is providing interactive group education during the prenatal phase, as well as establishing practice and referral opportunities for all health professionals. Evidence-based ongoing support of breastfeeding is necessary, and it is best at the point of care. Although this text focuses a lot on in-hospital care, it is important for other clinics serving families to host a variety of healthcare providers who have the skills to assist new parents with breastfeeding. As described in Chapter 7, supportive birthing practices have been found in BFHI facilities, which will in turn filter down to facilities in their support of breastfeeding overall. Paramount options that have not been discussed but deserve mention are providing teleconferencing options for families in rural or isolated communities and remembering to include pharmacists in lactation education.

It is interesting to note similarities and differences internationally between specific cultural beliefs about colostrum (the early human milk), breastfeeding, and barriers and facilitators to parents feeling supported in their decision making and journey. We hope this chapter has helped you to focus on some of the approaches to care rather than interventions. When it comes to cultural differences, it is best to ask parents rather than assume their beliefs and preferences. Open-ended questions about parents' thoughts and goals surrounding infant feeding, finding out what they know and what they have heard, will open up communication to allow for sharing of information about the benefits of breastfeeding in a broad sense. Peer support is helpful, and health professionals' use of explanations about infants' needs and capabilities will be better received when providing rationale for EBF and avoiding early supplementation and solid foods.

The lack of detailed information provided to parents that is consistent and specific is a problem. Health professionals stating "exclusive breastfeeding for six months," without understanding parents' attitudes, beliefs, and goals for infant feeding, is not sufficient to support parents. This is why guidelines like those provided in the Ten Steps and the BFHI (WHO, 2018) are so valuable, as they allow consistent information to be delivered in easily understandable terms. Overall, parents will appreciate feeling heard and understood, having their questions answered, and receiving evidence-based information so they can safely provide for their infants. Some of that basic information includes infant latch, milk production, feeding frequency, risk of use of human milk substitutes, and appropriate timing and use of supplements. Health professionals can promote, protect, and support breastfeeding in their communities by continued involvement in and support of local coalitions and social marketing campaigns. Being aware of global perspectives of barriers and facilitators to implementation provides insight that may be useful in your context, and it enhances our ability to scale up breastfeeding promotion programs worldwide.

Key Points to Remember

1. The strength of the impact of WABA (2020) and BFHI (WHO, 2018) in coordinating global efforts to protect, promote, and support breastfeeding lies in their consideration of the political will/support and in the recognition of other key factors.
2. Parental care practices and/or support for breastfeeding in the workplace are key components to support parents' decision making and ability to meet their infant-feeding goals.
3. Peer support is important in educating mothers about breastfeeding in a culturally sensitive and relevant manner and provides support in navigating the breastfeeding journey.
4. Healthcare professional support is dependent on parents' attitudes, beliefs, and education related to lactation as health promotion.
5. Media and social marketing can be important tools for or barriers to the protection, promotion, and support of breastfeeding.
6. Breastfeeding is a relationship between a parent and infant/child—it goes beyond the production of human milk as a product. Benefits for both parental, infant, and child health include a bond and connection that is formed when a parent is more in tune with the infant, starting with the ability to recognize the infant's feeding cues.

References

Alonso-Diaz, C., Utrera-Torres, I., de Alba-Romero, C., Flores-Anton, B., Lora-Pablos, D., & Pallas-Alonso, C. R. (2016). Breastfeeding support in Spanish neonatal intensive care units and the Baby-friendly Hospital Initiative. *Journal of Human Lactation*, 32(4), 613–626. https://doi .org/10.1177/0890334416658246

Banapurmath, C. R., Nagaraj, M. C., Banapurmath, S., & Kesaree, N. (1996). Breastfeeding practices in villages of Central Karnataka. *Indian Pediatrics*, 33, 477–479.

Bazzano, A. N., Oberhelman, R. A., Potts, K. S., Taub, L. D., & Var, C. (2015). What health service support do families need for optimal breastfeeding? An in-depth exploration of young infant feeding practices in Cambodia. *International Journal of Women's Health*, 7, 249–257. https://doi .org/10.2147/IJWH.S76343

BC Baby-Friendly Network. (2020). *About us*. http://bcbabyfriendly.ca/about

BC Women's Hospital + Health Centre. (2020). *BC Women's Provincial Milk Bank*. http://www .bcwomens.ca/our-services/labour-birth-post-birth-care/milk-bank

Benoit, B., & Semenic, S. (2014). Barriers and facilitators to implementing the Baby-friendly Hospital Initiative in neonatal intensive care units. *JOGNN: Journal of Obstetric, Gynecologic & Neonatal Nursing*, 43(5), 614–624. https://doi.org/10.1111/1552-6909.12479

Bharwani, S. K., Green, B. F., Pezzullo, J. C., Bharwani, S. S., Bharwani, S. S., & Dhanireddy, R. (2016). Systematic review and meta-analysis of human milk intake and retinopathy of prematurity: A significant update. *Journal of Perinatology*, 36(11), 913–920. https://doi.org/10.1038/jp .2016.98

Blomqvist, Y. T., Frölund, L., Rubertsson, C., & Hedberg-Nyqvist, K. (2013). Provision of Kangaroo Mother Care: Supportive factors and barriers perceived by parents. *Scandinavian Journal of Caring Sciences*, 27(2), 345–353. https://doi.org/10.1111/j.1471-6712.2012.01040.x

British Columbia Lactation Consultants Association. (2020, April 15). Breastfeeding and COVID-19: Time to patch the safety net. https://bclca.wildapricot.org/resources/Documents /BCLCA_COVID_statement_April_15.pdf

Bronner, Y. N., Barber, T., Vogelhut, J., & Resnik, A. K. (2001). Breastfeeding peer counseling: Results from the national WIC survey. *Journal of Human Lactation*, 17(2), 119. https://doi.org /10.1177/089033440101700205

Cartagena, D. C., Ameringer, S. W., McGrath, J., Jallo, N., Masho, S. W., & Myers, B. J. (2014). Factors contributing to infant overfeeding with Hispanic mothers. *JOGNN: Journal of Obstetric, Gynecologic & Neonatal Nursing, 43*(2), 139–159. https://doi.org/10.1111/1552-6909.12279

Chapman, D. J., Damio, G., & Pérez-Escamilla, R. (2004). Differential response to breastfeeding peer counseling within a low-income, predominantly Latina population. *Journal of Human Lactation, 20*(4), 389–396. https://doi.org/10.1177/0890334404269845

Chapman, D. J., Morel, K., Anderson, A. K., Damio, G., & Pérez-Escamilla, R. (2010). Review: Breastfeeding peer counseling: From efficacy through scale-up. *Journal of Human Lactation, 26*(3), 314–326. https://doi.org/10.1177/0890334410369481

Conde-Agudelo, A., & Díaz-Rossello, J. L. (2016). Kangaroo mother care to reduce morbidity and mortality in low birthweight infants. *Cochrane Database of Systematic Reviews,* (8). https:doi .org/10.1002/14651858.CD002771.pub4

Coutinho, S. B., Lima, M. d. C., Ashworth, A., & Lira, P. I. C. (2005). The impact of training based on the Baby-friendly Hospital Initiative on breastfeeding practices in the Northeast of Brazil. *Journal of Pediatrics, 81*(6), 471–477. https://www.scielo.br/pdf/jped/v81n6/en_v81n6a11.pdf

de Oliveira, R. R., Melo, E. C., Fujimori, E., & Mathias, T. A. d. F. (2016). The inner state differences of preterm birth rates in Brazil: A time series study. *BMC Public Health, 16*, 411. https://doi .org/10.1186/s12889-016-3087-9

Eckhardt, C. L., Lutz, T., Karanja, N., Jobe, J. B., Maupomé, G., & Ritenbaugh, C. (2014). Knowledge, attitudes, and beliefs that can influence infant feeding practices in American Indian mothers. *Journal of the Academy of Nutrition and Dietetics, 114*(10), 1587–1593. https://doi .org/10.1016/j.jand.2014.04.021

Family Larsson-Rosenquist Foundation. (2020). *Projects. Becoming breastfeeding friendly: A guide to global scale-up.* https://www.larsson-rosenquist.org/en/activities/projects/becoming -breastfeeding-friendly

Flores-Antón, B., Temboury-Molina, M. C., Ares-Segura, S., Arana-Cañedo-Argüelles, C., Nicolás-Bueno, C., Navarro-Royo, C., Pardo-Hernández, A., & Pallás-Alonso, C. R. (2012). Breastfeeding promotion plan in Madrid, Spain. *Journal of Human Lactation, 28*(3), 363–369. https://doi.org/10.1177/0890334412449516

Frieden, T. R. (2010). A framework for public health action: The Health Impact Pyramid. *American Journal of Public Health, 100*(4), 590–595. https://doi.org/10.2105/AJPH.2009.185652

Gill, S. L., Reifsnider, E., Mann, A. R., Villarreal, P., & Tinkle, M. B. (2004). Assessing infant breastfeeding beliefs among low-income Mexican Americans. *Journal of Perinatal Education, 13*(3), 39–50. http://www.ncbi.nlm.nih.gov/pmc/articles/PMC1595211/pdf/JPE130039.pdf

Global Breastfeeding Collective. (2017). *Nurturing the health and wealth of nations: The investment case for breastfeeding.* United Nation Children's Fund & World Health Organization. https:// www.who.int/nutrition/publications/infantfeeding/global-bf-collective-investmentcase/en/

Hernández-Aguilar, M. T., Lasarte-Velillas, J. J., Martín-Calama, J., Flores-Antón, B., Borja-Herrero, C., García-Franco, M., Navas-Lucen, V., & Pallás-Alonso, C. (2014). The Baby-Friendly Initiative in Spain: A challenging pathway. *Journal of Human Lactation, 30*(3), 276–282. https://doi .org/10.1177/0890334414531453

Hedberg-Nyqvist, K., Campbell, S. H., & Haiek, L. H. (2019). Breastfeeding a preterm infant. In S. H. Campbell, J. Lauwers., R. Mannel, & R. Spencer (Eds.), *Core curriculum for interdisciplinary lactation care* (pp. 215–236). Jones & Bartlett.

Hedberg-Nyqvist, K., Maastrup, R., Hansen, M. N., Haggkvist, A. P., Hannula, L., Ezeonodo, A., Kylberg, E., Frandsen, A. I., & Haiek, L. N. (2015). *The Neo-BFHI: The Baby-friendly Hospital Initiative for Neonatal Wards.* http://www.ilca.org/main/learning/resources/neo-bfhi

Human Milk Banking Association of North America (HMBANA). (2020). *About.* https://www .hmbana.org/about-us/overview.html

Lindenberger, J. H., & Bryant, C. A. (2000). Promoting breastfeeding in the WIC program: A social marketing case study. *American Journal of Health Behavior, 24*(1), 53–60. https://doi .org/10.5993/AJHB.24.1.8

MacMillan, K. L., Rendon, C. P., Verma, K., Riblet, N., Washer, D. B., & Volpe Holmes, A. (2018). Association of rooming-in with outcomes for neonatal abstinence syndrome: A systematic review and meta-analysis. *JAMA Pediatrics, 172*(4), 345-351. https://doi.org/10.1001 /jamapediatrics.2017.5195

Mannel, R. (2011). Defining lactation acuity to improve patient safety and outcomes. *Journal of Human Lactation, 27*(2), 163–170. https://doi.org/10.1177/0890334410397198

Mannel, R., Campbell, S. H., & Stehel, E. K. (2019). Interdisciplinary lactation services. In J. L. S. H. Campbell, R. Mannel, & R. Spencer (Eds.), *Core curriculum for interdisciplinary lactation care* (pp. 505–518). Jones & Bartlett.

Mannel, R., & Mannel, R. S. (2006). Staffing for hospital lactation programs: Recommendations from a tertiary care teaching hospital. *Journal of Human Lactation, 22*(4), 409–417. https://doi.org/10.1177/0890334406294166

Morris, Z. S., Wooding, S., & Grant, J. (2011). The answer is 17 years, what is the question: Understanding time lags in translational research. *Journal of the Royal Society of Medicine, 104*(12), 510–520. https://doi.org/10.1258/jrsm.2011.110180

Morse, J. M., Jehle, C., & Gamble, D. (1990). Initiating breastfeeding: A world survey of the timing of postpartum breastfeeding. *International Journal of Nursing Studies, 27*(3), 303–313. https://doi.org/10.1016/0020-7489(90)90045-k

Pérez-Escamilla, R. (2012). Breastfeeding social marketing: Lessons learned from USDA's "Loving Support" campaign. *Breastfeeding Medicine, 7*(5), 358–363. https://doi.org/10.1089/bfm.2012.0063

Pérez-Escamilla, R., Curry, L., Minhas, D., Taylor, L., & Bradley, E. (2012). Scaling up of breastfeeding promotion programs in low- and middle-income countries: The "Breastfeeding Gear" model. *Advances in Nutrition, 3*(6), 790–800. doi:10.3945/an.112.002873

Pound, C. M., Unger, S. L., & Canadian Paediatric Society, Nutrition and Gastroenterology Committee, Hospital Paediatrics Section. (2012). The Baby-Friendly Initiative: Protecting, promoting, and supporting breastfeeding. *Paediatric and Children's Health, 17*(6), 317–321. https://pubmed.ncbi.nlm.nih.gov/23730170/ ; PMCID: PMC3380749

Quigley, M., & McGuire, W. (2014). Formula versus donor breast milk for feeding preterm or low birth weight infants. *Cochrane Database of Systematic Reviews,* (4). https://doi.org/10.1002/14651858.CD002971.pub3

Rea, M. F. (2003). A review of breastfeeding in Brazil and how the country has reached ten months' breastfeeding duration. *Cad Saude Publica, 19 Suppl 1*, S37–S45. https://doi.org/10.1590/s0102-311x2003000700005

Read, K., & Rattenbury, L. (2018). Parents as partners in care: Lessons from the Baby Friendly Initiative in Exeter. *Journal of Neonatal Nursing, 24*(1), 17–20. https://doi.org/10.1016/j.jnn.2017.11.006

Renfrew, M., Craig, D., Dyson, L., McCormick, F., Rice, S., King, S., Misso, K., Stenhouse, E., & Williams, A. (2009). Breastfeeding promotion for infants in neonatal units: A systematic review and economic analysis. *Health Technology Assessment, 13*(40), 1–170. https://doi.org/10.3310/hta13400

Robinson, H., Buccini, G., Curry, L., & Pérez-Escamilla, R. (2019). The World Health Organization Code and exclusive breastfeeding in China, India, and Vietnam. *Maternal & Child Nutrition, 15*(1), e12685-n/a. https://doi.org/10.1111/mcn.12685

Rollins, N. C., Bhandari, N., Hajeebhoy, N., Horton, S., Lutter, C. K., Martines, J. C., Piwoz, E. G., Richter, L. M., & Victora, C. G. (2016). Why invest, and what it will take to improve breastfeeding practices? *The Lancet, 387*(10017), 491–504. https://doi.org/10.1016/S0140-6736(15)01044-2

Scochi, C. G. S., Castral, T., Rossetto, E., Gorete Vasconcelos, M., Eunice Dantas, M., Leite, A., Fonseca, L., Hedberg-Nyqvist, K., Haiek, L. N., Warnock, F., Campbell, S. H., & Seminic, S. (2014). *Breastfeeding of preterm infants: Impact of the neo-BFHI on neonatal units.* Bill & Melinda Gates Foundation Grant. (January 2014–December 2016).

Sloand, E., Lowe, V., Pennington, A., & Rose, L. (2018). Breastfeeding practices and opinions of Latina mothers in an urban pediatric office: A focus group study. *Journal of Pediatric Health Care, 32*(3), 236–244. https://doi.org/10.1016/j.pedhc.2017.11.001

Souza, S., Nascimdento, M. H. M., Castral, T. C., Hedberg-Nyqvist, K., Campbell, S. H., Scochi, C. G. S., Warnock, F., & Haiek, L. N. Health care providers perceived barriers and facilitators to implementing baby-friendly practices in neonatal practices in Brazil. Unpublished paper.

Sreedhara, M. S., & Banapurmath, C. R. (2014). A study of nutritional status of infants in relation to their complementary feeding practices. *Current Pediatric Research, 18*(1), 39–41.

Taylor, C., Gribble, K., Sheehan, A., Schmied, V., & Dykes, F. (2011). Staff perceptions and experiences of implementing the Baby Friendly Initiative in neonatal intensive care units in Australia. *JOGNN: Journal of Obstetric, Gynecologic & Neonatal Nursing, 40*(1), 25–34. https://doi.org/10.1111/j.1552-6909.2010.01204.x

UNICEF. (2005). *Innocenti Declaration 2005 on Infant and Young Child Feeding.* https://www.unicef-irc.org/publications/435

United Nations. (2020). *About the Sustainable Development Goals.* https://www.un.org/sustainabledevelopment/sustainable-development-goals/

World Alliance for Breastfeeding Action (WABA). (2020). *Home page.* https://waba.org.my

World Health Organization (WHO). (1981). *International Code of Marketing of Breast-Milk Substitutes.* https://www.who.int/nutrition/publications/infantfeeding/9789241594295/en/

World Health Organization (WHO). (2017). Global breastfeeding scorecard: Tracking progress for breastfeeding policies and programmes. *Breastfeeding.* https://www.who.int/nutrition/publications/infantfeeding/global-bf-scorecard-2017.pdf?ua=1

World Health Organization (WHO). (2018). Baby-friendly Hospital Initiative. *Nutrition.* http://www.who.int/nutrition/topics/bfhi/en

World Health Organization-United Nations International Children's Emergency Fund (WHO-UNICEF). (2009). *Baby-friendly Hospital Initiative: Revised, updated and expanded for integrated care.* http://www.who.int/nutrition/publications/infantfeeding/bfhi_trainingcourse/en/

Wieczorek, C. C., Schmied, H., Dorner, T. E., & Dür, W. (2015). The bumpy road to implementing the Baby-friendly Hospital Initiative in Austria: A qualitative study. *International Breastfeeding Journal, 10*(1), 3. https://doi.org/10.1186/s13006-015-0030-0

Wright, A. L., Naylor, A., Wester, R., Bauer, M., & Sutcliffe, E. (1997). Using cultural knowledge in health promotion: Breastfeeding among the Navajo. *Health Education & Behavior, 24*(5), 625–639. https://doi.org/10.1177/109019819702400509

CHAPTER 10

Equitable Lactation Health Promotion

Suzanne Hetzel Campbell, PhD, RN, IBCLC, CCSNE

"In winter, when the green earth lies resting beneath a blanket of snow, this is the time for storytelling. The storytellers begin by calling upon those who came before who passed the stories down to us, for we are only messengers."

— **Robin Wall Kimmerer**, *Braiding Sweetgrass: Indigenous Wisdom, Scientific Knowledge, and Teachings of Plants*

"Breastfeeding is not explicitly mentioned in the Sustainable Development Goals, but our Series (Lancet 2016) shows that improvements in breastfeeding would help achieve the targets for health, food security, education, equity, development, and the environment. Without commitment and active investment by governments, donors, and civil society, the promotion, protection, and support for breastfeeding will remain inadequate and the outcome will be major losses and costs that will be borne by generations to come."

— **Rollins et al.**, 2016, p. 50

LEARNING OBJECTIVES

1. Situate breastfeeding within a global perspective of health promotion.
2. Differentiate conceptual frameworks for health promotion of breastfeeding as related to equity and social determinants of health (SDOH).
3. Outline barriers and innovative strategies as potential opportunities for the support and promotion of breastfeeding and parents meeting their infant-feeding goals.
4. Reinforce the role of the interdisciplinary team for supporting and promoting breastfeeding through alignment of health equity system improvement.

KEY WORDS

- **Advocacy for Health Inequity:** "A deliberate attempt to influence decision makers and other stakeholders to support or implement policies that contribute to improving health equity using evidence" (Farrer et al., 2015, p. 396).
- **Allyship:** "[A]n active, consistent, and ongoing practice of unlearning and re-evaluating, in which a person in a position of privilege and power seeks to operate in solidarity with a targeted group. Practicing Allyship is not linear or constant and requires ongoing self-reflection and learning" (Anti-Oppression Network, n.d.).
- **Colonialism:** A controlling or governing influence of a nation acquiring full or partial political control of a dependent country, territory, or people, occupying it with settlers, and exploiting it economically.
- **Discrimination:** A prejudicial or unjust treatment of individuals based on a specific characterization, such as race, age, or sex.
- **Health Equality:** A state of being equal, in status and opportunities, with an aim to ensure that everyone gets fair and just access to enjoy full, healthy lives. Does not take into consideration privileges and rights afforded given one's race, gender, or social standing and that everyone does not start from the same place (EQUIP Health Care, 2017).
- **Health Equity:** Being fair and impartial takes into consideration that not everyone has similar privileges and contexts, so focuses on ensuring and treating those requiring care to have access to *what they need* to enjoy full, healthy lives. It aims to remove differences that may be unjust or unnecessary so resources or social institutions and policies can accommodate the needs of those requiring care (EQUIP Health Care, 2017).
- **Indigenous:** Native to or originating from a particular region or place.
- **Intersectionality:** A theoretical framework which posits that multiple social categories (e.g., race, ethnicity, gender, sexual orientation, socioeconomic status) intersect at the micro level of individual experience to reflect multiple interlocking systems of privilege and oppression at the macro, social–structural level (e.g., racism, sexism, heterosexism) (Bowleg, 2012).
- **Racism:** Discrimination, prejudice, or antagonism directed against a person or people based on their membership in a particular ethnic or racial group, typically a minority or marginalized group.
- **Settlers:** Persons who move with a group of others to live in a new area, country. May be co-conspirators with the powerful colonizing group, or consider themselves a visitor to the area or in allyship with the indigenous peoples inhabiting the new area.
- **Shared Decision Making:** A key component of patient-centered care that represents a collaborative process in which clinicians and patients work together to make decisions about health care, balancing risks and expected outcomes and considering patients' preferences and values (National Learning Consortium, 2013).
- **Social Determinants of Health (SDOH):** Effects of gender, poverty, trauma, race, status (immigrant, refugee), sexual orientation, and health literacy on one's ability to attain health and general well-being.
- **Social Justice:** Justice in terms of wealth, opportunities, and privileges in a society may represent the political–philosophical concept centered on equality among people along various social dimensions.
- **Stigma:** A mark of disgrace associated with a specific quality, circumstance, or person.

- **Systemic Racism:** Racism resulting from the inherent biases and prejudices of policies and practices of social and political organizations, groups, or institutions (The Free Dictionary, 2015); systemic racist practices (e.g., residential schools, continued influence today).
- **Trauma-Violence-Informed Care:** Takes into consideration the need for a complete picture of a patient's life situation, past and present, to provide effective care and healing; practices that promote a culture of safety, empowerment, and healing. Care is tailored to address interrelated forms of violence.

Overview

This chapter focuses on lactation within the context of equity and equitable health care, as statistics demonstrate that racial disparities persist in having an effect on breastfeeding rates, and race, history, class, and culture affect breastfeeding initiation, exclusivity, and duration. The author of this chapter identifies key concepts and areas of research but recognizes that, as an older, white, privileged, and educated female living in North America, capturing the voice of those who suffer from **systemic racism**. I oppose **racism** and hate through **allyship**, continuous unlearning, learning, and listening. Because pregnancy, birth, and lactation are for the most part a gendered experience, the voices of women throughout the ages have often been quieted and ignored. In this chapter, I provide tools for continued learning and unlearning and ask you to bring an open mind and broader vision of truth, health, and well-being to benefit our parent–infant dyads and families worldwide. I also ask for a level of cultural humility in which you take the opportunity to observe your own implicit biases and recognize our continued need for vigilance as health care providers committed to continuous lifelong learning and reflection.

Throughout the chapters in the first two sections of this text, the goal is to set a foundation for lactation as a strategy for health promotion. Global, national, and local initiatives have been examined as examples of health promotion theory in action, and the role of health care professionals has been identified. Chapters 1 and 2 outlined some of the key foundational theories and models addressing Collaboratives for Equity and Justice (Wolfe, 2020). The goal of this chapter is to summarize the role that inequities and **social determinants of health (SDOH)** play in parents' success with breastfeeding by examining the research in this area and knowledge-translation projects that have promoted access, equity, and **social justice** for all parents. Much work has yet to be done in this area, including more rigorous application of theory and research methods to identify outcomes, as well as support beyond private donors and volunteers.

We have situated breastfeeding as a "health promotion behavior" and asserted that public health issues surrounding breastfeeding go beyond the control of the individual and require a social, political, and community support system. Given the COVID-19 pandemic and global protests surrounding issues of racism that occurred within the midst of writing this text in early 2020, this chapter is supported by global evidence of the effects of these factors on breastfeeding families in the context of inequities. Although the health outcome costs have been identified in this text thus far (Rollins et al., 2016; Victora et al., 2016), the cost to the planet, and breastfeeding as an environmental imperative in the context of inequities cannot be disregarded (Joffe et al., 2019). The last five chapters of this text provide examples in specific areas, including populations that face issues of equity and injustice.

Author's Background

My own experience in supporting parents began in nursing school when I was drawn to maternal–child health and then lactation. I attended a La Leche League conference as a nursing student and was struck by how "natural" it all felt—I was surrounded by families with infants and other children. It actually took years to unlearn some of the patriarchal, post-colonial, hierarchical thought processes that baccalaureate nursing education and work in a tertiary-level academic-center obstetric unit had "taught" me along the way in the early 1980s. Through my own experience, having my first child 5 years after beginning to practice as a maternity nurse, and working with thousands of families since, I realized that parenthood and the transition to become a parent are fraught with a multitude of complexities. I found when working with parents that I needed to take into consideration the experience of their past history: everything that they have observed and seen (cultural factors that surround us all), constructs and definitions of family, community, society—the heritage of where they come from and how they were raised all have an impact. In addition, one's relationship with parents, siblings, and other family members all have an effect on who we become as parents.

Lactation is complicated by historical, industrialized, and socio-demographic components, including gender (breastfeeding as a female-dominated undertaking), race, a post-colonial era, and the pressures from a multibillion-dollar human milk substitutes (formula) marketing campaign that feeds on new parents' insecurities and their desire to be the best parents they can. A fundamental parental goal is to provide food to our children. Becoming a La Leche League leader, a WIC consultant, and working on a national peer counselor curriculum helped me to learn and incorporate human relationship enrichment (HRE) principles into my work with new parents by meeting individual parents and families "where they were" and helping them to proceed with the goals they had outlined. It wasn't that I did not do this as a nurse, but it was somehow different, being a lay person, peer counselor, and removing the artificial armor or "white coat" mentality of my hierarchical nursing role. Part of my growth professionally was recognizing my strength in the community, my preference for "public health nursing," my interest in population health supported by being with parents on their journey, and my desire to de-medicalize pregnancy, birth, and lactation from a pathological medical condition to a normal physiological developmental process. I was not able to articulate this desire for equity-oriented health care at the time and am grateful to colleagues at the University of British Columbia School of Nursing, who helped me find the language, theory, and understanding of that perspective. How global organizations have framed breastfeeding action to focus on parents' strengths and community responsibility and support are explored next.

World Alliance for Breastfeeding Action (WABA)

The World Alliance for Breastfeeding Action (WABA) is referenced frequently in this text. It is interesting to note how the organization's annual slogans fit the global context. In 2018, the WABA Slogan was "Breastfeeding – Foundation of Life." WABA embraced breastfeeding as the foundation of lifelong health for infants and parents, especially recognizing the inequality, crises, and poverty at a global level (WABA). Similarly, The WABA slogans for consecutive World Breastfeeding Weeks (WBWs) have included "Empower Parents, Enable Breastfeeding" (WABA, 2019) and "Support breastfeeding for a healthier planet!" (WABA, 2020). These slogans for WBW are a way for communities to come together and share the message about how breastfeeding requires empowerment of parents, including overcoming inequities, the connection between human health and nature's ecosystems, and how the protection, promotion and support of breastfeeding addresses inequalities, especially those standing in the way of meeting sustainable development goals (WBW, 2020). This empowerment of parents means ensuring that their rights are protected by advocating for policies and legislation to support parent-friendly workplaces and gender-equitable social norms (WABA, 2019). Social ecological theory as context for lactation health promotion helps us to identify the multitude of factors necessary for developing equitable programs and policies to support all parents in meeting their infant-feeding goals.

Not surprisingly, when there are specific social determinants of health (SDOH) that result in more tenuous situations—such as prematurity, substance use, poverty, unstable food supply or shelter, and the effects of racism and trauma—the ability for parents to meet their breastfeeding goals are often compromised. There is inequity in our breastfeeding outcomes, especially related to exclusive breastfeeding and breastfeeding duration to meet parents' anticipated goals. In these communities that would benefit most from breastfeeding, "desert-like conditions" for breastfeeding support and resources exist (Santhanam, 2019). Considering race as a social category and racism as a social process (Browne, 2017), within lactation we see negative impacts to health, access to care, and overall quality of life for women reflected by their race, class, and culture.

This is not something new—rather, it has been raised to the forefront in women's health more recently. Within breastfeeding, studies in the United States identified the discrepancies between exclusive breastfeeding (EBF) and duration differences based on race. Some of these inequities may be overcome by focusing on patient-centered care (PCC), which is identified as a significant priority for the health care system. Let's consider what this means for the breastfeeding family when we examine lactation as a foundation for health promotion especially considering a commitment to patient-centered care. (BCMOH, 2015).

The Ottawa Charter

In 1986, the World Health Organization (WHO) held an International Conference on Health Promotion in Ottawa, Canada. The Ottawa Charter was signed during the conference and suggested that the focus of public health policy and research needed to be on "upstream" factors like healthy environments and social context. This broader focus by Health Canada on a population health promotion (PHP) model focused on family, community, and socio-cultural health interventions based on the social determinants of health (SDOH). Beginning in1994, this broader focus on population health was criticized for its tendency to hold individuals responsible for their health outcomes, leading to **stigma**, victimization, personal fault, shame, and blame (Rootman et al., 2017). Public health and health promotion advocates—those working under models such as breastfeeding self-efficacy (BSE), theory of planned behavior (TPB), and theory of reasoned action (TRA)—look for ways to maintain patient-centered foci in care by incorporating **shared decision making**, strength-based support, and harm reduction. There is a connection between human well-being and economic costs for societies. In Canada, the government portfolios tend to reflect work within the areas of SDOH: health, education, income, housing, employment, and social safety, to name a few.

As outlined in previous chapters, infant feeding is a complex decision, and, historically, parents make choices based on the scientific knowledge and evidence available, societal expectations, and even political viewpoints. Advances in technology have made finding answers easier, but the information explosion means there is often conflicting advice. Understanding the influence of infant-feeding history, especially within the context of where parents live and work, can help healthcare professionals to better understand parents decision making around infant-feeding practices and to consider how best to support parents in setting goals and reaching them.

Factors that influence upstream health promotion include income disparities, early childhood development, social inclusion/exclusion, social safety nets, employment, and working conditions (Rootman et al., 2017). Situating lactation within the context of a gendered process involving intimate care (breasts), along with controversy over feminism and women's rights over their own bodies, adds an additional strain to conversation about breastfeeding. Given the historical context of women not having power over their own bodies in terms of physical and sexual abuse; violence against women; slavery and wet-nursing; and the objectification and over-sexualization of a woman's body through pornography and media, for many women, decision making around infant-feeding is not simple. Within this complexity, systemic racism in multiple forms in the health care system has led to a lack of respectful care during pregnancy, birth, and postpartum and incidences of maltreatment (Vedam et al., 2019; Vedam et al., 2017; Vedam, Stoll, Taiwo, et al., 2019).

Similarly, we recognize the impact of trauma and violence on women's pregnancy (Chisholm et al., 2017), birth, and postpartum adjustment (Kendall-Tackett, 2007) and have advocated for trauma-violence-informed care (BC Provincial Mental Health and Substance Use Planning Council, 2013; EQUIP Health Care, 2017). Similarly, traumatic birth experiences can affect breastfeeding outcomes (Beck & Watson, 2008) and result in a higher incidence of postpartum depression (PPD) or posttraumatic stress disorder (PTSD) (Kendall-Tackett, 2014; Modarres et al., 2012). Fortunately, health care professionals can play an important role in supporting families when they recognize risks and identify exposure to trauma, violence, or the impact of systemic racism.

As health care providers, **intersectionality** theory has been introduced as a framework by which the hierarchical nature of health care practice, originating from "white, middle class, post-colonial, patriarchal" perspectives that direct its education, practice, and research, can be debunked to attend to issues of oppression and privilege (Van Herk, 2010). Browne et al. (2018) have introduced key dimensions for equity-oriented care in their EQUIP health care model (2017) that include trauma-violence-informed care, Harm Reduction, and Culturally Safe Care (Browne et al., 2018, p. 154). There are 10 strategies for equity-oriented system improvement that are tailored to context and responsive to inequities to reduce the impacts of racism, **discrimination**, and stigma (Browne et al., 2018, p. 14). The goal is to reduce the disparities that individuals experience in conventional care to better meet people's needs by enhancing capacity for an equity-oriented system approach (Browne et al., 2018).

Chapter 9 examined some of the cultural variations in beliefs, attitudes, and intentions related to breastfeeding. In this chapter, we focus on the equity issues that arise and the impact on parents' ability to meet their infant-feeding goals.

Cultural Implications of Breastfeeding: Beliefs and Decision Making

Several studies examined some of the cultural beliefs affecting African American mothers in their experience with and decisions about breastfeeding. The historical influence of forced wet nursing has left generational legacies many black women in the United States fight to overcome. Some factors identified around breastfeeding that have an effect on mothers' experience may include a fear of pain, influence of partners or grandmothers, lack of privacy, and lack of role models (Lewallen & Street, 2010; Simpson, 2012). In the United States, racial disparities persist among breastfeeding mothers, with racism and bias identified as eroding factors to breast-feeding for women of color, compounded by hospital staff being less supportive, a need to return to work earlier, and their being less likely to receive accommodations for flexible hours or areas to pump (Santhanam, 2019). Fortunately, there are growing areas of support, including work by Seals Allers, author of *The Big Letdown: How Medicine, Big Business, and Feminism Undermine Breastfeeding* (2017), and social media applications that allow searching for practitioners who treat without bias (Santhanam, 2019).

Much research has examined the variety of breastfeeding experiences among different racial and ethnic groups in the United States. Although there was variability in women's experiences and large disparities in success with breastfeeding, when the BFHI strategies—skin-to-skin contact, breastfeeding early and often, and rooming-in—were followed, women tended to breastfeed exclusively and for longer durations (Ahluwalia et al., 2012; Bai et al., 2011; Cartagena et al., 2014; Sloand et al., 2018). Other countries incorporating the BFHI have reported dose-response relationships between the number of BFHI steps followed and the likelihood of improved breastfeeding outcomes according to a systematic review of 19 countries (Pérez-Escamilla et al., 2016). Long-term impacts of BFHI, such as duration and exclusivity of breastfeeding, are dependent upon community support (step 10) (Pérez-Escamilla et al., 2016).

In the past few years, a strong effort is occurring within professional organizations, such as the International Lactation Consultant Association, to enhance diversity, equity, and inclusion, and there have been more support systems put into place to work with the many diverse peer counselors to support these peer counselors to be paid and to become lactation consultants. Educational lactation programs are incorporating more support, and health care professional programs are alert to the need for more diversity, equity, and inclusion in teaching, mentoring, and advancing opportunities for professionals from a variety of backgrounds. Much of the research on breastfeeding support has come out of North America and examined effects of various ethnically diverse groups and immigrants. Throughout the previous chapters, we examined research theories and knowledge translation practices that support a global effort to scale up and support breastfeeding for all families.

It is important for healthcare professionals to have a solid foundation in evidence-based practices to support the benefits of breastfeeding. New in this area, we are learning about the effects of vaginal birth and breastfeeding on protection from trauma/toxic stress, epigenetics, and optimizing the microbiome (Fitzstevens et al., 2016; Gomez-Gallego, 2016). In addition, there are multiple parental health benefits (female/birth partner): (a) protection against postpartum hemorrhage; (b) lactation hormone protection against stress; (c) quicker return to pre-pregnancy weight and lower postpartum body mass index; (d) natural delay in return of fertility; (e) protection against breast and ovarian cancer; (f) protection against osteoporosis; (g) protection against type 2 diabetes; and (h) protection against hypertension, stroke, hyperlipidemia, and cardiovascular disease. For the infant, multiple health benefits also have been recorded, including (a) lifelong protection against upper- and lower-respiratory infections, otitis media, diarrheal disease, sepsis, rotavirus, meningitis, urinary tract infection, leukemia, lymphoma, and neuroblastoma; (b) increase in IQ, which is dose dependent, so the longer the infant breastfeeds, the higher the IQ; (c) protection against necrotizing enterocolitis, asthma, breast cancer, chronic and autoimmune diseases, hypertension, high cholesterol, and heart disease; (d) protection against sudden unexplained infant death (SUID); (e) decreased dental caries and promotion of better overall dental health; (f) protection against the common cold, fever, or more serious illness; and (g) protection against hypothyroidism (Rollins et al., 2016; Victora et al., 2016).

Given the evolution of conditions in early 2020, we now need to consider more seriously than ever the broader ramifications of not supporting breastfeeding as health promotion. In an age of questioning global catastrophes, such as the pandemic of 2020, we have outlined some of the basic premises of the "natural" aspect of feeding our babies from our breast. Biologically, mammals provide food to their offspring through lactation, however, for humans lactation includes both the product, 'human milk', and the 'process of breastfeeding'. First, human milk is individually suited and created for each child at the moment they are born. We are learning more everyday about the microbiome, its genetic components, and that there are living and genetic factors within human milk that are individually suited between the parent and infant. These factors should humble us toward the miraculous qualities of human milk, with research demonstrating the health benefits to both the mother/parents and the infant of breastfeeding, which are dose dependent (i.e., there are enhanced benefits with duration and exclusivity of breastfeeding) (Fitzstevens et al., 2016; Gomez-Gallego et al., 2016; Rollins et al., 2016; Victora et al., 2016). We now recognize the hormonal components of prolactin and oxytocin and that these mothering hormones lay down receptors in breast and brain tissue of both mother and infant during lactation. Thus, the breastfeeding experience is passed on through generations. The process of breastfeeding is affected by historical, cultural, and socio-demographic factors including the social determinants of health.

In addition to natural catastrophes, we are confronted with the damaging effect of racism, and within the health promotion frameworks we have examined, we can see the connections between racism, lack of privilege, and direct connections to lack of access to social determinants of health. Depending on one's gender, race, aboriginal status, and ability, there is a direct relationship with access to sustainable food sources, income and income distribution, education, job security, employment and safe working conditions, early childhood development, housing, social safety networks, and health services. Other factors, such as religion, immigrant/refugee status, sexual orientation, and political beliefs, can also result in a lack of respectful care and lack of access within health systems. Given the key areas where parents enter the system for pregnancy, birth, and post-birth follow-up care, there are many opportunities to identify and remedy these discrepancies. The EQUIP health care model (2017) was a framework introduced to build capacity for equity-oriented services in a way to provide culturally safe trauma-violence-informed care that uses a harm reduction approach incorporating shared decision making (Browne et al., 2018; Wathen et al., 2020).

There are many resources for taking action to combat racism and its effects on families' health and well-being. One stellar resource for maternal–child health is the BirthPlace Lab (University of British Columbia, Division of Midwifery, Birth Place Lab, 2020). The Academy of Breastfeeding Medicine released a statement on **health equity** that reminded us that racism, not race, is hazardous to the health of black, **indigenous** people of color (Stuebe & Lindhal, 2020). Advocating for a commitment to diversity, equity, and inclusion is paramount as we partner to promote justice in health care and educate our future healthcare providers in patient-centered care, cultural sensitivity/humility, and community engagement. In the ABM statement on health equity, it states, "Breastfeeding is the foundation of lifelong health and well-being. The events of the past few weeks are a potent reminder that racism, not race, is hazardous to the health of Black, Indigenous People of Color. We look forward to partnering with advocates and organizers to advance justice in healthcare across generations" (Stuebe & Lindahl, 2020).

This text provides examples of shared decision making, relational practice, and community programs to support breastfeeding parents and ideas for collaborations that address equity and justice issues surrounding lactation. Applying health communication principles to the promotion and protection of breastfeeding means that we need to consider the words we use in talking with parents about breastfeeding and to allow for open communication. We need to address the SDOH that may put them at risk and to assess for physical, mental, and emotional needs in a trauma-violence-informed manner. A lack of respect for women and their mistreatment in the health care system is not new. The medicalization of breastfeeding, pregnancy, and birth has led to women's significant distrust in their own bodies and trauma that lasts too long (Vedam, et al., 2019).

Examples of Policies or Programs in Support of Breastfeeding

Right to Breaks for Breastfeeding Women

An analysis of 182/193 member states of the United Nations tested the association between national policy for guaranteed breastfeeding breaks, the number of hours and the duration, and rates of exclusive breastfeeding (Heymann et al., 2013). They took into consideration potential confounding variables, such as national income level, urbanization, female percentage of the labor force, and female literacy rates. Findings revealed that there were 130 countries (71%) where breastfeeding breaks and parental leave from work with pay were guaranteed; 7 countries (4%) where unpaid breaks were guaranteed; and 45 countries (25%) without any policy for breastfeeding breaks. There was an 8.86% increase in exclusive breastfeeding rates when paid breastfeeding breaks for a duration of at least 6 months were reported ($p < 0.05$). The authors suggest that health outcomes could be improved by legislation that supports breastfeeding breaks, especially in those countries not supporting the right to breastfeed (Heymann et al., 2013, p. 398).

Health Communication (Individual/Interpersonal/Community Level of SEM Health Promotion)

Effective Parental Communication

1. Motivational interviewing
   a. Express empathy.
   b. Develop discrepancy.
   c. Avoid argument.
   d. Adjust to resistance.
   e. Support self-efficacy. (Galipeau et al., 2017)
2. Systematic review of interventions and their effect on breastfeeding self-efficacy (BSE) and low milk supply (LMS)

The Patient/Breastfeeding Family: At the Forefront of Their Health Care

Using a patient-centered-care framework at all levels, framing the inpatient health system within the individual/interpersonal/community levels of the socio-ecological framework of health promotion, one reflects on effective interprofessional communication to fully meet the needs of the patient.

The Collective Impact Framework was introduced in chapter 2 as a community health system approach that can be framed within the community/organizational levels of the socio-ecological framework of health promotion. It engages multiple players in working together to solve complex problems and addresses the cross-sector alignment necessary to impact breastfeeding. The development of coalitions and the successful work they accomplished has been outlined in Chapters 2, 4, 6, and 9.

We know that breastfeeding and lactation are physiological and psychological, and the percentage of women who actually do not have enough milk (whose bodies for physiological reasons cannot produce enough milk, not counting surgery, chemotherapy, and underlying biophysical issues) is actually quite low (see Chapter 14). Taking into consideration the supply and demand process of lactation, it would appear that "any breast that can make milk, can make more milk" (Christina Smillie, personal communication). When health care providers take the time to examine women's lives and the stressors they experience at this point in time, lactation is just another area where the stress of our society, the lack of support for new mothers in general, and the expectations for them on their lives are actually quite unrealistic. In addition, assessing for signs of anxiety, depression, and exposure to violence and trauma may be key to uncovering issues beyond the breastfeeding relationship. As a community, society, and global citizens, we need to recognize the importance of supporting parents in pregnancy, in labor and delivery, and in lactation for a better and healthier world. The effects of systemic racism, inequities, and lack of access to meet one's needs compound the risk of not meeting one's goals.

Finally, one of the most successful approaches in scaling up for breastfeeding promotion, support, and protection has been through the careful mentoring of peers in specific communities. Research has examined the usefulness and positive impact of peers within African American, Latinx, adolescent, neonatal intensive care units (NICUs), and Native American populations (Chapman et al., 2010). This will be explored next.

Peer Counseling

Chapter 9 identifies the important role of peer counseling, and when considering breastfeeding self-efficacy, the importance of vicarious experiences that reflect role models who you identify with is not a surprise. A review of the literature surrounding the effect of peer counseling reported its effectiveness in a Latinx low-income community (Anderson et al., 2005; Chapman et al., 2004), in neonatal intensive care units (Benoit & Semenic, 2014; Briere et al., 2014; Merewood et al., 2006), and the efficacy of a home-based peer counseling program (Morrow et al., 1999).

Other effects on breastfeeding initiation are in relation to the Affordable Care Act (Kapinos et al., 2017), which mandated coverage for lactation services but only seemed to impact privately insured mothers compared to those on Medicaid, representing an equity issue housed within a policy meant to decrease inequities.

Role of the Health Care Professional: Promote and Support Lactation

Considering all these factors, whose responsibility is it to support parents in their infant-feeding decisions? Is it an obligation of health care providers to be knowledgeable and support new parents? Given the role of lactation as intimate care, health care providers need support to communicate about this taboo around lactation. In mothering circles, one of the major controversies is the dialogue around breast and bottle feeding. There are national and international programs supporting the rights of parents and children related to breastfeeding.

As outlined in other chapters, the *International Code of Marketing of Breast-milk Substitutes* (World Health Organization [WHO], 1981) was created to protect parents from marketing by human milk substitute (formula) companies. The *Innocenti Declaration* (UNICEF, 1991) was then created, and many countries developed national policies as a result of compliance with the Innocenti Declaration. Some examples include New Zealand, U.S. Healthy People goals, and other global policies to protect the nutrition and development of children, as well as the United Nations Convention on the Rights of the Child (UNICEF, 1990) and the Global Strategy for Infant and Young Child Feeding (WHO, 2003).

When considering categories to manage inequities, the following have been successful on a global level:

- Baby-friendly Hospital Initiative (BFHI)–capitalize to synchronize efforts
- Supporting human milk banks, media campaigns for an increase in milk depots and donations

- Setting national public health care goals and benchmarks with evaluation of outcomes
- Community-based EBF promotion/support (e.g., World Breastfeeding Week)
- Parental leave policies
- Education/support for healthcare professionals
- Coalition development

Student Questions for Consideration

1. *How might you engage with a person to explore their health promotion needs related to lactation? Use the EQUIP health care model to uncover any health-equity concerns.*
2. *How can health care practitioners overcome barriers exacerbated by stigma and the consequential mistrust an individual might have for engaging in health care (e.g., conflicting advice, previous prejudice or maltreatment, trauma)?*
3. *What would a strengths-based approach to health promotion for lactation look like in your everyday practice?*

Group Activity

Break-out to consider (share and report out) the following.
   In your role, identify a concrete step you can take:

- *Knowledge translation*
- *Community engagement*
- *Intersectoral and transdisciplinary collaboration in your own community*

   Identify one area related to BFHI that you think could be conducive to knowledge translation in your area.

- *What resources would be needed?*
- *What is the first step?*
- *How would using an intersectoral framework help you identify any health inequities for your parents and their families?*

For health care professionals interested in further lactation education, there are many other resources that will enhance knowledge, practice, and understanding of lactation as a specialty discipline in health care (Mannel et al., 2019; Sanders et al., 2019). The International Board Certified Lactation Consultant (IBCLC) is certified through the International Board of Lactation Consultant Examiners (IBLCE) and represents 32,500 practitioners in over 122 countries worldwide (IBCLE, 2020). Some ways identified to increase the visibility of the IBCLC role in interdisciplinary practice include the following:

- *Work collaboratively with the health care team*
- *Develop professionally mediated and/or peer support programs*
- *Provide information to health care practitioners when patients are referred*
- *Provide ongoing support*
- *Use evidence-based practices in the hospital and at home*
- *Baby-friendly Hospital Initiative–capitalize to synchronize efforts*

- *Participate in development and implementation of national public health care goals*
- *Provide community-based exclusive breastfeeding (EBF) promotion/support (World Breastfeeding Week)*
- *Advocate for parental leave policies*
- *Provide health care professionals with education and support*
- *Participate in state and provincial think tanks and policy reinforcement*

Key Points to Remember

1. Consideration for equitable breastfeeding health promotion programs involves political will/support; parental care practices; peer support; educating parents; professional support; media and social marketing; and support for breastfeeding in the workplace. Taking action toward equity-oriented system improvements to address contexts that present inequities is paramount.
2. Human milk is a sustainable food source that every infant has a right to access, and it is a free, natural, renewable, safe food source uniquely suitable for human infants. There are environmental and economic advantages to supporting breastfeeding and long-term health benefits.
3. It benefits all health care providers to have a BFHI elevator speech prepared: education for family and other providers; skin-to-skin contact, nurse first hour; room-in → feed infant frequently and exclusively based on infant cues; educate and assist using EBP consistent messages; supplement for medical indication only; follow the WHO Code; corporate compliance; know your community breastfeeding support and resources.

Additional Resources

- Being an Ally https://opentextbc.ca/indigenizationcurriculumdevelopers /chapter/being-an-ally/#navigation
- EQUIP Health Care www.equiphealthcare.ca
- Implementation Toolkit https://decisionaid.ohri.ca/implement.html
- National Learning Consortium, Fact Sheet: Shared Decision Making https:// www.healthit.gov/sites/default/files/nlc_shared_decision_making_fact_sheet .pdf
- Patient Decision Aids https://decisionaid.ohri.ca/AZlist.html
- Promoting and Supporting the Initiation, Exclusivity, and Continuation of Breastfeeding in Newborns, Infants and Young Children https://rnao.ca/bpg /guidelines/breastfeeding-promoting-and-supporting-initiation-exclusivity -and-continuation-breast
- Summary: The Direct Economic Burden of Socio-Economic Health Inequalities in Canada https://www.canada.ca/en/public-health/services/reports-publications /health-promotion-chronic-disease-prevention-canada-research-policy-practice /vol-36-no-6-2016/report-summary-direct-economic-burden-socioeconomic -health-inequalities-canada-analysis-health-care-costs-income-level.html
- What is Health Equity? A Tool for Health & Social Service Organizations and Providers https://equiphealthcare.ca/resources/toolkit/
- World Alliance for Breastfeeding Action. https://waba.org.my/

References

Ahluwalia, I. B., Morrow, B., D'Angelo, D., & Li, R. (2012). Maternity care practices and breastfeeding experiences of women in different racial and ethnic groups: Pregnancy Risk Assessment and Monitoring System (PRAMS). *Maternal and Child Health Journal, 16*(8), 1672–1678. https://doi.org/10.1007/s10995-011-0871-0

Anderson, A. K., Damio, G., Young, S., Chapman, D. J., & Pérez-Escamilla, R. (2005). A randomized trial assessing the efficacy of peer counseling on exclusive breastfeeding in a predominantly Latina low-income community. *Archives of Pediatrics & Adolescent Medicine, 159*(9), 836–841. https://doi.org/10.1001/archpedi.159.9.836

Anti-Oppression Network. (n.d.). *Allyship.* https://theantioppressionnetwork.com/allyship

Bai, Y., Wunderlich, S. M., & Fly, A. D. (2011). Predicting intentions to continue exclusive breastfeeding for 6 months: A comparison among racial/ethnic groups. *Maternal and Child Health Journal, 15*(8), 1257–1264. https://doi.org/10.1007/s10995-010-0703-7

British Columbia (BC) Provincial Mental Health and Substance Use Planning Council. (2013, May). *Trauma-informed practice guide.* http://bccewh.bc.ca/wp-content/uploads/2012/05/2013_TIP-Guide.pdf

Beck, C. T., & Watson, S. (2008). Impact of birth trauma on breast-feeding: A tale of two pathways. *Nursing Research, 57*(4), 228–236. https://doi.org/10.1097/01.NNR.0000313494.87282.90

Benoit, B., & Semenic, S. (2014). Barriers and facilitators to implementing the Baby-Friendly Hospital Initiative in neonatal intensive care units. *JOGNN: Journal of Obstetric, Gynecologic & Neonatal Nursing, 43*(5), 614–624. https://doi.org/10.1111/1552-6909.12479

Bowleg, L. (2012). The problem with the phrase *women and minorities*: Intersectionality—an important theoretical framework for public health. *American Journal of Public Health, 102*(7), 1267–1273. https://doi.org/10.2105/AJPH.2012.300750

Briere, C. E., McGrath, J., Cong, X., & Cusson, R. (2014). An integrative review of factors that influence breastfeeding duration for premature infants after NICU hospitalization. *JOGNN: Journal of Obstetric, Gynecologic & Neonatal Nursing, 43*(3), 272–281. https://doi.org/10.1111/1552-6909.12297

British Columbia Ministry of Health (BCMOH). (2015). *The British Columbia patient-centered care framework.* https://www.health.gov.bc.ca/library/publications/year/2015_a/pt-centred-care-framework.pdf

Browne, A. J. (2017). Moving beyond description: Closing the health equity gap by redressing racism impacting indigenous populations. *Social Science & Medicine, 184*, 23–26. https://doi.org/10.1016/j.socscimed.2017.04.045

Browne, A. J., Varcoe, C., Ford-Gilboe, M., Nadine Wathen, C., Smye, V., Jackson, B. E., Wallace, B., Pauly, B., Herbert, C. P., Lavoie, J. G., Wong, S., & Blanchet Garneau, A. (2018). Disruption as opportunity: Impacts of an organizational health equity intervention in primary care clinics. *International Journal for Equity in Health, 17*(1), 154. https://doi.org/10.1186/s12939-018-0820-2

Cartagena, D. C., Ameringer, S. W., McGrath, J., Jallo, N., Masho, S. W., & Myers, B. J. (2014). Factors contributing to infant overfeeding with Hispanic mothers. *JOGNN: Journal of Obstetric, Gynecologic & Neonatal Nursing, 43*(2), 139–159. https://doi.org/10.1111/1552-6909.12279

Chapman, D. J., Damio, G., & Pérez-Escamilla, R. (2004). Differential response to breastfeeding peer counseling within a low-income, predominantly Latina population. *Journal of Human Lactation, 20*(4), 389–396. https://doi.org/10.1177/0890334404269845

Chapman, D. J., Morel, K., Anderson, A. K., Damio, G., & Pérez-Escamilla, R. (2010). Breastfeeding peer counseling: From efficacy through scale-up. *Journal of Human Lactation, 26*(3), 314–326. https://journals.sagepub.com/doi/10.1177/0890334410369481

Chisholm, C. A., Bullock, L., & Ferguson, J. E., II. (2017). Intimate partner violence and pregnancy: Epidemiology and impact. *American Journal of Obstetrics & Gynecology, 217*(2), 141–144. https://doi.org/10.1016/j.ajog.2017.05.042

EQUIP Health Care. (2017). *What is health equity? A tool for health & social service organizations and providers.* https://equiphealthcare.ca/resources/toolkit/

Farrer, L., Marinetti, C., Cavaco, Y. K., & Costongs, C. (2015). Advocacy for health equity: A synthesis review. *The Milbank Quarterly, 93*(2), 392–437. https://doi.org/10.1111/1468-0009.12112

Fitzstevens, J. L., Smith, K. C., Hagadorn, J. I., Caimano, M. J., Matson, A. P., & Brownell, E. A. (2016). Systematic review of the human milk microbiota. *Nutrition in Clinical Practice, 32*(3), 354–364. https://doi.org/10.1177/0884533616670150

Galipeau, R., Baillot, A., Trottier, A., & Lemire, L. (2017). Effectiveness of interventions on breastfeeding self-efficacy and perceived insufficient milk supply: A systematic review and meta-analysis. *Maternal & Child Nutrition.* https://doi.org/10.1111/mcn.12607

Gomez-Gallego, C., Garcia-Mantrana, I., Salminen, S., & Collado, M. C. (2016). The human milk microbiome and factors influencing its composition and activity. *Seminars in Fetal and Neonatal Medicine, 21*(6), 400–405. https://doi.org/10.1016/j.siny.2016.05.003

Heymann, J., Raub, A., & Earle, A. (2013). Breastfeeding policy: A globally comparative analysis. *Bulletin of the World Health Organization, 91,* 398–406. https://www.ncbi.nlm.nih.gov/pmc /articles/PMC3777140/

International Board of Lactation Consultant Examiners (IBLCE) (2020). *IBLCE exam facts & figures.* https://iblce.org/about-iblce/iblce-exam-facts-figures/

Joffe, N., Webster, F., & Shenker, N. (2019). Support for breastfeeding is an environmental imperative. *BMJ, 367,* l5646. https://doi.org/10.1136/bmj.l5646

Kapinos, K. A., Bullinger, L., & Gurley-Calvez, T. (2017). Lactation support services and breastfeeding initiation: Evidence from the Affordable Care Act. *Health Services Research, 52*(6), 2175–2196. https://doi.org/10.1111/1475-6773.12598

Kendall-Tackett, K. (2014). Childbirth-related posttraumatic stress disorder: Symptoms and impact on breastfeeding. *Clinical Lactation, 5*(2), 51–55. https://doi.org/10.1891/2158-0782.5.2.51

Kendall-Tackett, K. A. (2007). Violence against women and the perinatal period: The impact of lifetime violence and abuse on pregnancy, postpartum, and breastfeeding. *Trauma, Violence, & Abuse, 8*(3), 344–353. https://journals.sagepub.com/doi/10.1177/1524838007304406

Kimmerer, R. W. (2013). *Braiding sweetgrass: Indigenous wisdom, scientific knowledge, and teachings of plants.* Milkweed Editions.

Lewallen, L. P., & Street, D. J. (2010). Initiating and sustaining breastfeeding in African American women. *JOGYNN: Journal of Obstetric, Gynecologic, & Neonatal Nursing, 39*(6), 667–674. http:// doi.org/10.1111/j.1552-6909.2010.01196.x

Mannel, R., Campbell, S. H., & Stehel, E. K. (2019). Interdisciplinary lactation services. In S. H. Campbell, J. Lauwers, R. Mannel, & R. Spencer (Eds.), *Core curriculum for interdisciplinary lactation care* (pp. 505–518). Jones & Bartlett.

Merewood, A., Chamberlain, L. B., Cook, J. T., Philipp, B. L., Malone, K., Bauchner, H. (2006). The effect of peer counselors on breastfeeding rates in the neonatal intensive care unit: Results of a randomized controlled trial. *Archives of Pediatrics and Adolescent Medicine, 160*(7), 681–685.

Modarres, M., Afrasiabi, S., Rahnama, P., & Montazeri, A. (2012). Prevalence and risk factors of childbirth-related post-traumatic stress symptoms. *BMC Pregnancy and Childbirth, 12,* 88. https://doi.org/10.1186/1471-2393-12-88

Morrow, A. L., Guerrero, M. L., Shults, J., Calva, J. J., Lutter, C., Bravo, J., Ruiz-Palacios, G., Morrow, R., & Butterfoss, F. D. (1999). Efficacy of home-based peer counselling to promote exclusive breastfeeding: A randomised controlled trial. *Lancet, 353*(9160), 1226–1231. https://doi .org/10.1016/S0140-6736(98)08037-4

National Learning Consortium. (2013, December). *Fact sheet: Shared decision making.* https://www .healthit.gov/sites/default/files/nlc_shared_decision_making_fact_sheet.pdf

Pérez-Escamilla, R., Martinez, J. L., & Segura-Pérez, S. (2016). Impact of the Baby-friendly Hospital Initiative on breastfeeding and child health outcomes: A systematic review. *Maternal & Child Nutrition, 12*(3), 402–417. https://doi.org/10.1111/mcn.12294

Rollins, N. C., Bhandari, N., Hajeebhoy, N., Horton, S., Lutter, C. K., Martines, J. C., Piwoz, E. G., Richter, L. M., & Victora, C. G. (2016). Why invest, and what it will take to improve breastfeeding practices? *The Lancet, 387*(10017), 491–504. https://www.thelancet.com /journals/lancet/article/PIIS0140-6736(15)01044-2/fulltext

Rootman, I., Pederson, A., Frohlich, K., & Dupere, S. (2017). *Health promotion in Canada: New perspective on theory, practice, policy, and research* (4th ed.). Canadian Scholars.

Sanders, A., Ferrarello, D., & Judge, A. B. (2019). Lactation education for health professionals. In S. H. Campbell, J. Lauwers, R. Mannel, & R. Spencer (Eds.), *Core Curriculum for Interdisciplinary Lactation Care* (pp. 477–485). Jones & Bartlett.

Santhanam, L. (2019). Racial disparities persist for breastfeeding moms. Here's why. PBS Newshour: Health. https://www.pbs.org/newshour/health/racial-disparities-persist-for-breastfeeding-moms-heres-why

Seals Allers, K. (2017). *The big letdown: How medicine, big business, and feminism undermine breastfeeding.* St. Martin's Press.

Simpson, A. C. (2012). *Sociocultural barriers to breast feeding in African American women with focused intervention to increased prevalence.* (MS). Georgia State University, Atlanta, Georgia. https://scholarworks.gsu.edu/nutrition_theses/41

Sloand, E., Lowe, V., Pennington, A., & Rose, L. (2018). Breastfeeding practices and opinions of Latina mothers in an urban pediatric office: A focus group study. *Journal of Pediatric Health Care, 32*(3), 236–244. https://doi.org/10.1016/j.pedhc.2017.11.001

Stuebe, A. & Lindahl, J. (2020). *ABM statement on health equity.* https://abm.memberclicks.net/abm-statement-on-health-equity

The Free Dictionary. (2015). *Systemic racism.* https://idioms.thefreedictionary.com/systemic+racism

UNICEF. (1991). *Innocenti Declaration. On the protection, promotion and support of breastfeeding.* https://www.unicef.org/nutrition/index_24807.html

UNICEF. (1990). *Convention on the Rights of the Child.* https://www.unicef.org/child-rights-convention/convention-text

University of British Columbia, Division of Midwifery, Birth Place Lab. (2020). *Resources for taking action.* https://www.birthplacelab.org/resources-for-taking-action/

Vedam, S., Stoll, K., McRae, D. N., Korchinski, M., Velasquez, R., Wang, J., Partridge, S., McRae, L., Martin, R. E., Jolicoeur, G., & BC Steering Committee. (2019). Patient-led decision making: Measuring autonomy and respect in Canadian maternity care. *Patient Education and Counseling, 102*(3), 586–594. https://doi.org/10.1016/j.pec.2018.10.023

Vedam, S., Stoll, K., Rubashkin, N., Martin, K., Miller-Vedam, Z., Hayes-Klein, H., & Jolicoeur, G. (2017). The Mothers on Respect (MOR) index: Measuring quality, safety, and human rights in childbirth. *SSM - Population Health, 3*, 201–210. https://doi.org/10.1016/j.ssmph.2017.01.005

Vedam, S., Stoll, K., Taiwo, T. K., Rubashkin, N., Cheyney, M., Strauss, N., McLemore, M., Cadena, M., Nethery, E., Rushton, E., Schummers, L., Declercq, E., & the GVtM-US Steering Committee. (2019). The Giving Voice to Mothers Study: Inequity and mistreatment during pregnancy and childbirth in the United States. *Reproductive Health, 16*(1), 77. https://doi.org/10.1186/s12978-019-0729-2

Van Herk, K. A., Smith, D., & Andrew, C. (2011). Examining our privileges and oppressions: Incorporating an intersectionality paradigm into nursing. *Nursing Inquiry, 18*(1), 29–39. https://doi.org/10.1111/j.1440-1800.2011.00539.x

Victora, C. G., Bahl, R., Barros, A. J. D., França, G. V. A., Horton, S., Krasevec, J., Murch, S., Sankar, M. J., Walker, N., Rollins, N. C., & Lancet Breastfeeding Series Group. (2016). Breastfeeding in the 21st century: Epidemiology, mechanisms, and lifelong effect. *The Lancet, 387*(10017), 475–490. https://doi.org/10.1016/S0140-6736(15)01024-7

Wathen, C.N., Bungay, V., Wilson, E., Browne, A. J., & Varcoe, C. (2020). Equity-Oriented Health Systems Improvement: A Policy Brief. *EQUIP Health Care,* https://nursing.ubc.ca/sites/nursing.ubc.ca/files/files/news/attachments/EQUIP%20Equity%20System%20Improvement%20Policy%20Brief%20Spring2020.pdf

Wolfe, S. M., Long, P. D., & Brown, K. K. (2020). Using a principles-focused evaluation approach to evaluate coalitions and collaboratives working toward equity and social justice. *New Directions for Evaluation, 2020*(165), 45–65. https://doi.org/10.1002/ev.20404

World Alliance for Breastfeeding Action (WABA). (2018). *Breastfeeding: Foundation for Life.* http://worldbreastfeedingweek.org/2018/

World Alliance for Breastfeeding Action (WABA). (2019). *Empower parents: Enable breastfeeding.* https://worldbreastfeedingweek.org/2019/

World Alliance for Breastfeeding Action (WABA). (2020). *Support breastfeeding for a healthier planet!* https://worldbreastfeedingweek.org/

World Health Organization (WHO). (1981). *International Code of Marketing of Breast-milk Substitutes.* https://www.who.int/nutrition/publications/code_english.pdf

World Health Organization (WHO). (2003). *Global strategy for infant and young child feeding.* https://www.who.int/nutrition/publications/infantfeeding/9241562218/en

PART 3

Lactation as Health Promotion Under Challenging Circumstances

Breastfeeding: An Essential Link in Healthy Weight Promotion and Obesity Prevention

Cecilia Jevitt, RM, CNM, APRN, PhD, FACNM

LEARNING OBJECTIVES

1. Apply new definitions of obesity as a disease and people-first language to breastfeeding support.
2. Identify socio-economic disparities that exacerbate obesity.
3. Develop techniques to support breastfeeding based on the physiology of obesity.
4. Promote the health benefits and obesity-preventing effects of breastfeeding during lactation counseling.

KEY WORDS

- **Obesity:** A chronic, relapsing, multi-factorial, neurobehavioral disease, wherein an increase in body fat promotes adipose tissue dysfunction and abnormal fat mass physical forces, resulting in adverse metabolic, biomechanical, and psychosocial health consequences. Obesity is measured by a body mass index of > 30.
- **Body mass index (BMI):** A weight-to-height ratio used to measure underweight, normal weight, overweight, and obesity (**Table 11-1**). BMI = kg/m^2. BMI is an imperfect measure but is used in international research.
- **Delayed Lactogenesis II:** The onset of copious milk production later than 72 hours postpartum.
- **Depuration:** The removal of impurities from bodily fluids or tissues. Toxins are depurated from breast adipose tissue during weight loss.

Acknowledgement: The author thanks Juliette Mudra, RN, for her assistance in formatting this chapter.

- **Lactational Programming:** Programming that stems from an exposure that occurs during the period when the mother is nursing her infant, which may lead to changes in the nutrients, hormones, or bioactive components in the milk and epigenetic changes in the infant.
- **Postpartum Weight Retention:** The difference in prepregnancy weight and weight at 1 year postpartum.

Overview

This chapter reviews **obesity** as a chronic disease caused by and provoked by multiple socio-economic disparities and environmental disadvantages. The metabolic and mechanical changes that obesity imposes on the body can negatively affect breastfeeding; however, breastfeeding can be a powerful tool in ameliorating the metabolic impacts of obesity and reducing future risk for obesity in both the mother and infant.

Introduction

The difficulties women with obesity have with lactation and breastfeeding are well documented (Anstey & Jevitt, 2011). To understand how lactation and breastfeeding promote healthy weights for mothers and infants, an understanding of the complexity of obesity as a disease and its physiological effects on lactation and breastfeeding are needed. Obesity became a recognized epidemic across the postindustrialized world beginning about 1980 with obesity rates for adult women now ranging from 20% to 30% in middle- and high-income countries (World Health Organization [WHO], 2017). Currently in Canada and the United States, the prevalence of obesity in adult women ranges from 18% to 40% (Centers for Disease Control [CDC], 2018a; Statistics Canada, n.d.). Research into the roots of the epidemic has produced new understandings of obesity, which is now redefined as "a chronic, relapsing, multifactorial, neurobehavioral disease, wherein an increase in body fat promotes adipose tissue dysfunction and abnormal fat mass physical forces, resulting in adverse metabolic, biomechanical, and psychosocial health consequences" (Bays et al., 2019, p. 13). Obesity has multiple causes, including adverse medication reactions, nutritional imbalances, and unfavorable environmental factors (Bays et al., 2019). The WHO cites the absence of optimal fetal nutrition, unhealthy infant feeding practices, and the increasing availability and promotion of unhealthy foods as components of broken food systems, the foundation for the obesity epidemic (WHO, 2019). Repairing broken food systems includes providing access to adequate calories for energy and nutritious foods for growth, both necessary to attain Sustainable Development Goal #2, *No Hunger* (United Nations, n.d.). Fixing broken food systems will require broad public health and government support. Ensuring access to human milk is the first step in repairing broken food systems and promoting future healthy weights in mothers and newborns.

Obesity as Adipose Tissue Disease

Obesity is associated with multiple perinatal morbidities, including infertility, increased rates of miscarriage, gestational diabetes, hypertensive disorders of pregnancy, prolonged pregnancy, prolonged labor, cesarean birth, postpartum hemorrhage, and stillbirth (American College of Obstetricians and Gynecologists [ACOG], 2015). Most important to this chapter, obesity is associated with **delayed lactogenesis II**, reduced milk quantity, and early weaning (Antsey & Jevitt, 2011).

Obesity-Associated Inflammation

Obesity was classically conceptualized as excessive intake coupled with inadequate physical activity with unused calories being stored as adipose tissue. **Body mass index (BMI)** is the international measurement used to categorize weights and standardize obesity as a BMI > 30 (**Table 11-1**) (Bays et al., 2019). Although not a perfect measure of adiposity, BMI is a more useful measure during pregnancy as the abdomen grows during pregnancy and during the early postpartum period as it takes time to decrease in size. Forty years of research demonstrate that obesity is not simply a phenotype resulting from overeating but a disease of white adipose tissue (Coelho et al., 2013). White adipose tissue is the largest metabolically active organ producing and storing hormones, such as estrogen, and inflammatory proteins, including TNFα, IL-6, IL-1B, and Cox2 (Cinti, 2018; Coelho et al., 2013). These inflammatory factors are linked to other diseases associated with obesity such as diabetes, cardiac disease, and cancers (Cinti, 2018; Coelho et al., 2013).

The inflammatory environment in the mammary gland is evidenced by increased levels of inflammatory cytokines, such as TNFα, IL-1B, and Cox2, and increased macrophage infiltration (Lee & Kelleher, 2016). Mammary inflammation may reduce initial colostrum production and impede lactogenesis II. Excess breast adipose tissue results in elevated estrogen levels that may reduce the effectiveness of prolactin in initial milk production (Babendure et al., 2015; Brown, 2014; Lee & Kelleher, 2016). Insulin is needed for milk synthesis, and women with obesity are prone to insulin resistance. Oxytocin acts on myoepithelial cells to stimulate

Table 11-1 **Body Mass Index Categories for Adults**

Category	BMI Range
Underweight	< 18.5
Normal weight	18.5–24.9
Overweight	25.0–29.9
Obese Class I	30.0–34.9
Obese Class II	35.0–39.9
Obese Class III	> 40

Modified from Bays, H. E., McCarthy, W., Christensen, S., Wells, S., Long, J., Shah, N. N., & Primack, C. (2019). Obesity Algorithm. Retrieved from Obesity Medicine Association website: https://obesitymedicine.org/wp-content/uploads/2019/05/Obesity-Algorithm-2019.pdf

the contractions required for milk ejection during lactation (Lee & Kelleher, 2016). Leptin and visfatin, both elevated in obesity, counteract oxytocin and thereby diminish milk letdown and ejection (Mumtaz et al., 2015). While the average time to lactogenesis II is 72 hours, women with obesity self-reported an average onset of lactogenesis II of 85 hours in one prospective study (Preusting et al., 2017). Thirteen hours of reduced human milk intake could impact infant satiety and growth and push the maternal–newborn dyad toward early human milk substitute (formula) supplementation or weaning. Excess breast adipose tissue may also enlarge and flatten the nipple, making latch more challenging for the newborn, although fat deposition varies from woman to woman and not all women with obesity have large breasts.

Microbiome Alterations in Obesity

The gut microbiomes of those with obesity are different from individuals of normal weights (Li, 2018). The gut microbiome has roles in nutrient and satiety sensing and inflammatory responses in addition to energy harvesting (Bliss & Whitesie, 2018; Chu et al., 2016a; Li, 2018; Sanmiguel et al., 2015). High-carbohydrate, high-fat diets support a pro-inflammatory microbiome that promotes increased permeability in the interstitial layer of gut (Bliss & Whitesie, 2018; Chu, Anthony, et al., 2016a; Li, 2018; Sanmiguel et al., 2015). The cytokines produced by adipose tissue added to this pro-inflammatory environment alter gut-to-brain signaling, promoting the hyperphagia associated with obesity (Bliss & Whitesie, 2018; Chu et al., 2016a; Li, 2018; Sanmiguel et al., 2015). Infant microbiomes are altered when mothers consume high-fat diets independent of maternal BMI (Chu et al., 2016a). Encouraging lower-fat and lower-carbohydrate diets for mothers during lactation may decrease pro-inflammatory microbiome responses, thereby improving nutrient and satiety sensing in both mothers and newborns.

Obesity-Related Epigenetic Changes

The concept of fetal programming in utero started with Barker's research demonstrating a child's propensity to overweight, obesity, hypertension, and cardiovascular disease following maternal undernourishment during pregnancy (Fleming et al., 2018; Kwon & Kim, 2017). Maternal nutrition during pregnancy may cause histone modification or deoxyribonucleic acid (DNA) methylation that produces obesity-promoting epigenetic changes in the fetus. Epigenetic changes alter gene expression and resist later dietary or lifestyle interventions, partially explaining the difficulty in maintaining weight loss (Fleming et al., 2018; Kwon & Kim, 2017; Vickers, 2014). Maternal diet may influence epigenetic changes in maternal ova, the zygote, and the developing ova contained within a female fetus. Epigenetic propensities for obesity may be transmitted from grandmother to granddaughter (Vickers, 2014), highlighting the importance of public health efforts toward more accessible and more nutritious foods. The potential for epigenetic changes in ova highlights the importance of the prenatal period and maternal nutrition during this period as preparation for successful lactation not only during the current pregnancy but for another generation.

Socio-Economic Disparities That Contribute to Obesity

Multiple socio-economic disparities in education, employment, and the environment contribute to obesity (**Figure 11-1**) (Jevitt, 2019). These disparities cause other inequities in nutrition and housing and chronic stressors, including racism. Attention to socio-economic disparities shifts the focus of obesity causation from poor individual choices to broader public health problems. Obesity is an intergenerational adaptation to multiple socio-economic disparities; social and physical environments that alter the hypothalamic–pituitary–adrenal axis (HPA) through exposure to chronic stress and endocrine-disrupting chemicals; and broken, nonnutritive food systems (**Figure 11-2**).

Education and Employment

Obesity is associated with lower levels of formal education with an inverse relationship between education and BMI. There is a positive relationship between education

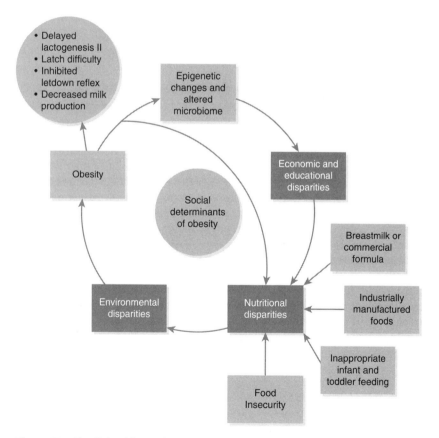

Figure 11-1 The Role of Breastfeeding in Healthy Weight Promotion and Obesity Prevention.

© Cecilia Jevitt 2020.

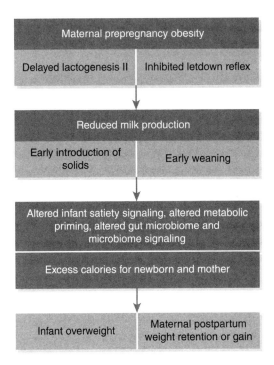

Figure 11-2 Obesity-related breastfeeding alterations and consequences.
© Cecilia Jevitt 2020.

and income across racial and ethnic groups in the United States (Centers for Disease Control [CDC], 2018b; Rubin, 2018). These relationships have been used to explain higher levels of obesity in groups with lower incomes because there is less income to purchase nutritious foods (Darmon & Drewnowski, 2015; Gordon-Larsen, 2014; Wilde et al., 2017). Lower levels of education are associated not only with reduced income but also with jobs that have little schedule flexibility to accommodate breastfeeding, such as night-shift jobs or those with rotating shifts. Night and rotating shift work are associated with obesity (Dashti et al., 2015; Liu et al., 2018). Rotating shifts alter sleep and circadian-based hormonal cycles, affecting insulin, melatonin, and leptin, which are also key hormones in human milk production (Dashti et al., 2015). In the United States, low-wage workers do not usually have paid parental leave, forcing women to choose between being available for infant-led feedings or balancing milk pumping with work hours (Dashti et al., 2015). Fifty percent of low-wage-earning mothers leave their jobs shortly after giving birth, further eroding family purchasing power (Fleming et al., 2018). Lactation support in many societies may involve assisting women to plan how to maximize infant contact for breastfeeding, effectively pump milk at work for breast stimulation, and adjust their work/home schedules to accommodate breastfeeding.

Access to Nutritious Food

Gaps in ability to purchase sufficient food lead to food insecurity and patterns of increased consumption when food is available (Caamaño et al., 2019; Wilde et al., 2017). Fruits and vegetables are more expensive than industrially manufactured, high-caloric-density, low-nutrition foods (Darmon & Drewnowski, 2015; Gordon-Larsen, 2014; Wilde et al., 2017). Additionally, low-income families may lack transportation to stores that feature low-cost fruits and vegetables, may lack adequate refrigerator storage for them; and may also lack cooking equipment to prepare them into palatable meals (Darmon & Drewnowski, 2015; Gordon-Larsen, 2014; Wilde et al., 2017). Providers must use caution in assuming that women with obesity have adequate nutrition. They may have an overabundance of nonnutritive, high-calorie foods at times but lack foods with health-promoting vitamins, minerals, and other ingredients. Choices for high-quality foods may be limited by income. For some women with obesity, lactation support might include referrals to public food programs with a nutrition counseling component, such as the U.S. Supplemental Nutrition Program for Women, Infants, and Children (WIC).

Families with low income may have different values regarding human milk or formula feeding. If families have experienced food insecurity, an overfed plump infant may seem healthy and satisfied. Women with prepregnancy obesity give infants age-inappropriate foods more often, introduce juices and foods such as cereals earlier, and wean to formula more often than women of normal prepregnancy BMIs (Gross et al., 2014; Preusting et al., 2017; Thompson & Bentley, 2013). Including education about appropriate infant feeding and introduction of solid foods is an important component of family education about breastfeeding. Education about breastfeeding and the introduction of other foods may need to consider the large number of women returning to work during the first year postpartum and their needs related to integrating breastfeeding into their daily schedules.

Environment

Although endocrine-disrupting chemicals (EDCs) are pervasive in indoor and outdoor environments, low-wage earners are more likely to do work that exposes them to EDCs and live and work in neighborhoods polluted with EDCs (Nelson et al., 2012). Bisphenol A, phthalates, organochlorines, parabens, polybrominated diphenylethers, and phytoestrogens are EDCs known to have obesogenic potential (Darbe, 2017; Ranjit et al., 2010). These chemicals are found in plastics, insecticides, flame retardants, canned food liners, dental sealants, and detergents (Darbe, 2017; Ranjit et al., 2010). Changes in hormonal control of hunger and satiety may be the obesity-supporting mechanism of EDCs, which are also known to interfere with steroid synthesis, thyroid function, and insulin sensitivity (Darbe, 2017; Ranjit et al., 2010). These hormonal perturbations increase adipose cell numbers and size. Endocrine-disrupting chemicals are stored in adipose tissue and are released through **depuration** during weight loss and lactation; however, no current recommendations advise against breastfeeding due to concerns about EDC depuration (Darbe, 2017; Ranjit et al., 2010).

Neighborhoods populated with low-wage earners are perceived as being less safe than the communities of higher-wage earners. The chronic stresses from fearing harm (Whitfield et al., 2018), the threat of overpolicing (McFarland et al., 2018), and racism (Hicken et al., 2018) may push the HPA axis toward elevated levels of cortisol, which increases adipose deposition. Women may be threatened by sexual violence (Hoffman et al., 2018) and have reduced physical activity from fear of walking in their own neighborhoods (Whitfield et al., 2018). Stress has long been credited with reducing human milk production (Niwayama, 2017). One study of 100 women doc umented this relationship by showing that mothers who experienced pain, exhaustion, and negative feelings in a stressful and long labor had delayed onset of lactation. These women, particularly primiparas, were rated by caregivers as having more negative emotional affects and scored higher on a posttraumatic stress inventory than women with easier labors (Dimitraki et al., 2016). Long-term societal improvements are needed to reduce overall social stress, but smaller stress-relieving exercises or programs may enable a woman to have improved milk production.

Breastfeeding as Healthy Weight Promotion and Obesity Prevention

The Lactation Window

That breastfeeding might be a tool to promote healthy weight and prevent obesity when obesity negatively affects lactation and breastfeeding seems paradoxical; however, breastfeeding has numerous actions that can improve future weight-related metabolic factors (Figure 11-2). These actions include promoting healthy newborn weight, priming glucose metabolism in the infant, supporting a healthy gut microbiome in the infant, setting patterns for infant satiety, and promoting postpartum weight loss in mothers. To take advantage of the metabolic benefits of breastfeeding, women with obesity must first be assisted to establish breastfeeding and lactogenesis II. Conversations with women with obesity are less awkward when patient-first language is used (**Table 11-2**). Patient-first language demonstrates attention to the

---

Table 11-2 **People-First Language Use in Obesity and Breastfeeding**

Examples of encouraged language	Examples of discouraged language
1. Your weight is increased and might be unhealthy.	1. You are morbidly obese, and this puts you at risk for breastfeeding problems.
2. Your body mass index is in the obese range.	2. Your fat is making your nipple difficult for the baby's latch.
3. You have excess energy stores that your body could use as fuel during breastfeeding.	3. She is obese, and that's delaying milk production.
4. Your first days of breastfeeding might be affected by obesity, but there are things we can do to help.	4. Big girls, women of size
5. She has Class III obesity (instead of, "She is morbidly obese").	

Note: People-first language recognizes the potential disrespect and harm that result from labeling individuals by their disease. Just as the phrase "diabetic patient" has been replaced by the "patient with diabetes," the "obese patient" has been replaced by the "patient with obesity."

Data from Bays, H. E., McCarthy, W., Christensen, S., Wells, S., Long, J., Shah, N. N., & Primack, C. (2019). Obesity Algorithm. Retrieved from Obesity Medicine Association website: https://obesitymedicine.org/wp-content/uploads/2019/05/Obesity-Algorithm-2019.pdf

©Cecilia Jevitt 2020

woman as an individual, not as an obese person, and acknowledges that obesity is a disease. A recent Cochrane review found that no large or reliable studies give evidence-based guidance toward effectively and consistently assisting women with obesity to breastfeed (Fair et al., 2019). **Table 11-3** outlines traditional methods for assisting women with obesity who have lactation and breastfeeding problems and the obesity-related metabolic perturbations that underlie those problems.

Table 11-3 Breastfeeding Problems Associated with Obesity and Ameliorating Techniques

Obesity-Related Physiology	Manifestation During Breastfeeding	Ameliorating Techniques
Insulin resistance decreasing secretory activation	Delayed lactogenesis II, reduced milk production	1. Infant-led feeding 2. Pump to stimulate breasts between feedings until lactogenesis II has occurred 3. Warm compresses to breasts before feedings 4. Assessment of newborn for hypoglycemia 5. Assessment of newborn for weight loss 6. Teaching of mothers to monitor infant urine and stool output 7. Supplementation with donor human milk if needed 8. Postpartum follow-up every 48 hours until lactogenesis II is established and infant weight is increasing
Hyperleptinemia reducing oxytocin stimulation of myocyte contraction	Reduced letdown reflex	
Adipose producing inflammation-causing cytokines	Reduced milk production	
Decreased prolactin response to suckling	Reduced milk production	
Adipocyte proliferation and increased size	Increased breast adipose tissue and size, making infant latch more difficult	1. Assess and assist infant latch and suck
Altered microbiome	Inflammation, altered satiety signaling	2. Microbiome diets: low fat, low glycemic index, low processed sugars

Data from Anstey, E. H., & Jevitt, C. (2011). Maternal Obesity and Breastfeeding: A Review of the evidence and implications for practice. Clinical Lactation, 2(3), 11–16; Fair, F. J., Ford, G. L., & Soltani, H. (2019). Interventions for supporting the initiation and continuation of breastfeeding among women who are overweight or obese. Cochrane Database of Systematic Reviews, 17(9), CD012099; Jevitt, C. M. (2019). Obesity and socioeconomic disparities: Rethinking causes and perinatal care. Journal of Perinatal & Neonatal Nursing, 33(2), 126–135

Promoting Healthy Weight in Newborns and Other Children

Breastfeeding has been associated with reduced infant obesity in multiple studies (Dunger et al., 2007; Robinson et al., 2015; Stuart & Panico, 2016). A 2-year prospective study of 450 mother–infant pairs found that rapid weight gain during the first week of life was associated with later overweight (defined as a BMI > 85th percentile for age) (Feldman-Winter et al., 2018). Newborns who gained more than 100 g during the first week of life were 2.3 times more likely to be overweight at 2 years of age compared to infants who lost weight (p = .02). Exclusively breastfed infants were least likely to gain > 100 g in the first week, therefore being at the lowest risk for future overweight (Feldman-Winter, 2018).

In one population-based study of more than 9,600 children in the United Kingdom, the influence of breastfeeding on preventing childhood obesity was so evident that the authors labeled lack of breastfeeding as a socio-economic disparity that promoted obesity (Stuart & Panico, 2016). In a large study examining the relationship of breastfeeding to childhood weight, the WHO collected height and weight data from children ages 6 to 9 years living in 22 countries (Rito et al., 2019). Breastfeeding practice and duration were recorded through recall. Data were pooled and a multivariate analysis by Rito et al. showed the following:

Compared to children who were breastfed for at least 6 months, the odds of being obese were higher among children never breastfed or breastfed for a shorter period, in cases of both general (adjusted odds ratio [adjOR] [95% CI] 1.22 [1.16–1.28] and 1.12 [1.07–1.16], respectively) and exclusive breastfeeding (adjOR [95% CI] 1.25 [1.17–1.36] and 1.05 [0.99–1.12], respectively) (p. 227).

In a multicenter European study of more than 16,000 children, exclusive breastfeeding for 4 to 6 months was protective of overweight and obesity when compared with children never exclusively breastfed (OR 0·73, 95% CI 0·63, 0·85) (Hunsberger & IDEFICS Consortium, 2014). How breastfeeding reduces the risk for obesity is not completely understood but is likely to be mediated by olfactory and gustatory priming through human milk, learned hunger and satiety cues, glucose metabolism priming, and gut microbiome optimization. Rapid weight gain in the first 6 months of life, even in infants born with growth restriction, is strongly associated with later childhood obesity (Perng et al., 2016; Rito et al., 2019). Leptin is produced by the placenta and is a fetal growth hormone during pregnancy. In children and adults, leptin is produced in adipose tissue and signals the hypothalamus that enough fat is stored and there is no need to eat more. In animal studies, prenatal leptin exposure facilitates normal maturation of appetite-regulating neurons in the hypothalamus (Boeke et al., 2013). In one study, higher levels of leptin at 3 years of age were associated with higher BMIs from ages 3 to 7 (Boeke et al., 2013). Women with obesity are leptin resistant and may expose the fetus to hyperleptinemia that causes epigenetic changes in leptin regulation leading to childhood obesity.

Breastfeeding is an essential link between passive intrauterine nourishment and early food selection by toddlers. Gustatory and olfactory senses begin to develop during the first trimester, allowing the flavors of the mother's diet to be transmitted through the amniotic fluid and human milk. Hetherington (2017) calls this exposure "chemical continuity" (p. 118), explaining that it teaches the infant the flavors of foods that are safe to eat. Human milk containing flavors from maternal foods continues to expose infants to flavors that will become preferred tastes. The flavors of human milk vary with the constituents of maternal meals. If the maternal diet consists of nutritious foods, including fruits, vegetables, and proteins, the infant is more likely to choose nutritious foods that are less associated with obesity (Ventura, 2017). In contrast, manufactured formulas have the same taste feeding after feeding and provide less stimulation for olfactory and gustatory sensory development. Formula-fed infants are more likely to reject novel tastes, such as those from vegetables and proteins. Newborns have an innate preference for sweet and savory food and shun bitter or sour foods (Marlier & Schaal, 2005; Steiner, 1979). This preference is adaptive as toxins and rancid foods are bitter or sour; however, when toddlers have no gustatory experience with varied flavors through breastfeeding, they are likely to default to sweet or blandly flavored foods that tend to be obesogenic foods, high in processed sugars and fats (Ventura, 2017).

The early introduction of solids has repeatedly been linked with increased risk for obesity. In one study, the introduction of solids before 4 months in previously formula-fed infants was associated with a six-fold increase in the odds of obesity at age 3 years (Huh et al., 2011). Studies of breastfeeding and subsequent obesity have many confounding variables, including the lack of a standard definition of breastfeeding doses. In spite of confounders, the American Academy of Pediatrics (AAP) cites a 15% to 30% reduction in adolescent and adult obesity rates if any breastfeeding occurred in infancy compared with no breastfeeding (Johnston et al., 2012). Evidence from investigations of early and inappropriate feeding linked with childhood obesity inform the AAP recommendation that infants should be exclusively breastfed for the first 6 months of life (Johnston et al., 2012).

Newborn Metabolic Programming

Lactation has been described as an essential period of organ and tissue development and susceptibility to lifelong injury, including obesity, insulin resistance, and diabetes (Ellsworth et al., 2018). Altered glucose homeostasis priming during lactation may underpin those three pathologies. Ellsworth et al. (2018) defines **lactational programming** as "programming that stems from an exposure that occurs during the period when the mother is nursing her infant, which may lead to changes in the nutrients, hormones or bioactive components in the milk" (p. R24). The lactational period can be impacted by maternal health status, nutrition, and environmental exposures. Bartol et al. (2013) proposed that milk composition can reprogram the development of organs leading to altered health outcomes in adult life, making the lactational period a unique opportunity to promote future health. Exposures during lactational programming may amplify the effects of in utero exposures on the risk for adult metabolic diseases. Although human studies are lacking, research in rats and nonhuman primates demonstrates that overnourishment during the period of lactational programming produces hyperinsulinemia and impaired insulin signaling with subsequent insulin resistance, increased weight, and fat mass (Ellsworth et al., 2018). Australian researchers followed 20 mother/infant pairs prospectively for 12 months, recording feedings and 24-hour intake and calculating total carbohydrates and lactose to analyze the relationships between human milk carbohydrate, infant growth, and fat mass. Higher concentrations of carbohydrate were associated with increased fat mass in the children at 12 months of age (Gridneva et al., 2019). Another study found higher glucose concentrations in the colostrum of women with obese BMIs, with total protein and triglyceride levels similar when compared to the colostrum of women with normal BMIs (Fujimori et al., 2017).

Low-protein diets have been studied in lactating rats with low-protein diets leading to increased plasma insulin levels in the sucklings. Insulin levels normalized after feeding with a normal diet but increased again when protein was removed from the suckling diet. The researchers concluded that programmed abnormalities may be latent, becoming evident only when a subsequent stressor is experienced (Koletzko et al., 2009; Moura et al., 2002).

The protein content of infant formulas was studied in a multicenter, double-blind trial in Europe with 1,090 infants fed formulas with varied protein levels (Koletzko et al., 2009). Breastfed infants ($n = 588$) provided the reference values. Children who were fed infant formulas with higher protein levels had higher fat mass at 2 and 6 years. Researchers concluded that lowering the protein content of commercial formulas might result in healthier body composition in later childhood (Koletzko et al., 2009). The same German research team projected the savings that might be associated with the use of low-protein formulas as an obesity reduction strategy by estimating the costs associated with childhood obesity that could be averted if low protein formulas were used by the 19% of German infants who were formula fed (Sonntag et al., 2019). They projected €2.5 billion could be saved over the children's lifetimes if this lactational programming intervention were used. The evidence showing that increased human milk carbohydrates and low protein content in formula feedings are associated with increased fat mass must lead to consideration of the current obesity epidemic being fueled by two to three generations of formula-fed infants. Exclusive breastfeeding as a lactational programming intervention could provide the greatest health benefits and cost savings in future weight and metabolic health optimization.

Research has shown that rats preferentially choose foods high in sugar or high in fats (Morris et al., 2015). Studies of human food choices have demonstrated the same preferences. High-sugar and/or high-fat diets change neurotransmitter responses in reward and stress pathways with subsequent addictive-like behavior in seeking these foods (Morris et al., 2015). Excess dietary lipids alter hypothalamus-pituitary-adrenal (HPA) axis function (Hryhorczuk et al., 2017). The carbohydrate and lipid formulation of human milk may temper early preference imprinting for high-sugar and high-lipid foods, thereby increasing the likelihood that the child will choose foods with lower obesogenic potential.

Newborn Microbiome Support

Infants build their gut microbiome. Although microbiome differences between newborns born vaginally compared to those born by cesarean section have been studied more than differences between breastfed and formula-fed infants, numerous studies demonstrate a difference with *Bifidobacteria* more common in the microbiota of breastfed infants and *Bacteroides* and *Clostridium coccoides* more common in formula-fed infants (Fallani et al., 2010). A Swedish study of 83 infants born vaginally at term (> 37 weeks gestation) analyzed stool samples from 4 to 12 months of age. The microbiomes of newborns who were exclusively breastfed did not differ from those who received mixed human milk and formula feedings ($p > 0.05$) (Fallani et al., 2010). However, at 4 months exclusively breastfed infants had increased levels of taxa that are used as probiotics such as *L. johnsonii/L.gasseri*, *L. paracasei/L. casei*, and *B. longum*. Four-month-old formula-fed infants had elevated levels of *Clostridium difficile*, *Granulicatella adiacens*, *Citrobacter spp.*, *Enterobacter cloacae*, *Bilophila wadsworthia* (Fallani et al., 2010). The Swedish researchers concluded that breastfeeding is important in the shaping and the succession of gut microbial communities during the first year of life (Fallani et al., 2010). Once children were weaned, their microbiota were enriched in species belonging to *Clostridia* that are prevalent in adults, such as *Roseburia*, *Clostridium*, and *Anaerostipes* (Fallani et al., 2010). The gut microbiota of breastfed infants at 12 months of age were still dominated by *Bifidobacterium* and *Lactobacillus*, both considered probiotic, suggesting that cessation of breastfeeding rather than introduction of solid foods is the major driver in the development of an adult microbiota (Fallani et al., 2010).

The role of a maternal high-fat diet in the formation of the infant gut microbiome has also been investigated (Chu et al., 2016). Maternal fat intake from the intrapartum period through 4 to 6 weeks postpartum was estimated using the Dietary Screener Questionnaire validated during the United States National Health and Examination Survey. Maternal dietary fat intake ranged from 14% to 55%. Women were divided into two groups: those above (high-fat group) and those below (low-fat group) the mean fat intake of 33% (Chu et al., 2016). Infants who were exposed to a high-fat diet had microbiomes that varied from infants with low-fat diets at 6 weeks postpartum with notable depletion in *Bacteriodes* even when maternal prepregnancy BMI and mode of birth were controlled between the groups (Chu et al., 2016). Numerous genes in skeletal muscle and adipose tissue have demonstrated changes in DNA methylation after exposure to a high-fat diet (van Dijk et al., 2015). *Bacteteriodes* levels have been shown to be higher in individuals with overweight and obesity. Thus, these researchers recommend counseling women to follow low-fat diets during lactation to optimize resident taxa in the infant gut microbiome (Chu et al., 2016).

Individuals with obesity are known to have microbiomes distinct from individuals of normal weights (Gerard, 2016). Like previous studies, a Canadian study detected lower bacterial diversity in infants who were breastfed. The oligosaccharides found in human milk provide a selective metabolic substrate for a limited number of gut microbes that seem to limit gut inflammation (Azad et al., 2013). The infant gut microbiome shifts to a more adult microbiome when breastfeeding is stopped, not when solid food is introduced (Backhed et al., 2015). The probiotic-rich microbiome of breastfed infants may more appropriately signal satiety and hunger in a way that optimizes metabolic pathways during the lactation window, thereby lowering risk for obesity.

Newborn Satiety Signaling

Postulating that infants receiving human milk might have different hormonal satiety cues, Mexican researchers followed 167 mother–newborn dyads for 16 weeks postpartum (Onaka et al., 2012). Dyads were divided into groups in which infants received only human milk, were partially breastfed, and received only human milk substitutes (formula). Serum levels of ghrelin, leptin, peptide YY, and glucagon-like peptide were measured in the infants 4 hours after fasting. Ghrelin, peptide YY, and glucagon-like peptide levels were all elevated in exclusively breastfed infants compared to those who were formula fed (Onaka et al., 2012). Ghrelin, peptide YY, and glucagon-like peptide decrease gastric acid secretion and delay gastric emptying, thereby prolonging feelings of satiety. Breastfeeding is likely to prime hormonal pathways, giving infants more appropriate satiety feedback.

Hetherington (2017) summarizes numerous studies that document a behavioral mechanism for overfeeding and overweight prevention. Studies found that breastfeeding infants engage and disengage from the breast more frequently than bottle-fed infants using more facial cues to indicate interest in feeding (Hetherington, 2017). These stop and start behaviors require greater maternal responsiveness during feeding. When the breasts are empty, the infant must wait for additional milk production. Bottle-fed infants have a steady source of formula and can overeat, particularly if mothers use assertive prompts to continue eating. Assertive maternal prompts and maternal intrusiveness with infant satiety cues have been associated with higher adiposity in toddlers (Jankowski et al., 2016). Hormonal, chemical, and behavioral cues that occur during breastfeeding may work synergistically to improve recognition of satiety by breastfed infants. A satisfied infant is less likely to fuss or cry, which are signals that a parent might interpret as hunger or insufficient human milk. An important part of lactation education is teaching normal infant breastfeeding behavior and recognition of infant satiety cues.

Reduced Maternal Stress Pathways

Breastfeeding is known to promote relaxation through oxytocin pathways and reduce infections through the inclusion of mononuclear phagocytes in human milk. Could these mechanisms ameliorate the inflammation and hormonal dysregulation associated with obesity? Oxytocin has been shown to have anxiety-reducing and pro-social effects (Morais et al., 2019). Additionally, intranasal oxytocin administered in controlled studies has been shown to increase energy expenditure, reduce hedonic eating, and reduce body weight (Katzer et al., 2016). The oxytocin produced during milk ejection may produce not only maternal stress relief but may have an effect on maternal postpartum weight reduction through its role in hormonal energy expenditure and appetite pathways.

In a study of 50 lactating women of normal BMIs and 50 lactating women with obese BMIs, Brazilian researchers found that women with obesity had higher levels of melatonin in their milk (Vásquez-Gariby et al., 2019). Melatonin, produced by the pineal gland, is an important hormone essential to the regulation of circadian rhythms. Human milk samples have been found to have higher levels of melatonin when collected at night (Katzer et al., 2016). Studies have associated reduced melatonin with dyslipidemia and obesity. Exposure to artificial light at night reduces melatonin levels (Katzer et al., 2016). This could be a mechanism for the increased obesity associated with night-shift work. Melatonin and its metabolites are capable of detoxifying free radicals. Melatonin has antioxidant potential; reduces oxidative stress, which may prolong the life of phagocytes; and plays a role in the maturation of the newborn intestinal mucosal barrier (Katzer et al., 2016). The elevated levels of melatonin found in the colostrum of women with obesity may help the newborn overcome exposure to obesity-related inflammatory proteins in human milk.

Maternal Postpartum Weight Loss

The most visible healthy weight promotion strategy to be obtained through breastfeeding is maternal postpartum weight loss. Lactation has an average energy cost of 2092 kJ (500 calories) per day, depending on maternal BMI, activity, and infant intake (Lovelady, 2011). In societies where available food is scarce, adipose stores accumulated during pregnancy can be burned as fuel during lactation. This mechanism usually brings women back to their prepregnancy weights. When women bottle-feed or continue high consumption postpartum, adipose tissue accumulated during pregnancy is not lost and additional accumulation may occur. A meta-analysis of 11 studies demonstrated that women with high gestational weight gain retained 3.21 kilograms (7 lbs) at 1 to 15 years postpartum (Widen et al., 2015). Similar associations observed in another meta-analysis of 9 studies focused on longer-term **postpartum weight retention** showed similar findings with women who had high gestational weight gain retaining 4.7 kilograms (10 lbs) after 15 years postpartum (Nehring et al., 2011). Excess gestational weight gain is defined as exceeding the Institute of Medicine (2009) Guidelines for Prenatal Weight Gain. In one international systematic review and meta-analysis of more than 1 million pregnant women, 47% had gestational weight gain greater than Institute of Medicine guidelines (Goldstein et al., 2017). Obesity is associated with the development of type 2 diabetes, hypertension, and cardiac disease (Gilmore et al., 2015). Lactation could be used as a gradual weight-reduction strategy to improve future maternal health.

That moderate weight loss has no effect on lactation performance, milk volume, or milk protein, lipid, or carbohydrate concentration had been known since the 1990s (Lovelady, 2011; Lovelady et al., 1990; McCrory et al., 1999). Moderate maternal intake restriction of 2092 kJ (500 calories) without an increase in physical activity will provide a .45 kilograms (1 lbs.) weight loss per week during exclusive breastfeeding (Lovelady et al., 1990). Moderate levels of physical activity have an additive effect on weight loss and do not affect the quantity of milk production, milk composition, or infant growth (Lovelady et al., 1990). Many women have difficulty finding the time for purposeful physical activity around the demands of childcare and breastfeeding. They can be counseled that calorie restriction alone will assist with postpartum weight loss. Ideally, women with obesity are counseled to reduce dietary fats while increasing intake of fruits and vegetables to maximize the effects of epigenetic foods, olfactory and metabolic programming, and support of the infant gut microbiome (Chu et al., 2016a; Chu et al., 2016b; Dunger, 2007). Postpartum weight loss is likely to be most effective when paired with intermittent support from clinicians or a structured weight-loss support program.

Public Health Promotion Toward Obesity Prevention

Broad, macrolevel, public health measures are effective obesity-prevention tools. When obesity is decreased, the chances for successful lactation and breastfeeding are increased. Public health policies that reduce obesity indirectly include reducing endocrine-disrupting chemicals manufacture and use, reducing environmental pollution, promoting farm subsidies for local growth and distribution of fresh fruits and vegetables, improving neighborhood safety, reducing work stress, increasing the minimum wage, and promoting paid postpartum parental leaves. Public health policies that promote better nutrition include imposing special taxes on nonnutritious foods such as sodas, limiting nonnutritious foods and sodas in school meal programs, and improving the quality of foods available through public nutrition programs. Because of breastfeeding's multiple roles in obesity prevention, breastfeeding promotion policies are obesity prevention policies.

Key Points to Remember

1. Obesity is a chronic, adipose tissue disease that alters metabolic, endocrine, and immune pathways and changes the gut microbiome.
2. People-first language should be used when discussing obesity; thus people have obesity rather than people are obese. Morbid obesity is more correctly labeled class III obesity.
3. Poverty, chronic stress, racism, endocrine-disrupting chemicals, disturbed sleep, industrially manufactured foods and manufactured infant formulas are all identified as causative factors in obesity.
4. Techniques that support breastfeeding based on the physiology of obesity include early and frequent breastfeeding on demand; maternal breast stimulation between feedings; and low-fat, epigenetic diets for the breastfeeder.
5. The health benefits and obesity-preventing effects of breastfeeding to be discussed during prenatal care and lactation counseling include reduction in postpartum maternal stress; support of maternal postpartum weight loss; reduction in maternal risk for type II diabetes, hypertension, and cardiac disease; optimization of infant weight gain with reduction of risk for future overweight and obesity; reduced risk for type II diabetes, hypertension, and cardiac disease in the child through adulthood; and gut microbiome normalization for both mother and child.

Case Study

Talina is a 27-year-old first-time mother who had an uncomplicated vaginal birth of a 4309 gram (9 pounds, 8 ounces) boy at 41 weeks and 3 days. Talina's prepregnancy BMI was 38 (obesity class II). Her blood pressure was normal at her first prenatal visit. Talina's medical and surgical histories were normal. Talina told her midwife that she had been overweight as long as she could remember. The midwife offered early glucose screening that was normal. She encouraged Talina to avoid sugar-sweetened drinks and to increase the number of low glycemic index foods she ate. She also encouraged Talina to limit her prenatal weight gain to 5 to 9 kilograms (11 to 20 lbs.). Talina followed this suggestion and added 30 minutes of walking during her lunch break. Talina gained a total of 5.9 kilograms (13 lbs.). Talina's 28-week glucose screen was normal, and her blood pressure remained normal throughout pregnancy and labor.

Immediately following birth, Talina brought the baby to her chest. The baby was covered with warm blankets, and the family was given quiet time so that the newborn could find the breast. Talina's son was alert and breathing easy. He rooted and crawled, thrusting his tongue but unable to locate a nipple. Talina's large breasts fell toward the side of her body away from the baby. The midwife assisted Talina into a sitting position so that the baby could be held near a nipple. The newborn latched well on both breasts and passed meconium after the initial feed.

The newborn slept briefly after feedings during the first 36 hours and seemed to want the breast continually. Wetting and stooling were normal. By the time of discharge at 40 hours, the newborn was sleeping 2 hours between feedings. Talina called the midwife on postpartum day three (65 hours postpartum) and said that the baby wasn't satisfied after feeding and she didn't feel like there was any milk in her breasts. The midwife asked Talina to bring the baby to the office.

In the office, the newborn was alert. His mouth was moist, and his anterior fontanel was level. Talina said he had wet about six diapers the day before and was having brown stool. Talina said the baby spent about 45 minutes feeding every 2 hours. He slept for a 3-hour period during the night. Talina said she was exhausted even though her mother helped with the baby. Her mother had never breastfed her children and was urging Talina to give the baby some formula. His weight was 4211 g, a 98 g or 9.6% weight loss. The midwife reassured Talina, saying that it might be another day before her milk came in (lactogenesis II) and that she might never have a feeling of fullness. She also reassured Talina that the weight loss was within a usual range and that many newborns don't regain their birthweights until a week after birth.

The midwife assisted Talina in planning extra breast stimulation. First, Talina was encouraged to rest as much as she could between feedings. The midwife arranged for Talina to borrow a breast pump from the hospital and ordered a large shield for the pump so that the large areolas would be fully covered by the shield. Talina was also encouraged to use warm compresses on the breast during pumping to encourage letdown. Talina had heard about mother's milk teas and wondered about their use. She was encouraged to try a tea that contained fenugreek and blessed thistle and cautioned that she might need 3 to 4 days to see an effect after tea use.

By 1 week postpartum, Talina's baby had regained his birthweight and another 25 grams. He was sleeping 3 hours between nighttime feedings. Talina had continued her low glycemic index diet and wondered if she might lose weight and how safe that would be for her newborn. The midwife counseled Talina to continue choosing low glycemic index foods and avoiding sugared drinks. She could reduce to target 0.5 kilogram (1 lb) weekly weight loss. Talina also planned to walk with the baby in a stroller for 20 to 30 minutes a day. At her annual family planning a year later, Talina's BMI was 36, approximately a weight loss from her prepregnancy weight of 4.5 kilograms (10 lbs). Talina had breastfed her son for 9 months and was now trying to decrease her daily calories to maintain her lower weight. Although still within an obese BMI range, Talina's weight loss lowered her risk for future metabolic diseases, including diabetes and hypertension.

Talina's case demonstrates the impact of breastfeeding support that begins with preparation during the prenatal period, including screening for diabetes and nutrition counseling. In this case, a midwife was the primary maternity provider; however, Talina's care could have been provided by a team including nurses, obstetricians or family practice physicians, nutritionists, and lactation consultants. The key to success is that all maternity providers have an up-to-date understanding of the multiple origins of obesity, obesity as a chronic disease, the important role of breastfeeding in improving the health of those with obesity, and obesity prevention for future generations.

Case Study Questions

1. What elements of prenatal counseling in this scenario helped Talina prepare for successful breastfeeding?
2. What factors might have contributed to Talina's feeling that her newborn wasn't getting enough milk on postpartum day #3.
3. Using the case study as an example, write a plan to support breastfeeding and increase milk supply for women with obesity.

Additional Resources

Obesity Algorithm
https://obesitymedicine.org/wp-content/uploads/2019/05/Obesity-Algorithm-2019.pdf
Body Mass Index Calculator
https://www.nhlbi.nih.gov/health/educational/lose_wt/BMI/bmicalc.htm
Health Effects of Obesity, and the Genetics of Obesity
https://obesitycanada.ca/public-resources/videos-and-infographics/.
5 As of Health Pregnancy
https://obesitycanada.ca/5as-pregnancy
MyPlate Nutrition
https://www.choosemyplate.gov
https://www.fns.usda.gov/tn/myplate

References

American College of Obstetricians and Gynecologists (ACOG). (2015). Practice Bulletin No. 156: Obesity in pregnancy. *Obstetrics & Gynecology, 126*(6), e112–e126.

Anstey, E. H., & Jevitt, C. (2011). Maternal obesity and breastfeeding: A review of the evidence and implications for practice. *Clinical Lactation, 2*(3), 11–16. https://doi.org/10.1891/215805311807010422

Azad, M. B., Konya, T., Maughan, H., & Guttman, D. S. (2013). Gut microbiota of healthy Canadian infants: Profiles by mode of delivery and infant diet at 4 months. *CMAJ, 185*(5), 385–394. https://doi.org/10.1503/cmaj.121189

Babendure, J. B., Reifsnider, E., Mendias, D., Moramarco, M. W., & Davila, Y. R. (2015). Reduced breastfeeding rates among obese mothers: A review of contributing factors, clinical considerations and future directions. *International Breastfeeding Journal, 10*, 1–11. https://doi.org/10.1186/s13006-015-0046-5

Backhed, F., Roswall, J., Peng, Y., Feng, Q., Jia, H., Kovatcheva-Datchary, P., Li, Y., Xie, H., Zhong, H., Khan, M. T., Zhang, J., Li, J., Xiao, L., Al-Aama, J., Zhang, D., Lee, Y. S., Kotowska, D., Colding, C., Tremaroli, V., . . . Wang, J. (2015). Dynamics and stabilization of the human gut microbiome during the first year of life. *Cell Host & Microbe, 17*(5), 690–703. https://doi.org/10.1016/j.chom.2015.04.004

Bartol, F. F., Wiley, A. A., Miller, D. J., Silva, A. J., Roberts, K. E., Davolt, M. L., Chen, J. C., Frankshun, A.-L., Camp, M. E., Rahman, K. M., Vallet, J. L., & Bagnell, C. A. (2013). Lactation Biology Symposium: Lactocrine signaling and developmental programming. *Journal of Animal Science, 91*(2), 696–705. https://doi.org/10.2527/jas.2012-5764

Bays, H. E., McCarthy, W., Christensen, S., Wells, S., Long, J., Shah, N. N., & Primack, C. (2019). *Obesity algorithm.* Obesity Medicine Association. https://obesitymedicine.org/wp-content/uploads/2019/05/Obesity-Algorithm-2019.pdf

Bliss, E., & Whitesie, E. (2018). The gut-brain axis, the human gut microbiota and their integration in the development of obesity. *Frontiers in Physiology, 9,* 900. https://doi.org/10.3389/fphys.2018.00900

Boeke, C. E., Mantzoros, C. S., Hughes, M. D., Rifas-Shiman, S., Vallamor, E., Zera, C. A., & Gillman, M. W. (2013). Differential associations of leptin with adiposity across early childhood. *Obesity (Silver Spring), 21*(7), 1430–1437. https://doi.org/10.1002/oby.20314

Brown, K. A. (2014). Impact of obesity on mammary gland inflammation and local estrogen production. *Journal of Mammary Gland Biology & Neoplasia, 19*(2), 183–189. https://doi.org/10.1007/s10911-014-9321-0

Caamaño, M. C., Garcia, O. P., Paras, P., Palacios, J. R., & Rosado, J. L. (2019). Overvaluation of eating and satiation explains the association of food insecurity and food intake with obesity and cardiometabolic diseases. *Food & Nutrition Bulletin, 40*(4), 432–443. https://doi.org/10.1177/0379572119863558

Centers for Disease Control (CDC). (2018a). *Adult obesity facts.* https://www.cdc.gov/obesity/data/adult.html

Centers for Disease Control (CDC). (2018b). *Obesity and socioeconomic status.* https://www.cdc.gov/obesity/data/adult.html

Chu, D. M., Anthony, K. M., Ma, J., Prince, A. L., Showalter, L., Moller, M., & Aagaard, K. M. (2016a). The early infant gut microbiome varies in association with a maternal high-fat diet. *Genome Medicine, 8*(1), 77. https://doi.org/10.1186/s13073-016-0330-z

Chu, D. M., Meyer, K. M., Prince, A. L., & Aagaard, K. M. (2016b). Impact of maternal nutrition in pregnancy and lactation on offspring gut microbial composition and function. *Gut Microbes, 7*(6), 459–470. https://doi.org/10.1080/19490976.2016.1241357

Cinti, S. (2018). Adipose organ development and remodeling. *Comprehensive Physiology, 8*(4), 1357–1431. https://doi.org/10.1002/cphy.c170042

Coelho, M., Oliveira, T., & Fernandes, R. (2013). Biochemistry of adipose tissue: An endocrine organ. *Archives of Medical Science, 9*(2), 191–200. https://doi.org/10.5114/aoms.2013.33181

Darbe, P. (2017). Endocrine disruptors and obesity. *Current Obesity Reports, 6,* 18–27. https://doi.org/10.1007/s13679-017-0240-4

Darmon, N., & Drewnowski, A. (2015). Contribution of food prices and diet cost to socioeconomic disparities in diet quality and health: A systematic review and analysis. *Nutrition Reviews, 73*(10), 643–660. https://doi.org/10.1093/nutrit/nuv027

Dashti, H. S., Scheer, F. A., Jacques, P. F., Lamon-Fava, S., & Ordovas, J. M. (2015). Short sleep duration and dietary intake: Epidemiologic evidence, mechanisms, and health implications. *Advances in Nutrition, 13*(6), 648–659. https://doi.org/10.3945/an.115.008623

Dimitraki, M., Tsikouras, P., Manav, B., Gioka, T., Koutlaki, N., Zervoudis, S., & Galazios, G. (2016). Evaluation of the effect of natural and emotional stress of labor on lactation and breast-feeding. *Archives of Gynecology & Obstetrics, 293,* 317–328. https://doi.org/10.1007/s00404-015-3783-1

Dunger, D. B., Salgin, B., & Ong, K. K. (2007). Session 7: Early nutrition and later health early developmental pathways of obesity and diabetes risk. *Proceedings of the Nutrition Society, 66*(3), 451–457. https://doi.org/10.1017/S0029665107005721

Ellsworth, L., Harman, E., Padmanabhan, V., & Gregg, B. (2018). Lactational programming of glucose homeostasis: A window of opportunity. *Reproduction, 156*(2), R23–R42. https://doi.org/10.1530/REP-17-0780

Fair, F. J., Ford, G. L., & Soltani, H. (2019). Interventions for supporting the initiation and continuation of breastfeeding among women who are overweight or obese. *Cochrane Database of Systematic Reviews, 17*(9), CD012099. https://doi.org/10.1002/14651858.CD012099.pub2

Fallani, M., Young, D., Scott, J., Norin, E., Amarri, S., Adam, R., Khanna, S., Gil, A., Edwards, C. A., & Doré, J. (2010). Intestinal microbiota of 6-week-old infants across Europe: Geographic influence beyond delivery mode, breast-feeding, and antibiotics. *Journal of Pediatric Gastroenterology & Nutrition, 51*(1), 77–84. https://doi.org/10.1097/MPG.0b013e3181d1b11e

Feldman-Winter, L., Burnham, L., Grossman, X., Matlak, S., Chen, N., & Merewood, A. (2018). Weight gain in the first week of life predicts overweight at 2 years: A prospective cohort study. *Maternal Child Nutrition, 14*(1). https://doi.org/10.1111/mcn.12472

Fleming, T. P., Watkins A. J., Velasquez, M. A., Mathers J. C., Prentice, A. M., Stephenson, J., Barker, M., Saffery, R., Yajnik, C. S., Eckert, J. J., Hanson, M. A., Forrester, T., Gluckman, P.

D., & Godfrey, K. M. (2018). Origins of lifetime health around the time of conception: Causes and consequences. *Lancet, 391*, 1842–1852. https://doi.org/10.1016/S0140-6736(18)30312-X

Fujimori, M., França, E. L., Morais, T. C., Fiorin, V., Abreu, L. C., & Honorio-França, A. C. (2017). Cytokine and adipokine are biofactors can act in blood and colostrum of obese mothers. *BioFactors, 43*(2), 243–250. https://doi.org/10.1002/biof.1339

Gerard, P. (2016). Gut microbiota and obesity. *Cellular & Molecular Life Sciences, 73*(1), 147–162.

Gilmore L. A., Klempel-Donchenko, M., & Redman, L. M. (2015). Pregnancy as a window to future health: Excessive gestational weight gain and obesity. *Seminars in Perinatology, 39*(4), 296–303. https://doi.org/10.1053/j.semperi.2015.05.009

Goldstein, R. F., Abell, S. K., Ranasinha, S., Misso, M., Boyle, J. A., Black, M. H., Li, N., Hu, G., Corrado, F., Rode, L., Kim, Y. J., Haugen, M., Song, W. O., Kim, M. H., Bogaerts, A., Devlieger, R., Chung, J. H., & Teede, H. J. (2017). Association of gestational weight gain with maternal and infant outcomes: A systematic review and meta-analysis. *JAMA, 317*(21), 2207–2225. https://doi.org/10.1001/jama.2017.3635

Gordon-Larsen, P. (2014). Food availability/convenience and obesity. *Advances in Nutrition, 5*, 809–817. https://doi.org/10.3945/an.114.007070

Gridneva, A., Rea, A., Tie, W. J., Lai, C. T., Kugananthan, S., Ward, L. C., & Geddes, D. T. (2019). Carbohydrate in human milk and body composition of term infants during the first 12 months of lactation. *Nutrients, 11*(7), pii:E1472. https://doi.org/10.3390/nu11071472

Gross, R. S., Mendelsohn, A. L., Fierman, A. H., Hauser, N. R., & Messito, M. J. (2014). Maternal infant feeding behaviors and disparities in early child obesity. *Childhood Obesity, 10*(2), 145–151. https://doi.org/10.1089/chi.2013.0140

Hetherington, M. M. (2017). Understanding infant eating behaviour – Lessons learned from observation. *Physiology & Behavior, 176*, 117–124. https://doi.org/10.1016/j.physbeh.2017.01.022

Hicken, M., Lee, H., & Hing, A. (2018). The weight of racism: Vigilance and racial inequalities in weight-related measures. *Social Science & Medicine, 199*, 157–166. https://doi.org/10.1016/j.socscimed.2017.03.058

Hoffman, E. E., Mair, T. T. M., Hunter, B. A., Prince, D. M., & Tebes, J. K. (2018). Neighborhood sexual violence moderates women's perceived safety in urban neighborhoods. *Journal of Community Psychology, 46*(1), 79–94. https://doi.org/10.1002/jcop.21917

Hryhorczuk, C., Decarie-Spain, L., Sharma, S., Daneault, C., Rosiers, C. D., Alquier, T., & Fulton, S. (2017). Saturated high-fat feeding independent of obesity alters hypothalamus-pituitary -adrenal axis function but not anxiety-like behaviour. *Psychoneuroendocrinology, 83*, 142–149. https://doi.org/10.1016/j.psyneuen.2017.06.002

Huh, S. Y., Rifas-Shiman, S. L., Taveras, E. M., Oken, E., & Gillman M. W. (2011). Timing of solid food introduction and risk of obesity in preschool-aged children. *Pediatrics, 127*, e544–e551. https://doi.org/10.1542/peds.2010-0740

Hunsberger, M., & IDEFICS Consortium. (2014). Early feeding practices and family structure: Associations with overweight in children. *Proceedings of the Nutrition Society, 73*(1), 132–136. https://doi.org/10.1017/S0029665113003741

Institute of Medicine and National Research Council. (2009). *Weight gain during pregnancy: Reexamining the guidelines*. National Academies Press. https://doi.org/10.17226/12584

Jankowski, M., Broderick, T., & Gutkowska, J. (2016). Oxytocin and carioprotection in diabetes and obesity. *BMC Endocrine Disorders, 16*(1), 34. https://doi.org/10.1186/s12902-016-0110-1

Jevitt, C. M. (2019). Obesity and socioeconomic disparities: Rethinking causes and perinatal care. *Journal of Perinatal & Neonatal Nursing, 33*(2), 126–135. https://doi.org/10.1097/JPN.0000000000000400

Johnston, M., Landers, S., Noble, L., Szucs, K., & Viehmann, L. (2012). American Academy of Pediatrics. (2012). Breastfeeding and the use of human milk. *Pediatrics, 129*(3), e827–841. https://doi.org/10.1542/peds.2011-3552

Katzer, D., Pauli, L., Mueller, A., Reutter, H., Reinsberg, J., Fimmers, R., Bartmann, P., & Bagci, S. (2016). Melatonin concentrations and antioxidative capacity of human breast milk according to gestational age and the time of day. *Journal of Human Lactation, 32*(4), NP105–NP110. https://doi.org/10.1177/0890334415625217

Koletzko, B., von Kries, R., Closa, R., Escribano, J., Scaglioni, S., Giovannini, M., Beyer, J., Demmelmair, H., Gruzfeld, D., Dobrzanska, A., Sengier, A., Langhendries, J., Cachera, M. R., Grote,

V., & European Childhood Obesity Trial Study Group. (2009). Lower protein in infant formula is associated with lower weight up to age 2 y: A randomized clinical trial. *American Journal of Clinical Nutrition, 89*(6), 1836–1845. https://doi.org/10.3945/ajcn.2008.27091

Kwon, E. J., & Kim, Y. J. (2017). What is fetal programming?: A lifetime of health is under the control of in utero health. *Obstetrics & Gynecology Science, 60*(6), 506–519. https://doi.org/10.5468/ogs.2017.60.6.506

Lee, S., & Kelleher, S. L. (2016). Biological underpinnings of breastfeeding challenges: The role of genetics, diet, and environment on lactation physiology. *American Journal of Physiology, Endocrinology & Metabolism, 311*(2), e405–e422. https://doi.org/10.1152/ajpendo.00495.2015

Li, Y. (2018). Epigenetic mechanisms link maternal diets and gut microbiome to obesity in the offspring. *Frontiers in Genetics, 9,* 342. https://doi.org/10.3389/fgene.2018.00342

Liu, Q., Shi, J., Duan, P., Liu, B., Li, T., Wang, C., Li, H., Yang, T., Gan, Y., Wang, X., Cao, S., & Lu, Z. (2018). Is shift work associated with a higher risk of overweight or obesity? A systematic review of observational studies with meta-analysis. *International Journal of Epidemiology, 47*(6), 1956–1971. https://doi.org/10.1093/ije/dyy079

Lovelady, C. (2011). Balancing exercise and food intake with lactation to promote post-partum weight loss. *Proceedings of the Nutrition Society, 70,* 181–184. https://doi.org/10.1017/S002966511100005X

Lovelady, C. A., Lonnerdal, B., & Dewey, K. G. (1990). Lactation performance of exercising women. *The American Journal of Clinical Nutrition, 52*(1), 103–109. https://doi.org/10.1093/ajcn/52.1.103

Marlier, L., & Schaal, B. (2005). Human newborns prefer human milk: Conspecific milk odor is attractive without postnatal exposure. *Child Development, 76*(1), 155–168. https://doi.org/10.1111/j.1467-8624.2005.00836.x

McCrory, M. A., Nommsen-Rivers, L. A., Mole, P. A., Lonnerdal, B., & Dewey, K. G. (1999). Randomized trial of the short-term effects of dieting compared with dieting plus aerobic exercise on lactation performance. *The American Journal of Clinical Nutrition, 69,* 959–967. https://doi.org/10.1093/ajcn/69.5.959

McFarland, M. J., Taylor, J., & McFarland, C. A. S. (2018). Weighed down by discriminatory policing: Perceived unfair treatment and black-white disparities in waist circumference. *SSM-Population Health, 5,* 210–217. https://doi.org/10.1016/j.ssmph.2018.07.002

Morais, T. C., Honorio-França, A. C., Fujimori, M., de Quental, O. B., Pessoa, R. S., Franca, E. L., & de Abreu, L. C. (2019). Melatonin action on the activity of phagocytes from the colostrum of obese women. *Medicina, 55*(10), E625. https://doi.org/10.3390/medicina55100625

Morris, M. J., Beilharz, J. E., Maniam, J., Reichelt, A. C., & Westbrook, R. F. (2015). Why is obesity such a problem in the 21st century? The intersection of palatable food, cues and reward pathways, stress, and cognition. *Neuroscience & Biobehavioral Reviews, 58,* 36–45. https://doi.org/10.1016/j.neubiorev.2014.12.002

Moura, A. S., Franco de Sa, C. C., Cruz, H. G., & Costa C. L. (2002). Malnutrition during lactation as a metabolic imprinting factor inducing the feeding pattern of offspring rats when adult. The role of insulin and leptin. *Brazilian Journal of Medical & Biological Research, 35*(5), 617–622. https://doi.org/10.1590/s0100-879x2002000500016

Mumtaz, S., AlSaif, A., Wray, S., & Noble, D. (2015). Inhibitory effect of visfatin and leptin on human and rat myometrial contractility. *Life Sciences, 125,* 57–62. https://doi.org/10.1016/j.lfs.2015.01.020

Nehring, I., Schmoll, S., Beyerlein, A., Hauner, H., & von Kries, R. (2011). Gestational weight gain and long-term postpartum weight retention: A meta-analysis. *The American Journal of Clinical Nutrition, 94,* 1225–1231. https://doi.org/10.3945/ajcn.111.015289

Nelson, J. W., Scammell, M. K., Hatch, E. E., & Webster, T. F. (2012). Social disparities in exposure to bisphenol A and polyfluoroalkyl chemicals: A cross-sectional study within NHANES 2003–2006. *Environmental Health, 11,* 10. https://doi.org/10.1186/1476-069X-11-10

Niwayama, R., Nishitani, S., Takamura, R., Shinohara, K., Honda, S., Miyamura, T., Nakao, Y., & Araki-Nagahashi, M. (2017). Oxytocin mediates a calming effect on postpartum mood in primiparous mothers. *Breastfeeding Medicine, 12*(2), 103–109. https://doi.org/10.1089/bfm.2016.0052

Onaka, T., Takayanagi, Y., & Yoshida, M. (2012). Roles of oxytocin neurons in the control of stress, energy metabolism, and social behaviour. *Journal of Neuroendocrinology, 24*(4), 587–598. https://doi.org/10.1111/j.1365-2826.2012.02300.x

Perng, W., Rifas-Shiman, S. L., Kramer, M. S., Haugaard, L. K., Oken, E., Gillman, M. W., & Belfort, M. B. (2016). Early weight gain, linear growth, and mid-childhood blood pressure novelty and significance. *Hypertension, 67*(2), 301–308. https://doi.org/10.1161/HYPERTENSIONAHA.115.06635

Preusting, I., Brumley, J., Odibo, L., Spatz, D. L., & Louis, J. M. (2017). Obesity as a predictor of delayed lactogenesis II. *Journal of Human Lactation, 33*(4), 684–691. https://doi.org/10.1177/0890334417727716

Ranjit, N., Siefert, K., & Padmanabhan, V. (2010). Bisphenol-A and disparities in birth outcomes: A review and directions for future research. *Journal of Perinatology, 30*(1), 2–9. https://doi.org/10.1038/jp.2009.90

Rito, A. I., Buoncristiano, M., Spinelli, A., Salanave, B., Kunešová, M., Hejgaard, T., Solano, G., Fijalkowska, A., Sturua, L., Hyska, J., Kelleher, C., Duleva, V., Mialnović, M. S., Sant'Angelo, V. F., Abdrakhmanova S., Kujundzic E., Peterkova, V., Gualtieri, A., Pudule, I., . . . Breda, J. (2019). Association between characteristics at birth, breastfeeding and obesity in 22 countries: The WHO European childhood obesity surveillance initiative-COSI 2015/2017. *Obesity Facts, 12*(2), 226–243. https://doi.org/10.1159/000500425

Robinson, S. M., Crozier, S. R., Harvey N. C., Barton, B. D., Law, C. M., Godfrey, K. M., Cooper, C., & Inskip, H. M. (2015). Modifiable early-life risk factors for childhood adiposity and overweight: An analysis of their combined impact and potential for prevention. *American Journal of Clinical Nutrition, 101*(2), 368–75. https://doi.org/10.3945/ajcn.114.094268

Rubin, R. (2018). Obesity tied to income, education, but not in all populations. *JAMA, 319*(6), 540. https://doi.org/10.1001/jama.2018.0381

Sanmiguel, C., Gupta, A., & Mayer, E. (2015). Gut microbiome and obesity: A plausible explanation for obesity. *Current Obesity Reports, 4*(2), 250–261. https://doi.org/10.1007/s13679-015-0152-0

Sonntag, D., De Bock, F., Totzauer, M., & Koletzko, B. (2019). Assessing the lifetime cost-effectiveness of low-protein infant formula as an early obesity prevention strategy: The CHOP randomized trial. *Nutrients, 11*(7), 1653. https://doi.org/10.3390/nu11071653

Statistics Canada. (n.d.). *Body mass index, overweight or obese, self-reported, adult, age groups (18 years and older)*. https://www150.statcan.gc.ca/t1/tbl1/en/tv.action?pid=1310009620

Steiner, J. E. (1979). Human facial expressions in response to taste and smell stimulation. *Advances in Child Development Behaviour, 13*, 257–295. https://doi.org/10.1016/S0065-2407(08)60349-3

Stuart, B., & Panico, L. (2016). Early-childhood body mass index trajectories: Evidence from a prospective, nationally representative British cohort study. *Nutrition & Diabetes, 7*(6), e198. https://doi.org/10.1038/nutd.2016.6

Thompson, A. L., & Bentley, M. E. (2013). The critical period of infant feeding for the development of early disparities in obesity. *Social Science & Medicine (1982), 97*, 288–296. https://doi.org/10.1016/j.socscimed.2012.12.007

United Nations. (n.d.). *Sustainable development goals*. https://sustainabledevelopment.un.org/?menu=1300

van Dijk, S. J., Tellam, R. L., Morrison, J. L., Muhlhausler, B. S., & Mollo, P. L. (2015). Recent developments on the role of epigenetics in obesity and metabolic disease. *Clinical Epigenetics, 7*, 66. https://doi.org/ https://doi.org/10.1186/s13148-015-0101-5

Vásquez-Gariby, E. M., Larrosa-Haro, A., Guzmán-Mercado, E., Muñoz-Esparza, N., García-Arellano, S., Muñoz-Valle, F., & Romero-Velarde, E. (2019). Serum concentration of appetite-regulating hormones of mother-infant dyad according to the type of feeding. *Food, Science & Nutrition, 7*(2), 869–874. https://doi.org/10.1002/fsn3.938

Ventura, A. K. (2017). Does breastfeeding shape food preferences linked to obesity. *Annals of Nutrition & Metabolism, 70*(suppl 3), 8–15. https://doi.org/10.1159/000478757

Vickers, M. (2014). Developmental programming and transgenerational transmission of obesity. *Annals of Nutrition & Metabolism, 64*, 26–34. https://doi.org/10.1159/000360506

Whitfield, G. P., Carlson, S. A., Ussery, E. N., Watson, K. B., Brown, D. R., Berrigan, D., & Fulton, J. E. (2018). Racial and ethnic differences in perceived safety barriers to walking, United States National Health Interview Survey–2015. *Preventative Medicine, 114*, 57–63. https://doi.org/10.1016/j.ypmed.2018.06.003

Widen, E. M., Whyatt, R. M., Hoepner, L. A., Ramirez-Carvey, J., Oberfield, S. E., Hassoun, A., Perera, F. P., Gallagher, D., & Rundle, A. G. (2015). Excessive gestational weight gain is associated with long-term body fat and weight retention at 7 y postpartum in African American and Dominican mothers with underweight, normal, and overweight prepregnancy BMI. *The American Journal of Clinical Nutrition, 102*(6), 1460–1467. https://doi.org/10.3945/ajcn.115.116939

Wilde, P., Steiner, A., & Ver Ploeg, M. (2017). For low-income Americans, living < 1 mile (< 1.6 km) from the nearest supermarket is not associated with self-reported household food security. *Current Developments in Nutrition, 1*(11), e001448. https://doi.org/10.3945/cdn.117.001446

World Health Organization. (2017). *Prevalence of obesity among adults, BMI > 30, age-standardized.* http://apps.who.int/gho/data/view.main.REGION2480A?lang=en

World Health Organization. (2019, September 23). *Broken food systems and poor diets are increasing rates of obesity.* http://www.emro.who.int/media/news/broken-food-systems-and-poor-diets -are-increasing-rates-of-obesity.html

CHAPTER 12

Infant Feeding in Emergencies: Where the Safety Net Falls Away

Michelle Pensa Branco

"Exclusively breastfed infants have food security and immunological protection against the illnesses most likely to make them sick in a humanitarian setting."

All of the things that are bad for babies and young children get worse in an emergency. And breastfeeding protects against them all.

LEARNING OBJECTIVES

1. Explain how breastfeeding health promotion protects infant and maternal health during the emergency and recovery period.
2. Describe examples of interventions that protect breastfeeding and appropriate infant feeding practices in emergency settings.
3. List six key areas for optimal Infant Youth Child Feeding Emergency (IYCF-E) response.

KEY WORDS

- **Global Strategy on Infant and Young Child Feeding (2003):** The Global Strategy on Infant and Young Child Feeding, jointly created by the World Health Organization (WHO) and the United National International Children's Emergency Fund (UNICEF), is a global guidance document with the aim of promoting, protecting, and supporting IYCF. It has been adopted by the World Health Assembly (WHA), the decision-making body of the WHO, and forms the basis for IYCF policy globally, with the objective of raising awareness of the importance of IYCF, increasing government commitment to funding IYCF programs and services, and creating an enabling environment for parents and caregivers.
- **Emergency:** An emergency is any situation with the potential to cause life-threatening or significant harm to an individual, household, community,

nation, or multiple nations and which does or could outstrip the capacity of local resources to respond. Emergencies can take many forms and typically do not impact all members of affected groups equitably. The term *emergency* is often used interchangeably with the term *disaster*, though the latter more often refers to a sudden-onset emergency affecting a specific geographic area, such as a tornado.

- **IFE Core Group:** The Infant Feeding in Emergencies Core Group is a collaborative interagency expert group created to review and issue guidance on IYCF-E for policy makers and program managers.
- **Infant and Young Child Feeding (IYCF):** Global term for nutrition guidance and programs from pregnancy through 23 months of age. IYCF includes breastfeeding, complementary feeding and nutrition for the non-breastfed child, and maternal nutrition through pregnancy and lactation. In some documents, Maternal, Infant & Young Child Nutrition (MIYCN) is also used to refer to similar guidance and programs.
- **Infant and Young Child Feeding in Emergencies ("IYCF-E"):** Global term for nutrition guidance and programs from pregnancy through 23 months of age during emergencies.
- **Infant and Young Child Feeding in Emergencies: Operational Guidance for Emergency Relief Staff and Programme Managers v 3.0 (Ops Guidance):** Resource developed for policy makers, program managers, and staff providing support to children 0 to 23 months of age and their parents and caregivers in emergencies. This is the core reference document for the development and implementation of evidence-based IYCF-E policies and practices.
- **International Code of Marketing of Breast-milk Substitutes (the Code):** Passed as a resolution of the WHA in 1981 and updated periodically through subsequent WHA resolutions, the Code is a key mechanism for preventing the inappropriate distribution and promotion of human milk substitutes (formula) in emergency and humanitarian settings. Resolutions WHA49.15, WHA55.25, WHA59.21, and WHA63.23 are of particular relevance to emergency and humanitarian settings.
- **Sphere Standards:** The Sphere Standards are the most commonly recognized set of minimum humanitarian standards, which are widely used by nongovernmental organizations in humanitarian response.

Overview

In an **emergency**, infant and maternal morbidity and mortality typically rise faster than in the general population. Infants and young children (< 24 months) who are not breastfed in an emergency face significantly higher risks of illness and death, primarily from diarrheal disease and respiratory infections and aggravated by preexisting malnutrition or other chronic illnesses. A breastfed child is a food secure child in an emergency. Protecting existing breastfeeding practices and supporting initiation and continued exclusivity through an emergency and recovery period are critical to mitigating the risks on this vulnerable population. However, the effectiveness of interventions often depends largely on preemergency practices and capacity. An effective response requires coordination between functional areas. Targeted health promotion messages and evidence-based support interventions at each stage of the emergency preparedness, response, and recovery process can improve outcomes and protect life and long-term well-being.

I. Why are Infants and Young Children at Increased Risk in Emergencies?

Infants and young children are at increased risk in emergencies due to their unique physiological and developmental characteristics as well as their dependency on caregivers for basic care (Council & Committee on Pediatric Emergency Medicine, 2015). Vulnerabilities include increased surface and permeability of skin, more rapid respiration rate, inability to take protective action or flee and immaturity of the immune system (Council & Committee on Pediatric Emergency Medicine, 2015). Infants and young children have specific dietary requirements met by human milk and a greater intake per kilogram of body weight than older children or adults (Council & Committee on Pediatric Emergency Medicine, 2015). Although infants over 6 months and children may consume many table foods, their developmental and nutritional needs may not be met by foods available in an emergency, particularly where those foods are not aligned to the prevailing cultural practices.

Crowded unhygienic conditions coupled with stress increase the risk of the illnesses most likely to cause severe morbidity and mortality in infants and young children. Such conditions should be expected regardless of the broader macroeconomic context, though preexisting food insecurity, poverty, and underdeveloped local, regional and national infrastructure aggravate risks further. Breastfeeding rates are usually eroded during emergencies, which is when human milk is most critical.

> *The belief that stress causes breastmilk to "dry up" or "spoil" is common across many cultures, including among some health care workers. Unsettled infant behaviour during an emergency may reinforce this belief and lead to erosion of breastfeeding. For example:*
>
> - *Fussiness at the breast that did not occur before is likely due to delayed letdown.*
> - *Increased cueing to feed is normal in disrupted circumstances as children seek closeness for comfort and reassurance.*
> - *Delaying or shortening feeds to attend to emergency-related tasks may cause temporary down-regulation of supply.*

While much of the research in emergency response has focused on low- and middle-income countries, increased risks are also born by infants and young children in high-income countries. There remains relatively little **IYCF-E** focused research in high-income contexts, but erosion of breastfeeding practices is a common theme across multiple settings (DeYoung et al., 2018; Gribble, Peterson, & Brown, 2019; Summers & Bilukha, 2018; Theurich & Grote, 2017).

II. How Breastfeeding Helps

Globally, almost half of the deaths of children under age 5 years are nutrition related, with malnutrition, respiratory infection, and diarrheal disease accounting for the majority of deaths, particularly in children under the age of 1 year (Liu et al., 2016). These risks of death are increased in emergencies. Breastfeeding mitigates many of the most common dangers that infants and young children face in disaster and humanitarian settings.

Breastfeeding provides complete nutrition for the infant under 6 months and continues to provide a substantial proportion of calories and nutrients through the first year. Initiation of breastfeeding within the first hour of life ensures that breastfeeding gets off to the right start and supports continued exclusivity to 6 months, followed by continued breastfeeding alongside complementary foods to age 2 and beyond (WHO, 2003). Births that occur in emergency settings benefit from this early initiation and the practices that surround it, such as skin to skin (Saxton et al., 2014). Early frequent feeding of colostrum and skin-to-skin contact help to prevent low blood sugar and stabilize infant temperature, while also reducing the risk of postpartum hemorrhage (WHO, 2017).

Infants under 6 months are among the most vulnerable in emergencies. Exclusively breastfed infants have food security and immunological protection against the illnesses most likely to make them sick in a humanitarian setting. While complementary foods are needed after the first 6 months, short-term return to exclusive breastfeeding when other acceptable food sources are not available is viable, and weaned older children may also return to drinking human milk as a survival food.

At the family unit level, infants who are not exclusively breastfed require significant resources on the part of the caregiver to obtain and prepare a consistent supply of human milk substitutes, such as infant formula. These resources, which include financial costs and time spent seeking, obtaining, and preparing human milk substitutes, can be preserved for other family needs. Breastfeeding primarily requires a contribution of time and care on the part of women, whose needs should be prioritized in order for them to focus on breastfeeding and care of their children. Women are at increased risk of gender-based violence during emergencies and bear much of the burden of household disruptions. In addition, to provide protection against postpartum hemorrhage (Saxton et al., 2014), breastfeeding provides a buffer against stress responses (Altemus et al., 1995) and suppresses menstruation and fertility (McNeilly, 2001), protecting both maternal health and the mother's ability to care for her infant and fulfill other family needs.

At the community level, the costs of nonbreastfed children are multiplied during emergencies. Procurement and distribution of human milk substitutes are only part of the cost because parents and caregivers must also have access to education on the safe use of substitutes in the emergency context as well as access to facilities, such as washing stations, to permit an acceptable level of hygiene. Moreover, even with controlled distribution and adequate levels of hygiene, infants and young children who are not breastfed will be at greater risk of illness and are more likely to require assessment and medical treatment.

Populations who have robust breastfeeding practices and knowledge are able to help themselves and each other, with far fewer external resources. While the aim is for children to be breastfed by their own parents, disasters may lead to separation of the breastfeeding dyad and some infants and young children will have been fed with human milk substitutes prior to the occurrence of the disaster. Shared or co-nursing by available healthy mothers, either directly at the breast or expressed into cups for feeding, is practiced by many cultures. In a disaster, this practice can serve as a critical lifeline and support for both the donor, and recipient families can be a cornerstone of a successful response (Azad et al., 2019). In the Philippines, where natural disasters regularly disrupt communities, Innes Fernandez and the national mother support organization Arugaan have developed a breastfeeding support program that includes shared breastfeeding and relactation. The interventions have been successfully deployed in multiple major disasters, including Typhoon Haiyan in 2015 (Garg et al., 2016).

Parents, support people, and health care providers who have the knowledge and skills to initiate and maintain exclusive breastfeeding for 6 months and then continue breastfeeding through the second year and beyond are critical to the survival of infants and young children in emergencies. Breastfeeding support is a disaster risk reduction (DRR) activity, increasing individual resilience to emergencies as well as reducing the resources required at the community level to keep vulnerable infants and young children safe and healthy through an emergency and recovery.

III. Protecting and Supporting Breastfeeding

Investment in breastfeeding support ensures that breastfeeding is maximized within each population and provides for an informed and trained workforce of health care providers and helpers who can provide education and skilled support before, during, and after a disaster. The Operational Guidance for **Infant and Young Child Feeding** in Emergencies v. 3.0 (ENN & UNICEF, IFE Core Group, 2017) is the primary global guidance document for policy makers, program managers, and field operations staff. The Ops Guidance is evidence based and expert developed to provide practical guidance and resources at all levels, endorsed at the WHA (WHO, 2018a) and referenced in the **Global Strategy on Infant and Young Child Feeding** as well as the Sphere Standards (Sphere Association, 2018).

1. Endorse or develop IYCF-E policies.
2. Train staff in IYCF-E interventions and best practices.
3. Coordinate activities in a multi-sectoral approach.
4. Assess and monitor IYCF-E needs and response.
5. Protect, promote, and support optimal practices, including breastfeeding.
6. Minimize the risks of artificial feedings. (IFE Core Group, 2017, p. 4)

The six steps are specific to IYCF-E, and the expectation is that they will also be integrated into wider maternal–child health and **IYCF** policies and programs. High-quality maternal–infant health services are supported by frameworks such as the Baby-friendly Hospital Initiative (BFHI), called the Baby-friendly Initiative (BFI) in Canada. In what is sometimes described as a handshake, comprehensive IYCF policies and programs enable effective IYCF-E responses, which in turn supports families through recovery without eroding healthy feeding practices. Integration of IYCF-E policy, training, and practices in IYCF and maternal–child health guidance as well as in relevant guidance in other sectors, such as logistics or communications, ensures comprehensive support and consistent messaging (See **Figure 12-1**).

Minimizing the risks of artificial feeding begins with maximizing supports for breastfeeding, including provision of donor human milk and support for relactation where possible. Safer procurement and distribution of human milk substitutes require the cooperation of several sectors to ensure that solutions are Acceptable, Feasible, Affordable, Sustainable, and Safe (AFASS). The risks of minimizing artificial feedings also includes eliminating look-alike products such as toddler milks

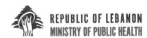 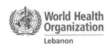

Infant and Young Child Feeding in Lebanon
A JOINT STATEMENT - December 2019

Amidst the economic crisis that Lebanon is going through and the various initiatives for help amongst community members, the Ministry of Public Health and partners and based on the **Infant and Young Child Feeding Policy**, remind of:

✓ The importance of promoting and supporting breastfeeding and protecting the right of children to be breastfed and of mothers to breastfeed to ensure appropriate care for infants and young children.

✓ The **importance of abiding by Law 47/2008** and the protection against unethical marketing of products that replace breastfeeding.

Rationale	Recommendations
Protecting and supporting exclusive breastfeeding in normal situations and particularly in economic crises is key, as breastfeeding provides a protective measure against the increased risks of illness among infants, ensures safe and available nutrition for the baby and provides a comforting environment for both the mother and baby.	**Exclusive breastfeeding** of infants during the first six months, with no introduction of other food or drinks even water, is the ideal natural nutrition, as it meets the nutritional requirements of the infant and provides valuable protection from disease and infection. After 6 months, the infants' requirements increase beyond what is provided by breast milk alone, and therefore infants should receive complementary foods in addition to breast milk up to two years and beyond.

What you can do to support and protect breastfeeding?

1. **Support exclusive breastfeeding for the first 6 months of life and continued breastfeeding up to 2 years or beyond**
   ✓ Prioritize access to food and safe water to mothers with infants less than 2 years of age
   ✓ Encourage and support mothers to continue breastfeeding. Mothers may be stressed; therefore, it is important to provide assurance and safe havens for them to exclusively breastfeed.
   ✓ Identify and refer mothers and babies who need more support with breastfeeding to a lactation consultant[1].

2. **Support complementary feeding** and ensure that it is age appropriate, nutritionally adequate, and safely prepared.

3. **Protect breastfeeding** and abide by Law 47/2008 based on the International Code of Marketing of Breast-Milk Substitutes including:
   ☒ **Never** include **infant formula or any other milk products** including powdered or Ultra High Temperature milk in the **general distribution of food or food baskets.**
   ☒ **Never** accept unsolicited **donations** of any milk products or distribute donations to the general population.

What can you do to help families with infants less than one year who are not breastfed?
   ✓ Refer to a health care center or to a lactation consultant.
   ✓ Support the family with food and other needed items or refer to existing support programs.

Breast-milk substitutes or infant formula should only be provided discretely to infants who need it and in accordance with Law 47/2008.

✓ Infant formula should only be sourced and provided when:
   o The need has been confirmed by a health professional i.e. the mother and baby have been assessed
   o There is access to adequate clean water and resources are available to continuously provide appropriate infant formula with safe preparation, with family support and access to health services,
   o The infant formula is purchased and in line with Law 47/2008 including being **unbranded.**

For more information please contact the Ministry of Public Health, Infant and Young Child Nutrition Program, Beirut - **Hotline: 1214**

---
[1] Refer to list of lactation specialists
This joint statement was developed with support from IOCC Lebanon

Figure 12-1 Joint Infant Feeding Statement. Early release of a joint statement clarifies applicable policy and provides interim situation-specific guidance and key messages. The IFE Core Group provides a model statement.

Reproduced from Republic of Lebanon Ministry of Public Health, Infant and young child feeding in Lebanon a joint statement - December 2019

as well as products that cannot be used safely, such as feeding and breast pumps (ENN & UNICEF, IFE Core Group, 2017). Donations of infant formula and related products are associated with increased use and morbidity and mortality among recipients of such donations (Hipgrave et al., 2012). Eliminating donation of products requires the coordinated efforts of policy makers, program managers, field staff, and communications experts, as well as ongoing monitoring and reporting in the field. The full implementation of the **International Code of Marketing of Breast-Milk Substitutes (the Code)** creates an environment that enables safer responses (WHO, 1981). The Code requires plain-language labeling that outlines the risks of use and requirements for safe preparation of human milk substitutes (formula) and prohibits the donation of covered products in emergency situations (WHO, 1981).

Supporting breastfeeding and appropriate complementary feeding in emergencies requires a multi-sectoral response. Hierarchical management protocols that create silos are particularly challenging for infants and young children because their needs cross functional areas. For example, registration of people in need is a major early-response function in a disaster. Registration must include the infant feeding information to trigger triage and appropriate referrals to services. Separate registration areas that are also set up to provide services to meet urgent, immediate needs are one solution. Priority registration areas also reduce the time spent in long waiting lines that may lead to delaying or replacement of breastfeeds due to family separation or a lack of privacy.

Parent–baby spaces, often called baby tents, form an important part of IY-CF-E response. Bringing breastfeeding mothers together allows for mutual emotional support and delivery of IYCF-E programming in a supportive safe space. Parent–baby spaces have been deployed successfully in multiple humanitarian settings, both for short- and long-term responses. Following the 2010 earthquake in Haiti, a network of baby tents provided comprehensive supports to women and their babies. Infant feeding practices prior to the earthquake were not optimal, with only 54% of mothers initiating breastfeeding and high rates of mixed feeding (Ayoya et al., 2013). Infants who participated in the baby tent program had a 70% exclusivity rate, with a further 10% moving from mixed to exclusive breastfeeding over the course of their participation (Ayoya et al., 2013). Comparatively, a postearthquake study found that fewer than 20% of infants under 6 months were exclusively breastfeeding (Dörnemann & Kelly, 2013). Parent–baby spaces have been used successfully in high-income settings (Hargest-Slade & Gribble, 2015) as well as for refugee populations (Alsamman, 2015).

Why are donations of human milk substitutes such as infant formula and feeding equipment, such as teats and breast pumps, prohibited in emergencies?

- Large quantities of donations overwhelm responders, leading to untargeted distribution and overuse.
- Donated products are frequently inappropriate and cannot be used safely.
- Labeling is often misleading and/or incomplete and may be in the wrong language for the affected population.

Communications are a critical function in emergency response, for both public-facing messages and responders. Health promotion messages about breastfeeding and complementary foods that are used in normal times are intended to provide a base of knowledge and skills within the targeted population. In an emergency, ensuring that public health messages reach affected populations requires planning for both communications and subject matter expertise.

Preventing myths or misinformation from taking hold requires public health messages to be deployed quickly because the public will fill in knowledge gaps with whatever is available. Using the Centers for Disease Control and Prevention (CDC) model for crisis and emergency response communications (CERC), the cycle of planning, deployment, recovery, and evaluation are ongoing activities that are adapted to respond to each emergency and then integrated into evaluation results for the next planning cycle. Communications in the acute phase of an emergency are focused on speed, accuracy, and specific calls to action, rather than on general information or education. To be useful, emergency messages must include actions that are feasible and targeted to the audience, taking into account language, literacy levels, and access to information sources.

Each emergency and affected community is unique and will require messages and supports specific to the circumstances on the ground. Because emergencies are situations that require a response beyond the normal capacity of the local community, having strong liaisons in place who are aware of local cultural practices is critical. Coordination of expertise is also strengthened when preparedness planning is multi-sectoral. The creation of interim guidance specific to the circumstances and population affected may require multiple areas of expertise and ongoing coordination as evidence evolves. For example, in areas with high levels of HIV infection, interim guidance to adapt general infant feeding recommendations may be necessary (WHO, 2018b).

Emergencies offer an opportunity for learning and policy change, if outcomes are evaluated and results disseminated. The recovery period following an emergency is a time of increased readiness to focus on preparedness and openness to education. Lessons learned from an emergency have the ability to impact not only preparedness activities but also wider policy approaches in support of quality improvement initiatives such as the Baby-Friendly Initiative or regulatory changes such as creation or strengthening of national legislation to align with the International Code of Marketing of Breast-Milk Substitutes. Ensuring that infant feeding outcomes are captured and reported in evaluations is critical to ensuring that IYCF-E policy and practices continue to improve.

Key Points to Remember

1. Infants and young children are uniquely vulnerable in emergencies, and breastfeeding protects them from several of the most significant risks.
2. Populations with high breastfeeding rates are more resilient to emergencies and require fewer resources during response and recovery.
3. Coordination with other sectors to meet the needs of families is critical to a successful response.

Additional Resources/Websites

Infant and Young Child Feeding in Emergencies Operational Guidance (version 3.0, 2017)
https://www.ennonline.net/operationalguidance-v3-2017
Crisis & Emergency Response Training (CERC)
https://emergency.cdc.gov/cerc
Infant and Young Child Feeding in Emergencies (IYCF-E) Toolkit: Rapid start-up for emergency nutrition personnel

https://resourcecentre.savethechildren.net/library/infant-and-young-child-feeding-emergencies-iycf-e-toolkit-rapid-start-emergency-nutrition
Infant Feeding in Emergencies (IFE) Core Group
www.ennonline.net/ife
SafelyFed Canada
http://safelyfed.ca/
Carolina Global Breastfeeding Institute (CGBI): Resources - Lactation & Infant Feeding in Emergencies
https://sph.unc.edu/cgbi/cgbi-resources-l-i-f-e-support-basic-kit

References

Aguayo, V. M., Sharma, A., & Subedi, G. R. (2015). Delivering essential nutrition service for children after the Nepal earthquake. *The Lancet Global Health, 3*(11), e665-e666.

Alsamman, S. (2015). Managing infant and young child feeding in refugee camps in Jordan. *Field Exchange 48*, 85.

Altemus, M., Deuster, P. A., Galliven, E., Carter, C. S., & Gold, P. W. (1995). Suppression of hypothalmic-pituitary-adrenal axis responses to stress in lactating women. *The Journal of Clinical Endocrinology and Metabolism, 80*(10), 2954-2959. https://doi.org/10.1210/jcem.80.10.7559880

Arvelo, W., Kim, A., Creek, T., Legwaila, K., Puhr, N., Johnston, S., Masunge, J., Davis, M., Mintz, E. & Bowen, A. (2010). Case–control study to determine risk factors for diarrhea among children during a large outbreak in a country with a high prevalence of HIV infection. *International Journal of Infectious Diseases, 14*(11), e1002-e1007. https://doi.org/10.1016/j.ijid.2010.06.014

Ayoya, M. A., Golden, K., Ngnie-Teta, I., Moreaux, M. D., Mamadoultaibou, A., Koo, L., Boyd, E., Beauliere, J. M., Lesavre, C., & Marhone, J. P. (2013). Protecting and improving breastfeeding practices during a major emergency: Lessons learnt from the baby tents in Haiti. *Bulletin of the World Health Organization, 91*, 612–617. https://www.who.int/bulletin/volumes/91/8/12-113936/en/

Azad, F., Rifat, M. A., Manir, M. Z., & Biva, N. A. (2019). Breastfeeding support through wet nursing during nutritional emergency: A cross sectional study from Rohingya refugee camps in Bangladesh. *PloS one, 14*(10). https://doi.org/10.1371/journal.pone.0222980

Callaghan, W. M., Rasmussen, S. A., Jamieson, D. J., Ventura, S. J., Farr, S. L., Sutton, P. D., Mathews, T.J., Hamilton, B.E. Shealy, K.R., Brantley, D. & Posner, S. F. (2007). Health concerns of women and infants in times of natural disasters: Lessons learned from Hurricane Katrina. *Maternal and Child Health Journal, 11*(4), 307–311.

Council & Committee on Pediatric Emergency Medicine. (2015). Ensuring the health of children in disasters. *Pediatrics, 136*(5), e1407–e1417.

DeYoung, S. E., Chase, J., Branco, M. P., & Park, B. (2018). The effect of mass evacuation on infant feeding: The case of the 2016 Fort McMurray wildfire. *Maternal and Child Health Journal, 22*(12), 1826–1833. https://doi.org/10.1007/s10995-018-2585-z

Dörnemann, J., & Kelly, A. H. (2013). 'It is me who eats, to nourish him': A mixed method study of breastfeeding in post-earthquake Haiti. *Maternal & Child Nutrition, 9*(1), 74–89. https://doi.org/10.1111/j.1740-8709.2012.00428.x

ENN & UNICEF (2017, October). *Operational guidance on infant feeding in emergencies (version 3.0).* https://www.ennonline.net/operationalguidance-v3-2017

Garg, A., Bucu, A. R., & Garela, R. G. (2016). Philippines Nutrition Cluster: Lessons learnt from the response to Typhoon Haiyan (Yolanda). *Field Exchange 52*, 61.

Gribble, K., Peterson, M., & Brown, D. (2019). Emergency preparedness for infant and young child feeding in emergencies (IYCF-E): An Australian audit of emergency plans and guidance. *BMC Public Health, 19*(1), 1278. https://doi.org/10.1186/s12889-019-7528-0

Hargest-Slade, A. C., & Gribble, K. D. (2015). Shaken but not broken: Supporting breastfeeding women after the 2011 Christchurch New Zealand earthquake. *Breastfeeding Review, 23*(3), 7.

Hipgrave, D. B., Assefa, F., Winoto, A., & Sukotjo, S. (2012). Donated breast milk substitutes and incidence of diarrhoea among infants and young children after the May 2006 earthquake in Yogyakarta and Central Java. *Public Health Nutrition, 15*(2), 307–315. https://doi.org/10.1017/S1368980010003423

Infant Feeding in Emergencies (IFE) Core Group. https://www.ennonline.net/ife

Ishii, K., Goto, A., Ota, M., Yasumura, S., Abe, M., & Fujimori, K. (2016). Factors associated with infant feeding methods after the nuclear power plant accident in Fukushima: Data from the Pregnancy and Birth Survey for the Fiscal Year 2011 Fukushima Health Management Survey. *Maternal and Child Health Journal, 20*(8), 1704–1712. DOI: 10.1007/s10995-016-1973-5

Liu, L., Oza, S., Hogan, D., Chu, Y., Perin, J., Zhu, J., Lawn, J. E., Cousens, S., Mathers, C., & Black, R. E. (2016). Global, regional, and national causes of under-5 mortality in 2000–15: An updated systematic analysis with implications for the Sustainable Development Goals. *The Lancet, 388*(10063), 3027–3035. https://doi.org/10.1016/S0140-6736(16)31593-8

McNeilly, A. S. (2001). Lactational control of reproduction. *Reproduction, Fertility and Development, 13*(8), 583–590. https://doi.org/10.1071/rd01056

Palmquist, A. E., & Gribble, K. D. (2018). Gender, displacement, and infant and young child feeding in emergencies. In *International Handbook on Gender and Demographic Processes* (pp. 341–355). Springer, Dordrecht.

Salvatori, G., De Rose, D. U., Concato, C., Alario, D., Olivini, N., Dotta, A., & Campana, A. (2020). Managing COVID-19-Positive Maternal–Infant Dyads: An Italian Experience. *Breastfeeding Medicine, 15*(5), 347-348.

Saxton, A., Fahy, K., & Hastie, C. (2014). Effects of skin-to-skin contact and breastfeeding at birth on the incidence of PPH: A physiologically based theory. *Women Birth, 27*(4), 250–253. https://doi.org/10.1016/j.wombi.2014.06.004

Shaker, Berbari, L., Ghattas, H., Symon, A. G., & Anderson, A. S. (2018). Infant and young child feeding in emergencies: Organisational policies and activities during the refugee crisis in Lebanon. *Maternal & child nutrition, 14*(3), e12576.

Sphere Association. (2018). *The Sphere handbook 2018: Humanitarian charter and minimum standards in humanitarian response.* Geneva, Switzerland. https://spherestandards.org/handbook-2018

Summers, A., & Bilukha, O. O. (2018). Suboptimal infant and young child feeding practices among internally displaced persons during conflict in eastern Ukraine. *Public Health Nutrition, 21*(5), 917–926. https://doi.org/10.1017/S1368980017003421

Svoboda, A. (2017). Retrospective qualitative analysis of an infant and young child feeding intervention among refugees in Europe. *Field Exchange 55,* 85.

Theurich, M. A., & Grote, V. (2017). Are commercial complementary food distributions to refugees and migrants in Europe conforming to international policies and guidelines on infant and young child feeding in emergencies? *Journal of Human Lactation, 33*(3), 573–577. https://doi.org/10.1177/0890334417707717

World Health Organization (WHO). (1981). *International Code of marketing of breast-milk substitutes.* https://www.who.int/nutrition/publications/infantfeeding/9789241594295/en

World Health Organization (WHO). (2003). *Global Strategy for Infant and Young Child Feeding.* http://www.who.int/nutrition/topics/global_strategy_iycf/en/

World Health Organization (WHO). (2017). *Guideline: Protecting, promoting and supporting breastfeeding in facilities providing maternity and newborn services.* Geneva, Switzerland. https://www.who.int/nutrition/publications/guidelines/breastfeeding-facilities-maternity-newborn/en/

World Health Organization (WHO). (2018a). *World Health Assembly Resolution 71.9, Agenda Item 12.6, Infant and young child feeding.* Geneva, Switzerland. https://apps.who.int/gb/ebwha/pdf_files/WHA71/A71_R9-en.pdf

World Health Organization (WHO). (2018b). *HIV and infant feeding in emergencies: Operational guidance. The duration of breastfeeding and support from health services to improve feeding practices among mothers living with HIV.* Geneva, Switzerland. https://www.who.int/nutrition/publications/hivaids/hiv-if-emergencies-guidance/en

CHAPTER 13

Breastfeeding for People Experiencing Criminalization and Incarceration

Martha Paynter, RN, MSc, PhD(c)

LEARNING OBJECTIVES

1. Identify how increasing numbers of women experiencing incarceration contributes to the growing public health problem of interference with lactation.
2. Consider the complex health and social histories of women experiencing criminalization and incarceration and how those intersect with the experience of justice system involvement and the carceral infrastructure to create multiple barriers to breastfeeding success.
3. Consider the unique benefits breastfeeding may afford women who experience criminalization and their children.
4. Outline the policy and legal protections available to people experiencing incarceration with respect to lactation.
5. Analyze best practices to supporting people experiencing incarceration and criminalization in their breastfeeding goals.

KEY WORDS

- **Criminalization:** The social, political, and economic process through which interaction with the (in)justice system occurs.
- **Incarceration:** The state of being confined in jail, prison, or another carceral facility, including immigration and youth detention.

People experiencing incarceration and criminalization is the term used in this chapter. No disparaging and incorrect terms for people experiencing incarceration and criminalization will be used, nor will individuals be defined by their experiences.

This chapter intends to be inclusive of trans and nonbinary people. While there is no research evidence to date that examines the breastfeeding/chestfeeding experiences of transgender and nonbinary people who experience incarceration, this is an important area for future research. There is evidence that transgender and nonbinary people experience disproportionate criminalization.

- **Children's Rights:** The United Nations Convention on the Rights of the Child (United Nations General Assembly, 1989) sets out 54 articles that define 18 human rights for all children around the world that define the standards in international law for how children must be treated to survive and thrive.
- **Reproductive Health:** The World Health Organization (WHO, n.d.) defines reproductive health as a state of complete physical, mental, and social well-being and not merely the absence of disease or infirmity, in all matters relating to the reproductive system and to its functions and processes.

Overview

Women are the fastest-growing population in prisons around the world. The increasing **incarceration** of women affects **reproductive health**, including the right to breastfeed, breastfeeding intentions, and success and experiences for lactating people and children. Most women experiencing incarceration are mothers. Although perinatal health generally among this population has been the subject of several systematic reviews, breastfeeding is under-researched among people experiencing incarceration. This chapter begins with a review of the literature about breastfeeding among women experiencing incarceration. Key cases known to the public regarding how breastfeeding has been experienced in carceral spaces are described to set context for the chapter. Next, legal and policy protections that support breastfeeding for women experiencing incarceration are outlined. Last, recommendations are offered for how health care providers and others can support populations inside and outside of carceral facilities.

Introduction

Increasing Incarceration of Women

Decades of cumulative research demonstrates the benefits of breastfeeding to both mother and child (Victora et al., 2016). The World Health Organization (WHO) Ten Steps to Successful Breastfeeding, the foundation to the Baby-Friendly Hospital Initiative (BFHI), requires mothers and infants be kept together to support breastfeeding success (WHO, 2018). The increasing incarceration of women, and within that the increasing incarceration of mothers and potentially lactating people, creates dual risks of harm to mother and child. The routine separation of the mother–infant dyad required by incarceration and restrictions on breastfeeding education, clinical care, and support, to which incarcerated people are subjected, challenge breastfeeding success. To support breastfeeding among women experiencing **criminalization**, we must understand the context of the carceral environment, the histories of these women's lives, barriers and restrictions to accessing information and resources, and how to confront carceral systems to offer comprehensive breastfeeding support.

Rates of women's incarceration vary widely across the globe. In 2018, the Prison Policy Initiative found a worldwide average of 133 women experiencing incarceration per 100,000 women in the population (Kajstura, 2018). The rates vary wildly across countries: in Brazil, the rate was 45 per 100,000 (Kajstura,

2018). In Canada, it was 13 per 100,000 (Kajstura, 2018). In several countries in Africa, the rate was less than 1 per 100,000 (Kajstura, 2018). These variations demonstrate the constructedness of criminalization as a social process. Societies decide what is criminalized and how it is punished. In considering the phenomenon of breastfeeding, we must always consider alternatives to incarceration and criminalization.

Already marginalized populations including Black and Indigenous women, transgender and nonbinary persons, and newcomers experience disproportionate criminalization. In Canada, 40% of the women in prison are Indigenous, despite only 4% of the general population identifying as such.

Complex Health Histories and Needs of Women Experiencing Incarceration

Women experiencing incarceration have complex health histories and disproportionate burdens of disease and disability (Kouyoumdjian et al., 2018). Women in federal prisons in Canada report high rates of infectious disease (Nolan & Stewart, 2017). They are at greater than average risk of physical illnesses and of injury, particularly head injury (Nolan & Stewart, 2017). There is clear evidence of pervasive childhood abuse among people who are incarcerated, and higher rates among women than men (Bodkin et al., 2019). Childhood trauma also predisposes people in federal prisons to posttraumatic stress disorder, substance use, and self-harm (Tam & Derkzen, 2014). In Canada, 80% of women experiencing federal incarceration report a substance use disorder (MacDonald et al., 2015a). Among women in federal prisons in Canada, 46% are prescribed psychotropic medication (MacDonald et al., 2015b).

People in prison and those recently released from prison have higher usage of health care services, such as emergency departments, ambulatory care, psychiatric hospitalization, and medical–surgical hospitalization (Kouyoumdjian et al., 2018). As most are survivors of trauma, women experiencing incarceration have high rates of histories of substance use and may use substances while incarcerated or be treated with opioid replacement therapy.

Incarceration also has health impacts on the children of parents in prison. The attachment literature pioneered by Bowlby (1952) theorizes that mother–child attachment is an evolutionary, instinctive survival mechanism; disrupting this attachment to the primary parent, usually the mother, in the first 2 years of a child's life constitutes "maternal deprivation," with long-term emotional, cognitive, and social consequences for the child's development. Indeed, the canonical Adverse Child Event (ACE) study (Felitti et al., 1998)—a Centers for Disease Control and Prevention–funded survey of over 17,000 Americans about their childhood experiences of adversity—identified parental imprisonment as one of the key factors with which ill health in adulthood is correlated. This imprisonment is itself driven by such structural factors as racism and poverty.

Literature Review

International systematic review of the health research literature about maternal health found negligible examination of breastfeeding outcomes (Paynter et al., 2019);

only one of the 13 included studies mentioned breastfeeding, and in that study population only a single person out of 12 initiated breastfeeding (Chambers, 2009). One case study from the United States discusses the logistics of milk transport from a woman experiencing incarceration to her child in the community (Allen, 2017). Through a qualitative study in England with 28 women, researchers found high needs for support and mother–child cohabitation to be important (Abbott & Scott, 2017). Huang et al. (2012) interviewed pregnant women incarcerated in a New York facility and found that the participants felt positively about breastfeeding and believed it could offer a new start to their lives as mothers. Women who have experienced incarceration are a difficult population to follow longitudinally, and this study did not follow up with participants to determine if they realized their breastfeeding goals. In Minnesota, a funded doula program for incarcerated women was examined for its impact on breastfeeding (Shlafer et al., 2018). Of the 39 participants, over two-thirds talked with their doulas about breastfeeding, and nearly two-thirds initiated breastfeeding after delivery (Shlafer et al., 2018).

Potential Benefits of Breastfeeding to Mothers Experiencing Incarceration

While the benefits of breastfeeding generally are well established, the benefits of breastfeeding for mothers experiencing incarceration may be greater than average because of the health inequities these women experience prior to, during, and upon release from incarceration. Positive maternal health outcomes associated with breastfeeding include postpartum weight loss, bonding, and reduced risk of reproductive cancers, metabolic diseases including diabetes, and cardiovascular disease (Dieterich et al., 2013). Breastfeeding may be a protective factor against peripartum depression (Figueiredo et al., 2014). Systematic review of existing research has found women with a history of mental illness are predisposed to perinatal depression (Biaggi et al., 2016).

Withdrawal from Substance Exposure

Children of women who use substances have unique needs in relation to breastfeeding and contact with their mothers. Infant withdrawal from physical substance dependence includes gastrointestinal, neurological, and general symptoms of irritability, such as tremors, crying, and feeding intolerance. Withdrawal results from maternal substance use. Opioid agonist therapy (OAT) such as methadone is recommended for mothers experiencing opioid use disorders, as it reduces risk of exposure to infection and of miscarriage.

Opioids and opioid agonists will cross the placental barrier in pregnancy, and up to 80% of opioid-exposed babies will experience withdrawal. Systematic review of the evidence has found that breastfeeding reduces the severity of withdrawal symptoms, need for and length of pharmacological intervention, and hospital length of stay, and it delays onset of withdrawal symptoms (Bagley et al., 2014). The impact of breastfeeding on recovery is mediated by factors including skin-to-skin contact, the microbiome, and trace amounts of opioid agonists in human milk (Bogen & Whalen, 2019).

"Maternal therapy," whereby infants room-in with their mothers, enhances recovery as infants withdraw from substances to which they were exposed prenatally (Bagley et al., 2014). Skin-to-skin contact while breastfeeding and the dietetic quality of human milk may also relieve withdrawal symptoms.

Barriers to Breastfeeding for Women Experiencing Criminalization

Physical and Practical Barriers

Fundamentally, the separation of mother and child intrinsic to incarceration directly impedes breastfeeding success. Residential mother–child programs exist across the world; however, in North America these programs are rare. In the United States, there are approximately one dozen prison nursery programs. In Canada, only the federal prisons for women and one provincial jail, in British Columbia, have residential programs. Even in facilities with such programs, the majority of incarcerated women are ineligible due to strict participation criteria.

The institutional routines of carceral facilities, such as regular requirements to be in certain places at certain times for count, are at odds with breastfeeding. Women may require staff escort to clinical appointments or educational/supportive programming. Staff shortages affect ability to attend. Use of shackling and leg irons presents risks that the infant will be dropped.

Separation from the infant will impede success of the breastfeeding experience. Because breastfeeding is both hormonal and mechanical, presence of the child with direct stimulation of the breast significantly improves establishment and maintenance of milk supply. Breastfeeding operates through a positive feedback loop: more breastfeeding empties the breast, causing a prolactin (hormonal) response of faster filling of the breast. Skin-to-skin contact improves this hormonal response.

Pumping Is Not a Panacea

Pumping milk, a substitute process for feeding at the breast, is not necessarily adequate to maintain supply nor is it predictive of long-term success with breastfeeding (Flaherman et al., 2016). The feeling of stress and anxiety about being under surveillance and separated from one's infant could also inhibit pumping success. Lack of ability to drain the breast worsens engorgement and risk of mastitis. Pumping milk and feeding at the breast are not equal; the optimal solution is to keep mothers and breastfeeding children together. Pumping is logistically challenging in an environment that includes strict routines such as count, programs, yard time, and medication rounds. Consider how difficult it would be to pump eight or so times per day to maintain supply for an exclusively human milk-fed baby. When separated from children but provided with a pump, women need access to pump education, support, milk storage supplies and equipment such as clean bottles and a temperature-controlled refrigerator, ability to properly clean and store equipment, and clinical attention for difficulties such as engorgement, blocked ducts, and infection. Prisons are unhygienic environments in which infectious diseases spread rapidly. They may be inappropriate environments for milk expression and storage.

Women's Health Invisible in Prisons

Globally, women represent about 10% of the population in prison. As women form a small portion of this population, there is a likelihood of lack of attention and familiarity with reproductive and perinatal health needs among care providers. In many jurisdictions, women are a small population in a carceral facility, collocated with men. Incarceration in sites that do not prioritize or have familiarity with reproductive and perinatal health presents multiple challenges, including barriers to prenatal education, information seeking, and knowledge sharing with an external health care provider, peers, family, and friends in regard to breastfeeding.

Socio-economic Barriers

In addition to the direct challenges of maternal–infant separation, women experiencing incarceration face layers of socioe-conomic barriers, including poverty, racism, age, and lone parenting. Young, low-income, racialized, and single women face barriers to breastfeeding and comparably lower rates of breastfeeding (Jones et al., 2015; Moffitt & Dickinson, 2016). In Canada in 2009–2010, the rate of breastfeeding initiation among women ages 15 to 24 was 84%, compared with 89% among women over age 35; the rate among single women was 80% compared with married/common law women, who had a rate of 89% (Health Canada, 2012). At 6 months, 25.9% of women were breastfeeding their babies exclusively. However, this differed significantly between income quintiles: 23% of women in the lowest income quintile breastfed to 6 months, compared with 33% of those in the highest-income quintile (Health Canada, 2012).

Knowledge, attitudes, and social support are known factors in the decision to breastfeed (Casal et al., 2016). For women experiencing criminalization, uncertainty regarding maintenance of infant custody (Huang et al., 2012), policies of separation (Chambers, 2009), or lack of access to mother–child residential programs for cohabitation impact intention to breastfeed, initiation, and duration.

Trauma

Childhood and precarceral experiences of violence, trauma, and poverty are barriers to developing the intention to breastfeeding and comfort with the physical experience of breastfeeding. For victims of sexual trauma, breastfeeding and exposure of the breasts for breastfeeding can be retraumatizing (Elfgen et al., 2017). Institutional circumstances amplify trauma and discomfort. While incarcerated, women may experience punishment and violence, such as administrative segregation that causes stress and/or separation from their infants. Search policies, such as strip searching before and after appointments inside and outside of the carceral setting, are a barrier to access.

Minimum Needs

At a minimum, a breastfeeding client experiencing incarceration needs (a) prenatal education to familiarize themselves with breastfeeding benefits, how-to's, common minor problems and solutions, milk expression techniques, and where to go for help;(b) permission to breastfeed or pump as needed, not on an institutional schedule, and in privacy; and (c) adequate equipment and supplies for milk supply maintenance, milk storage, and prevention of bacterial and virus transmission into the milk, which includes a personal-use high-quality electrical pump, a personal mini fridge not shared with other people, bags for milk storage, soap and a sink and dry rack for cleaning the pump; (d) access to health care professionals with lactation expertise, who either come to them or to whom they may easily visit on the outside; (e) culturally appropriate supports for breastfeeding for Black, Indigenous, and women of color; and (f) appropriate supports for trans and nonbinary people wishing to chest or breastfeed. The unlikelihood of carceral contexts ever being able to meet these minimum requirements points to the need for alternatives to incarceration.

Issues on Release

On release, people are introduced to new types of threats to breastfeeding. They may be paroled to locations in which they lack support networks. They are likely to experience poverty, unemployment, and strain to meet the demands of parole or probation conditions. For example, some may face such requirements as mandatory attendance at Alcoholics Anonymous or Narcotics Anonymous sessions at which children are not allowed. These harms are rarely considered before sentencing or even as release is being planned.

Legal Protections

Bangkok Rules

While it is not possible to collate the legal protections for breastfeeding in carceral facilities in every country, the United Nations *Rules for the Treatment of Women Prisoners and Non-custodial Measures for Women Offenders,* called the Bangkok Rules, were unanimously accepted by member countries in 2010 and provide a critical foundation to examine the opportunities for legal protections in individual country human rights regimes. The first rule is that "the distinctive needs of women prisoners shall be taken into consideration and provided for in order to accomplish substantial gender equality" (United Nations Office on Drugs and Crime [UNODC], 2011, p. 12). Many of the 70 rules directly or indirectly apply to perinatal health and breastfeeding.

The Bangkok Rules stipulate that, whenever possible, alternatives to incarceration should be sought for pregnant women and mothers of young children because of the deleterious effects on children's well-being. "Rule 2: Prior to or on admission, women with caretaking responsibilities for children shall be permitted to make arrangements for those children, including the possibility of a reasonable suspension of detention, taking into account the best interests of the children" (UNODC, 2011, p. 12). Several countries have taken measures to keep out of prison pregnant women and parents with primary care of young children. These include Russia, Algeria, China, Iceland, Italy, Kazakhstan, Norway, and Sweden (Law Library of Congress, 2015).

The Bangkok Rules emphasize the need for data collection about reproductive health to inform decision making in regard to incarceration: "Rule 3.1: The number and personal details of the children of a woman being admitted to prison shall be recorded at the time of admission"; and "Rule 6.a: The health screening of women prisoners shall be comprehensive . . . including reproductive health history and primary health-care needs" (UNODC, 2011, pp. 12–14).

To make decisions that avoid incarceration in the first place, the court system must be aware of family structures and needs. This information is not routinely collected by either defense counsel or prosecution or presented in court. In 1992, then assistant editor of the *British Medical Journal*, Luisa Dillner, wrote that "only a few judges ever receive 'social' information on the women they sentence, even though a custodial sentence on a mother often means that her children are put into care" (Dillner, 1992, p. 933). A recent national report by the Quakers in Canada that examined every written sentencing decision across the country in 2016 found that not one mentioned the best interests of the child (Canadian Friends Service Committee [Quakers], 2018).

The Bangkok Rules do not require the child be collocated with the mother in the prison environment; however they do recognize the value of physical closeness to the child. "Rule 4: Women prisoners shall be allocated, to the extent possible, to prisons close to their home or place of social rehabilitation, taking account of their caretaking responsibilities" (UNODC, 2011, p. 13).

The Bangkok Rules require an appropriate environment and supplies for women's health maintenance: "Rule 5: The accommodation of women prisoners shall have facilities and materials required to meet women's specific hygiene needs" (UNODC, 2011, p. 13). While not specific to breastfeeding, this could include milk expression, storage, and transport.

Most relevant to breastfeeding, Rule 10 stipulates that "gender-specific health-care services at least equivalent to those available in the community shall be provided to women prisoners" (UNODC, 2011, p. 15). Prenatal and postpartum education and support for breastfeeding could fall under this requirement.

In regard to the punishment and restraints for the breastfeeding person, three rules are relevant. "Rule 22: Punishment by close confinement or disciplinary segregation shall not be applied to pregnant women, women with infants and breastfeeding mothers in prison" (UNODC, 2011, p. 15); "Rule 23: Disciplinary sanctions for women prisoners shall not include a prohibition of family contact, especially with children"; and "Rule 24: Instruments of restraint shall never be used on women during labour, during birth and immediately after birth" (UNODC, 2011, p. 12). In the United States, at least 22 states have legislation to ban the shackling of prisoners during labour and delivery (Ferszt et al., 2018). In Canada, federal legislation governing prisoners, the Corrections and Conditional Release Act (Government of Canada, 1992), does not include any mention of pregnancy; however, internal federal prison policy may protect from shackling in labor.

Mandela Rules

The United Nations General Assembly Mandela Rules, another example of international legal protections, are general standards governing the treatment of prisoners. They include rules that impose health care obligations on carceral facilities (United Nations General Assembly, 2015). Health care obligation rules include (a) Rule 24, which states that "the provision of health care for prisoners is a State responsibility. Prisoners should enjoy the same standards of health care that are available in the community" (United Nations General Assembly, 2015, p. 12); (b) Rule 45 makes plain the harm of segregation on health: "The imposition of solitary confinement should be prohibited in the case of prisoners with mental or physical disabilities when their conditions would be exacerbated by such measures"; (c) the Mandela Rules specify obligations for perinatal care. Rule 28 states that "in women's prisons, there shall be special accommodation for all necessary prenatal and postnatal care and treatment. Arrangements shall be made wherever practicable for children to be born in a hospital outside the prison" (United Nations General Assembly, 2015, p. 13).

The Mandela Rules further stipulate how health care providers must act in their care for incarcerated people: (a) Rule 32 states that "the relationship between the health-care professionals and the prisoners shall be governed by the same ethical and professional standards as those applicable to patients in the community" (United Nations General Assembly, 2015, p. 14); (b) Rule 32 imposes "an absolute prohibition on engaging, actively or passively, in acts that may constitute torture or other cruel, inhuman or degrading treatment or punishment" (United Nations General Assembly, 2015, p. 14); (c) Rule 34 explains that "if health-care professionals become aware of any signs of torture or other cruel, inhuman or degrading treatment or punishment, they shall document and report such cases to the competent medical, administrative or judicial authority" (United Nations General Assembly, 2015, p. 14); this rule would prohibit health care providers from participating in solitary confinement. In general, the Mandela Rules clearly state the obligation of the state to care for prisoners and the obligation of health care providers to treat imprisoned patients with the same dignity and care as they would patients on the outside.

Convention of the Rights of the Child

A third set of rules defined by the United Nations applies to the context of incarcerated mothers. The United Nations General Assembly *Convention on the Rights of the Child* (UNCRC), Article 7, asserts a child's right "to know and be cared for by his or her parents" (United Nations General Assembly, 1989, p. 3). Canada ratified the UNCRC in 1991. The United States signed it in 1995 but never ratified it (The Economist, 2013). The third article of the UNCRC is the principle of Best Interests of the Child, which is integrated in family law legislation, under provincial/territorial jurisdiction, across Canada. The UNCRC does not define "Best Interests of the Child," but Article 24 states that children have a right to "enjoyment of the highest attainable standard of health and to facilities for the treatment of illness and rehabilitation of health" (United Nations General Assembly, 1989, p. 7).

Key Cases

Inglis v. British Columbia (Public Safety), 2013 SCBC 2309

In British Columbia in 2006, Lisa Anne Whitford, an Indigenous woman, who had long endured abuse at the hands of her common law partner, was charged with killing him. She was sent to pretrial detention at the Alouette Correctional Centre provincial jail for women and gave birth while incarcerated (Cohen, 2016). Alouette had a mother–child program in which babies could remain with their incarcerated mothers; Whitford participated (Strickland, 2008). Approximately 100 infants used the Alouette program before Whitford (Mulgrew, 2013). The program or others like it had been in place in British Columbia since 1973 (*Inglis vs. BC*, 2013 SCBC 2309). Whitford's case received wide media attention, and criticism of the program accompanied that attention. The Alouette program closed in February 2008.

In 2008, two women who were formerly incarcerated at Alouette, and their children, sued the BC Minister of Public Safety, arguing that closing Alouette's mother–child program was a violation of the Canadian Charter of Rights and Freedoms (Government of Canada, 1982). When the case concluded in 2013, the judge ruled in their favor. She found that separating mothers and infants violated Section 7 of the charter, Security of the Person, because it interfered with bonding and breastfeeding. Several years later the Alouette program reopened, although participation reportedly remains low.

This case did not result in provinces across Canada opening mother–child programs. Legally, removing a program is a different violation than not having one in the first place. British Columbia remains the only province with such a program.

Lillian Desjarlais

An important case that shifts expectations and practices for police forces is that of Lillian Desjarlais in Saskatoon, Saskatchewan. At the time of her arrest in 2016, Desjarlais was 21 years old and exclusively nursing a 4-month-old son. Desjarlais is Indigenous. She was arrested after a physical altercation with her boyfriend. All Canadian provinces and territories have "pro-charging" or "pro-prosecution" policies in relation to domestic violence (Government of Canada, 2017). When police are called, there is a requirement to charge; this type of policy has resulted in the increasing criminalization of Black women, Indigenous women, and women of color (Kim, 2018).

Desjarlais was held in the Saskatoon police cells for more than 3 days. Police officers prohibited her from contact with her baby, and she was not provided with a breast pump or clean and dry clothes. She was given sanitary napkins to soak up leaking milk. She reported experiencing humiliation, pain, and signs of infection (Allen, 2017). Desjarlais filed a complaint against the police with the Public Complaints Commission. Her treatment was ruled "neglect of duty" evidenced by lack of documentation and communication about her health needs. The commission did not, however, require disciplinary action. Desjarlais received an apology from the Saskatoon police, who reportedly made several policy and practice changes in response to the case. These included always having a female commissionaire at the station, providing people in detention with blankets, having a paramedic available, and money to purchase breast pumps.

There are several challenges with making arrest and police detention compatible with breastfeeding. Individuals being held are not permitted privacy nor are they permitted to bring in any objects or belongings into the cell, such as their breast pump and milk storage supplies. Adults in police custody cannot be held with children under the age of 18 in the same cell. While police are empowered to release arrestees on their own recognizance to return to the court for hearings, they cannot release an alleged assailant into a home with an alleged victim. The continued enforcement of proarrest policies impacts women not only in relation to breastfeeding but in regard to childcare generally.

Hidalgo v. New Mexico Department of Corrections

In 2017, while incarcerated at the Western New Mexico Correctional Facility, Monique Hidalgo gave birth to a girl (Prison Legal News, 2018). Hidalgo experienced an opioid substance use disorder, and when the baby was born she required support, including breastfeeding, to withdraw from opioid exposure. The New Mexico Department of Corrections (DOC) denied Hidalgo access to methadone treatment after the birth. The mother and baby stayed together in the hospital for 2 weeks and then, recognizing the value to an infant in recovery, Dr. Lawrence Leeman prescribed continued breastfeeding as part of a treatment plan for the dyad. Hidalgo's fiancé was to bring the baby with him on daily visits to her in prison so the infant could breastfeed and to retrieve expressed milk. However, the DOC revoked her right to breastfeed based on an unconfirmed drug test that found trace Suboxone (buprenorphine) in her blood. Suboxone, like methadone, is a treatment for opioid use disorder.

Hidalgo filed a restraining order and a permanent injunction against the DOC (1st J.D. Ct. of Santa Fe County [NM], Case No. D-101-CV-2017-01658). The court held she could not be denied the right to breastfeed during visiting hours and to express milk at other times of the day to give to her baby. Supported by the New Mexico Breastfeeding Taskforce, Hidalgo sued the DOC (Sheppard, 2017). Judge David Thomson ruled the prohibition on breastfeeding and milk expression to be gender discrimination, in violation of NM's equal rights amendment (Haywood, 2017). Several months later, Hidalgo again tested positive for Suboxone (buprenorphine). Although a recommended treatment for opioid use disorder, her use was in violation of the court order. She again was prevented from breastfeeding (Prison Legal News, 2018). This case also illustrates the need for lactation specialists to support breastfeeding clients' needs for pharmacotherapy to treat substance use disorder.

Best Practices

Health care providers with experience and/or expertise in lactation are optimally positioned to educate not only patients who are incarcerated but also the stakeholders in their circumstances, including correctional officers, administrators, sheriffs, police, prosecution and defense counsel, and the judiciary. We health care providers have professional responsibility and privilege to advocate for individual women and their **children's rights** to breastfeed and breastfeeding resources. We also have professional platforms to advocate more broadly, such as for understanding among our colleagues of the Bangkok Rules and the Mandela Rules and how our practices should be responsive. More broadly still, we can use our positions to call for political attention to disproportionate criminalization and incarceration of Black, Indigenous and women of color and trans and nonbinary people.

In our care for this population, it is essential that our actions be trauma informed. We must seek consent and accept when our support is declined. Forced care is retraumatizing and dehumanizing. As we ought to with all clients, this population is at great need of education about milk expression techniques for infant feeding, maintenance of milk supply, and prevention of engorgement and infection. We must plan, foreseeing the potential for mother–child separation even if at this moment both are together. Incarceration is an experience of uncertainty. Life after release presents its own challenges, for which we must anticipate and prepare. For the population experiencing criminalization, lactation support means not only teaching breastfeeding but also securing resources for clients and navigating community services.

This is difficult work that challenges the odds. Be profoundly proud of success.

Key Points to Remember

1. Increasing incarceration of women affects reproductive health, including rights to breastfeed, breastfeeding intentions, success and experiences for lactating people and children, and risks of harm to both mother and child.
2. People in prison have experienced oppression that is likely to impact breastfeeding, including pervasive histories of poverty, childhood trauma, and high rates of substance use. These experiences have intergenerational impacts on their children. People experiencing incarceration lack access to support and have additional needs.
3. The policies, practices, and infrastructure of policing and corrections are not readily compatible with breastfeeding support. Advocates must know not only how to navigate these systems but also what local and international laws support breastfeeding as a right of incarcerated people.

Student Questions for Consideration

1. What are the practical, ethical, and clinical challenges associated with incarcerating infants and young children with their mothers to facilitate breastfeeding success? What alternatives can you imagine?
2. How would you define the best interests of the child in the situations described in this chapter? Where do you foresee conflicts in how that would be defined?
3. What does the corrections landscape look like where you live? How would you navigate that system to provide lactation support?

References

Abbott, L., & Scott, T. (2017). Women's experiences of breastfeeding in prison. *MIDIRS Midwifery Digest, 27*(2), 217–223.

Allen, B. (2017). *Saskatoon police chief apologizes for refusing young mom a breast pump while in custody.* CBC News. http://www.cbc.ca/news/canada/saskatchewan/saskatoon-police-chief-apologizes-for-refusing-young-mom-a-breast-pump-while-in-custody-1.4141326

Allen, D. (2013). Supporting mothering through breastfeeding for incarcerated women. Proceedings of the 2013 AWHONN Convention. *JOGNN: Journal of Obstetrical, Gynecologic, and Neonatal Nursing, 42*(Suppl 1), S103. https://doi.org/10.1111/1552-6909.12203

Bagley, S. M., Wachman, E. M., Holland, E., & Brogley, S. B. (2014). Review of the assessment and management of neonatal abstinence syndrome. *Addiction Sciences and Clinical Practice, 9*(1), 19. https://doi.org/10.1186/1940-0640-9-19

Biaggi, A., Conroy, S., Pawlby, S., & Pariante, M. (2016). Identifying the women at risk of antenatal anxiety and depression: A systematic review. *Journal of Affective Disorders, 191*, 62–77. https://doi.org/10.1016/j.jad.2015.11.014

Bodkin, C., Pivnick, L., Bondy, S., Ziegler, C., Martin, R., Jernigan, C., & Kouyoumdjian, F. (2019). History of childhood abuse in populations incarcerated in Canada: A systematic review and meta-analysis. *American Journal of Public Health, 109*(3), E1–E11. https://doi.org/10.2105/AJPH.2018.304855

Bogen, D., & Whalen, B. (2019). Breastmilk feeding for mothers and infants with opioid exposure: What is best? *Seminars in Fetal and Neonatal Medicine, 24*(2), 95–104. https://doi.org/10.1016/j.siny.2019.01.001

Bowlby, J. (1952). *Maternal care and mental health.* World Health Organization Monograph. http://darkwing.uoregon.edu/~eherman/teaching/texts/Bowlby%20Maternal%20Care%20and%20Mental%20Health.pdf

Canadian Friends Service Committee (Quakers). (2018). *Considering the best interests of the child when sentencing parents in Canada: Sample case law review.* https://quakerservice.ca/wp-content

/uploads/2018/12/Considering-the-Best-Interests-of-the-Child-when-Sentencing-Parents-in-Canada.pdf

Casal, C. S., Lei, A., Young, S. L., & Tuthill, E. L. (2016). A critical review of instruments measuring breastfeeding attitudes, knowledge, and social support. *Journal of Human Lactation, 31*(1), 21–47. https://doi.org/10.1177/0890334416677029

Chambers, A. (2009). Impact of forced separation policy on incarcerated postpartum mothers. *Policy, Politics, & Nursing Practice, 10*(3), 204–211. https://doi.org/10.1177/1527154409351592

Cohen, S. (2016). *Mother-baby unit at B.C. jail in-use for the first time in eight years.* Metro News. https://www.thestar.com/news/world/2016/07/17/mother-child-prison-program-giving-babies-mothers-a-better-chance.html

Dieterich, C. M., Felice, J. P., O'Sullivan, E., & Rasmussen, K. M. (2013). Breastfeeding and health outcomes for the mother–infant dyad. *Pediatric Clinics of North America, 60*(1), 31. https://doi.org/10.1016/j.pcl.2012.09.010

Dillner, L. (1992). Keeping babies in prison: Regime should be more compassionate. *British Medical Journal, 304,* 932–933. https://europepmc.org/backend/ptpmcrender.fcgi?accid=PMC1882308&blobtype=pdf

Elfgen, C., Hagenbuch, N., Gorres, G., Block, E., & Leeners, B. (2017). Breastfeeding in women having experienced childhood sexual abuse. *Journal of Human Lactation, 33*(1), 119–127. https://doi.org/10.1177/0890334416680789

Felitti, V. J., Anda, R. F., Nordenberg, D., Williamson, D. F., Spitz, A. M., Edwards, V., Koos, M. P., & Marks, J. S. (1998). Relationship of childhood abuse and household dysfunction to many of the leading causes of death in adults. The Adverse Childhood Experiences (ACE) Study. *American Journal of Preventive Medicine, 14*(4), 245–258. https://doi.org/10.1016/s0749-3797(98)00017-8

Ferszt, G., Palmer, M., & McGrane, C. (2018). Where does your state stand on shackling of pregnant women? *Nursing for Women's Health, 22*(1), 17–23. https://nwhjournal.org/article/S1751-4851(17)30335-5/pdf

Figueiredo B., Canário C., & Field T. (2014). Breastfeeding is negatively affected by prenatal depression and reduces postpartum depression. *Psychological Medicine, 44*(5), 927–936. https://doi.org/10.1017/S0033291713001530

Flaherman, V. J., Hicks, K. G., Huynh, J., Cabana, M. D., & Lee, K. A. (2016). Positive and negative experiences of breast pumping during the first 6 months. *Maternal Child Nutrition, 12,* 291–298. https://doi.org/10.1111/mcn.12137

Government of Canada. (1982). *Canadian Charter of Rights and Freedoms.* https://laws-lois.justice.gc.ca/eng/const/page-15.html

Government of Canada. (1992). *Corrections and Conditional Release Act.* https://laws-lois.justice.gc.ca/eng/acts/C-44.6

Government of Canada, Department of Justice. (2017). *Final report of the ad hoc federal-provincial-territorial working group reviewing spousal abuse policies and legislation.* https://justice.gc.ca/eng/rp-pr/cj-jp/fv-vf/pol/p2.html

Haywood, P. (2017). Judge: Breast-feed ban in state prison violates constitution. *Sante Fe New Mexican.* http://www.santafenewmexican.com/news/local_news/judge-breast-feed-ban-in-state-prison-violates-constitution/article_199084e1-bf2b-5381-b4ad-c37a5d9a5e95.html

Health Canada. (2012). *Breastfeeding initiation in Canada: Key statistics and graphics (2009/2010).* https://www.canada.ca/en/health-canada/services/food-nutrition/food-nutrition-surveillance/health-nutrition-surveys/canadian-community-health-survey-cchs/breastfeeding-initiation-canada-key-statistics-graphics-2009-2010-food-nutrition-surveillance-health-canada.html#a2

Hidalgo v. New Mexico. (2017). 1st J.D. Ct. of Santa Fe County (NM), Case No. D-101-CV-2017-01658

Huang, K., Atlas, R., & Parvez, F. (2012). The significance of breastfeeding to incarcerated pregnant women: An exploratory study. *Birth, 39*(2), 145–155. https://doi.org/10.1111/j.1523-536X.2012.00528.x

Inglis vs. BC. 2013. *SCBC 2309.* https://www.courts.gov.bc.ca/jdb-txt/SC/13/23/2013BCSC2309.htm

Jones, K. M., Power, M. L., Queenan, J. T., & Schulkin, J. (2015). Racial and ethnic disparities in breastfeeding. *Breastfeeding Medicine, 10*(4), 186–196. https://doi.org/10.1089/bfm.2014.0152

Kajstura, A. (2018). *States of women's incarceration: The global context 2018.* Prison Policy. https://www.prisonpolicy.org/global/women/2018.html

Kim, M. (2018). From carceral feminism to transformative justice: Women of colour feminism and alternatives to incarceration. *Journal of Ethnic and Cultural Diversity in Social Work, 27*(3), 219–233.

Kouyoumdjian, F., Cheng, S., Fung, K., Orkin, A., McIsaac, K., Kendall, C., Kiefer, L., Matheson, F. I., Green, S. E., & Hwang, S. (2018). The health care utilization of people in prison and after prison release: A population-based cohort study in Ontario, Canada. *PloS One, 13*(8), E0201592. https://doi.org/10.1371/journal.pone.0201592

Law Library of Congress. (2015). *Laws on children residing with parents in prison.* https://www.loc.gov/law/help/children-residing-with-parents-in-prison/foreign.php#_ftnref411

MacDonald, F. S., Gobeil, R., Biro, S. M., Ritchie, M. B., & Curno, J. (2015a). *Women offenders, substance use, and behaviour, Research Report R358.* Corrections Services Canada.

MacDonald, F. S., Keown, L. A., Boudreau, H., Gobeil, R., & Wardrop, K. (2015b). *Prevalence of psychotropic medications among federal offenders, Research Report R373.* Corrections Services Canada.

Moffitt, P., & Dickinson, R. (2016). Creating exclusive breastfeeding knowledge translation tools with First Nations mothers in Northwest Territories, Canada. *International Journal of Circumpolar Health, 75*(1), 32989. https://doi.org/10.3402/ijch.v75.32989

Mulgrew, I. (2013). Jailed mothers have right to be with their babies, B.C. Court rules. *The Vancouver Sun.* http://www.vancouversun.com/life/mulgrew+jailed+mothers+have+right+with+their+babies+court+rules/9293262/story.html

Nolan, A., & Stewart, L. (2017). Chronic health conditions among incoming Canadian federally sentenced women. *Journal of Correctional Health Care, 23*(1), 93–103.

Paynter, M. J., Drake, E., Cassidy, C., & Snelgrove-Clarke, E. (2019). Maternal health outcomes for incarcerated women: A scoping review. *Journal of Clinical Nursing, 28*(11–12), 2046–2060. https://doi.org/10.1111/jocn.14837

Prison Legal News. (2018). *New Mexico prisoner obtains court order to allow breastfeeding.* https://www.prisonlegalnews.org/news/2018/apr/2/new-mexico-prisoner-obtains-court-order-allow-breastfeeding

Sheppard, M. (2017). MDC among first to have inmate breastfeeding policy. *Albuquerque Journal.* https://www.abqjournal.com/1165424/mdc-among-first-to-have-inmate-breastfeeding-policy.html

Shlafer, R., Davis, L., Hindt, L., Goshin, L., & Gerrity, L. (2018). Intention and initiation of breastfeeding among women who are incarcerated. *Nursing for Women's Health, 22*(1), 64–78. https://doi.org/10.1016/j.nwh.2017.12.004 https://pubmed.ncbi.nlm.nih.gov/29433701/

Strickland, P. (2008). Mother allowed to serve prison time with baby. *The Globe and Mail.* https://beta.theglobeandmail.com/news/national/mother-allowed-to-serve-prison-time-with-baby/article18444303/?ref=http://www.theglobeandmail.com&

Tam, K., & Derkzen, D. (2014). *Exposure to trauma among women offenders: A review of the literature, Research Report R333.* Correctional Service of Canada.

The Economist. (2013). *Why won't America ratify the UN Convention on Children's Rights?* https://www.economist.com/the-economist-explains/2013/10/06/why-wont-america-ratify-the-un-convention-on-childrens-rights

United Nations General Assembly. (1989). *Convention on the Rights of the Child.* https://www.ohchr.org/Documents/ProfessionalInterest/crc.pdf

United Nations General Assembly. (2015). *United Nations Standard Minimum Rules for the Treatment of Prisoners (the Nelson Mandela Rules).* https://cdn.penalreform.org/wp-content/uploads/1957/06/ENG.pdf

United Nations Office on Drugs and Crime [UNODC]. (2011). *The Bangkok Rules: United Nations Rules for the Treatment of Women Prisoners and Non-custodial Measures for Women Offenders with their Commentary.* https://www.unodc.org/documents/justice-and-prison-reform/Bangkok_Rules_ENG_22032015.pdf

Victora, C. G., Bahl, R., Barros, A. J. D., França, G. V. A., Horton, S., Krasevec, J., Murch, S., Sankar, M. J., Walker, N., & Rollins, N. C. (2016). Breastfeeding in the 21st century: Epidemiology, mechanisms, and lifelong effect. *The Lancet, 387*(10017), 475–490. https://doi.org/10.1016/S0140-6736(15)01024-7

World Health Organization (WHO). (n.d.). *Reproductive health.* https://www.who.int/westernpacific/health-topics/reproductive-health#:~:text=Reproductive%20health%20is%20a%20state,to%20its%20functions%20and%20processes

World Health Organization (WHO) and United Nations Children's Emergency Fund (UNICEF) (2018). *Ten steps to successful breastfeeding.* https://www.who.int/nutrition/bfhi/ten-steps/en

CHAPTER 14

Domperidone to Treat Low Milk Supply: Drivers of Use, Efficacy, and Safety

Janet Currie, PhD(c), MSW
Suzanne Hetzel Campbell, Ph.D., RN, IBCLC, CCSNE

LEARNING OBJECTIVES

1. Describe the characteristics and key drivers of low milk supply (LMS).
2. Evaluate the efficacy and safety of domperidone prescribed off label to treat LMS.
3. Understand the value of a precautionary approach to using domperidone to treat LMS.

KEY WORDS

- **Low milk supply (LMS):** A perceived or physiologically based deficit of human milk that is considered to be insufficient to meet a baby's needs.
- **Off-label prescribing:** Occurs when a drug is prescribed for an indication, patient group, dose level, or method of administration that has not been approved by a national health regulator such as Health Canada. The use of domperidone to treat LMS is an off-label use.
- **Prolongation of the QT interval:** An alteration of the electrical activity in the ventricular chambers of the heart that can lead to fatal arrhythmias.

Overview

LMS is one of the main reasons why mothers stop breastfeeding early. This chapter examines the factors that contribute to a diagnosis of LMS and discusses the safety and efficacy of domperidone, a drug that is increasingly being prescribed off label in some jurisdictions to treat this condition. Domperidone has not been approved to treat LMS in any jurisdiction in the world. Its efficacy in significantly increasing milk supply has not been clearly established. Research has also established a link between the use of domperidone and its QT-prolonging effects, including the potential for serious ventricular arrhythmia (VA), cardiac arrest, or sudden cardiac death (SCD). In this chapter, weighing the evidence on domperidone's efficacy in relation to its potential harms is discussed.

Introduction

There is a strong global consensus on the importance of exclusive breastfeeding for a minimum of 6 months, followed by up to 2 years with complementary feedings because of the overwhelming advantages of breastfeeding for the health and well-being of infants and their mothers.

About 90% of new Canadian mothers intend to breastfeed and go on to initiate breastfeeding. However, by the time their babies are 3 months old, rates of breastfeeding are declining. By 6 months, the rate of exclusive breastfeeding among Canadian women has dropped to an average of 14.4% (Public Health Agency of Canada, 2009). The duration of exclusive breastfeeding in Canada is comparable to other countries but shows a decline when compared with earlier Canadian research (AlSahab et al., 2010). In order to reverse these trends, the challenges faced by breastfeeding families must be understood and addressed.

One of the most common reasons mothers cite for stopping breastfeeding early is their belief that they lack sufficient human milk to feed their babies (Ahluwalia et al., 2005; Gatti, 2008; Li et al., 2008). Based on a review of the literature on the determinants of breastfeeding cessation, Gatti (2008) found that for about 35% of the women who stopped breastfeeding early, milk supply was the primary concern.

Low milk supply (LMS) is defined as a perceived or physiologically based deficit of human milk that is considered to be insufficient to meet a baby's needs. However, despite LMS being one of the main reasons mothers stop breastfeeding early, there is still much that we do not understand about this condition. This chapter discusses the scope and characteristics of LMS, the factors that contribute to it, how it is diagnosed, and the growing use of domperidone to treat it. In British Columbia, domperidone is being increasingly prescribed off label to new mothers to treat LMS, despite this indication being unapproved by Health Canada (Smolina et al., 2016).

Domperidone is a dopamine D2-receptor antagonist that has been approved for use in Canada as an antiemetic to prevent nausea and vomiting and as a prokinetic to enhance gastric mobility. One of domperidone's actions is the elevation of serum prolactin levels, which can lead to the adverse effect of lactation in those not breastfeeding (Apotex Inc., 2015). This use of the drug is off label—in other words, domperidone has never been approved by a drug regulator such as Health Canada to treat LMS.

Off-label prescribing is common, representing about 11% to 20% of all prescriptions and up to 100% for some drug classes. It is legal for a health care provider to prescribe a drug off label, but research indicates that the majority of drugs that are prescribed off label lack evidence of effectiveness (Eguale et al., 2012; Radley et al., 2006).

Off-label prescribing can be beneficial, especially when no other effective treatment options exist. However, because off-label uses are not subject to standard regulatory approval processes, they may expose patients to an "uncontrolled experiment" and to potential harms (Eguale et al., 2016; Herring et al., 2010; Weda et al., 2018).

In British Columbia, the off-label prescribing of domperidone to treat LMS grew from 8% in 2002 to 19% in 2011 among women with full-term births and from 17% to 32% for women with preterm births. The median daily dose for initial prescriptions increased from 60 mg/day in 2002 to 80 mg/day in 2011. The duration of treatment with domperidone also increased (Smolina et al., 2016). To date, this study is the most comprehensive review of the off-label use of domperidone to treat LMS in one jurisdiction. Other recent research suggests that, while the prescribing of domperidone to treat LMS in England has been low, the rate of use is increasing (Mehrabadi et al., 2018).

Domperidone has never been approved to treat LMS by any health regulator in any jurisdiction. In the United States, it was initially approved to treat dyspepsia in 1978 prior to some of its potential cardiac effects being well recognized. In 1986, the intravenous use of the drug was withdrawn, and the drug is no longer approved, although it can be obtained under special access provisions (U.S. Food & Drug Administration [FDA], 2019).

Some breastfeeding support websites and Facebook groups recommend domperidone as a treatment for LMS. There are no data available on the number of mothers accessing domperidone through online prescriptions.

Characteristics and Drivers of LMS

There are two broad categories of LMS, although these conditions are not always clearly differentiated. *Primary lactation insufficiency* involves limitations in milk supply related to physiological problems of the mother and/or baby. Examples include mammary hypoplasia or lack of sufficient glandular tissue, sometimes resulting from previous health conditions or breast reduction surgery. Other causes include severe illnesses, endocrine problems, spinal cord injury, obesity, metabolic disorders or physiological issues affecting the baby's ability to breastfeed (Campbell et al., 2018; Galipeau et al., 2017; Marasco, 2014; Neifert et al., 1990).

There is no definitive data on the percentage of mothers who have LMS because of physiological problems. Some studies state the rate of prevalence as high as 15%, whereas other estimates range from 1% to 5% (Neifert et al., 1990). In addition, physiological factors, such as endocrine disorders or previous breast reductions, do not always represent an "absolute contraindication" to breastfeeding (Marasco, 2014; Neifert et al., 1990).

Secondary breastmilk insufficiency or *perceived breastmilk insufficiency* is the most common type of LMS and is the primary focus of this chapter. LMS occurs when normal physiological processes that affect milk supply occur and/or when a mother interprets a baby's behavior as indicating a lack of satiety, which is then attributed to LMS. The factors that influence this type of LMS are multifactorial and can include the mother's misinterpretation of baby cues, such as fussiness or cluster feeding, her misunderstanding of the lactation process, or a baby's normal feeding and sleeping patterns.

Other factors can influence a mother's perception of whether she has LMS, including the impact of some caregivers on a mother's confidence to breastfeed, hospital breastfeeding policies, and how and when LMS is determined. The early introduction of human milk substitutes (formula), as a response to LMS may affect the milk supply further. Mothers may also lack knowledge of how well babies are adapted to the early postpartum period when only small amounts of colostrum are available and may worry that the baby's early weight loss indicates a problem (Campbell et al., 2018; Gatti, 2008; Hookway, 2016; Kent et al., 2012; Li et al., 2008). These and other factors can work alone or in combination to reduce the level of breastfeeding and the stimulation of the breast necessary for the establishment of breastfeeding.

There is not always a clear delineation between *primary* and *secondary* LMS, and often the two terms are used interchangeably. Gatti (2008) believes that this lack of differentiation could limit research on LMS because each is affected by different dynamics and may require different interventions.

Mothers' concerns about milk supply can be exacerbated by the lack of support and information provided to them in the early postpartum period. Leurer and Misskey (2015) identified the types of information and support needed by mothers to support successful breastfeeding. These include more clarity on feeding frequency and length, understanding baby behavior, and accurate ways of gauging milk supply.

Institutional policies can affect the early establishment of milk supply. Policies that support the mother's self-efficacy, early initiation of breastfeeding, skin-to-skin contact between mothers and babies, and rooming-in are known to assist in this process (Brockway et al., 2017; Kent et al., 2012; Moore et al., 2016; Renfrew et al., 2012).

Impact of Methods Used to Assess LMS

The methods most commonly used to diagnose LMS and the way concerns are conveyed to the mother may affect the mother's confidence as well as lead to overdiagnosis of LMS and early interventions that can affect milk supply (Brockway et al., 2017; Galipeau et al., 2018; McCarter-Spaulding, 2001).

One of the most validated methods for assessing milk volume is weighing an infant before and after each breastfeeding session over a 24-hour period (Scanlon et al., 2002). However, Mannion and Mansell (2012) suggest that this method is rarely used: "Maternal perception of insufficient milk production is almost never validated by measured milk volume but is a prime influence in maternal decision making to supplement with formula, discontinue breastfeeding, or use products that stimulate milk supply" (pp. 2–3).

Tracking the infant's weight for the first few weeks postpartum is also commonly used to assess whether the baby is receiving sufficient human milk. All babies lose a percentage of body weight in the first few days postpartum while the mother is producing small amounts of colostrum. Healthy full-term babies are well adapted to survive on the fluid and energy reserves in their own bodies until their mothers begin to produce more copious amounts of milk.

Research suggests that there is a lack of clear consensus on the weight-loss patterns of babies after birth and that there is variability among infants. Babies who are fed human milk substitutes (formula) gain weight more quickly than breastfed babies. This can skew perceptions of what is normal (DiTomasso & Paiva, 2018; Macdonald et al., 2003; Noel-Weiss et al., 2008; Tawia & McGuire, 2014).

The intensive monitoring of weight loss and the application of narrow guidelines about weight gain can contribute to the early introduction of human milk substitutes (formula) and lead to early breastfeeding cessation. In a study of weight changes in full-term breastfeeding newborns during their first 2 weeks of life, DiTomasso and Paiva (2018) found that the majority of the infants lost over 7% of their body weight and that, in this group, the use of human milk substitutes (formula) increased markedly by 14 days in comparison to the babies who lost under 7%. Verd et al. (2018) found that in cases where weight loss was above the median (6%), breastfeeding was more likely to be discontinued at 15, 30, or 100 days of the baby's life.

DiTomasso & Paiva (2018) suggest that close monitoring of the newborn's weight and health care providers raising alarms that may be premature may contribute to undermining a mother's confidence that may lead to the eventual cessation of breastfeeding: "When a provider expresses concern about a newborn's weight loss, this has the potential to shake a woman's confidence in her ability to breastfeed. Women who lack confidence in breast feeding are then more likely to discontinue breastfeeding and/or supplement breastfeeding with formula" (p. 91).

Torres (2014) has explored the impacts of medicalization on breastfeeding. She believes that medicalization has profound effects on the self-confidence of mothers and contributes to their worries about milk supply. The components of medicalization she describes include defining "normal" breastfeeding concerns in medical terms or pathologizing them, the increasing monitoring/surveillance of mothers who are breastfeeding, the use of specialists to address breastfeeding problems, and an increasing reliance on medical treatments or technologies to address problems. Technologies include human milk substitutes (formula), breast pumps, feeding syringes, and pharmaceuticals.

The growing use of domperidone to treat LMS can be seen as an aspect of the medicalization of breastfeeding. In British Columbia, between 2002 and 2011, there was a dramatic increase in domperidone's use as a galactogogue as well as increases in the duration of use and dose levels. By 2011, one in three mothers with preterm births and one in five with full-term births were being prescribed domperidone off label (Smolina et al., 2016).

Efficacy and Safety of Domperidone When Used to Treat LMS

Given the rising use of domperidone to address LMS, what can we say about the drug's efficacy and safety for this unapproved use?

There is a lack of high-quality research evidence on the efficacy of domperidone in terms of significantly increasing a mother's milk supply. A systematic review of domperidone's efficacy and safety when used to treat LMS (unpublished) by Puil et al. (2016) found that the quality of randomized controlled trials (RCTs) examining domperidone's efficacy were limited in terms of sample size, had very short follow-up periods, often focused primarily on preterm births, and did not consider meaningful outcome such as impacts on the duration of breastfeeding. Of the 10 RCTs that explored domperidone's effectiveness in increasing human milk supply, 4 looked at domperidone versus placebo (Blank et al., 2003; Campbell-Yeo et al., 2010; da Silva et al., 2001; Rai et al., 2016). All involved preterm births, and the participant levels for these studies were low: in total, 53 in the domperidone group and 56 in the placebo group.

Two of the RCTs (Knoppert et al., 2013; Wan et al., 2008) involved preterm births and compared different doses of domperidone (30 vs 60 mg/day). There was no significant difference in the increase in milk volume when higher dose levels were used.

No research has indicated that higher dose levels of domperidone are more effective for treating milk supply although dose levels appear to be increasing. Research conducted in British Columbia (Smolina et al., 2016) showed that median dose levels of domperidone increased from 60 mg/day in 2002 to 80 mg/day in 2011.

EMPOWER was a Canadian Institutes of Health Research, Health Canada–approved trial that compared domperidone with placebo and was designed to assess whether preterm babies were able to achieve an increase in human milk supply if given domperidone on or before 21 days postdelivery (Asztalos et al., 2017). The study found that women using domperidone increased their milk supply, but the volume of increase was modest and not statistically significant. The EMPOWER trial intended to enroll 560 participants but was terminated in 2015 due to low enrollment. Enrollment decreased when potential trial participants were required to participate in an expanded consent process that included information about domperidone's cardiac risks.

One of the criticisms of current research on domperidone is that the measurement of milk volume as an indicator of domperidone's efficacy may not be the most meaningful outcome to measure. Outcomes such as the effect of domperidone on an infant's weight or whether it contributes to the exclusivity or duration of breastfeeding were either not measured or were measured only for a few weeks during the trials.

When the safety of domperidone is considered, the drug is associated with a number of potential harms. Domperidone has properties related to other neuroleptics resulting in potential adverse effects, including akathisia, restlessness, and depression due to its blockage of D2 receptors, which not only affect the gut but also the central nervous system (Prescrire Analysis, 2014). Some research indicates that dose levels between 30 mg/day and 160 mg/day could lead to the drug acting as an antipsychotic. This could expose patients to many adverse effects, including effects upon withdrawal from the drug (Champion et al., 1986).

These neuroleptic-type effects were reported in two case reports (Doyle & Grossman, 2018; Papstergiou et al., 2013) describing mothers who had taken domperidone to increase their milk supply. Both women had unremarkable medical histories. They had been prescribed domperidone at doses over 80 mg/day. Both initially tapered the drug when they decided to stop breastfeeding.

After an initial period of no symptoms, both mothers experienced multiple disturbing symptoms, including anxiety, agitation, panic attacks, and insomnia. These symptoms immediately disappeared when the previous dose of domperidone was reintroduced. Each recovered after a slow taper of domperidone lasting 8 to 12 weeks.

The most serious and well-documented adverse effect associated with domperidone is drug-induced **prolongation of the QT interval** of the heart (LQTS). The QT interval is considered to be a biomarker for sudden cardiac death (SCD) because, with prolongation, the cardiac polarization/repolarization cycle can become more chaotic and occur concurrently, leading to ventricular dysrhythmia and torsades de pointes, which has a high rate of SCD.

QT prolongation can be congenital, caused by electrolyte disorders or by the concurrent use of other QT prolonging medications (Giudicessi et al., 2018; Jolly et al., 2009; New Zealand Medicines and Medical Devices, 2010; Straus et al., 2005). Domperidone is a known QT-prolonging medication as are many other commonly used drugs, including some antidepressants, antipsychotics, gastrointestinal drugs, and antibiotics (Credible Meds, 2019).

Research has clearly established a link between the use of domperidone and its QT-prolonging effects, including the potential for serious ventricular arrhythmia (VA), cardiac arrest, or SCD (Arana et al., 2015; Buffery, 2015; Doggrell & Hancox, 2014; Johannes et al., 2010; Hill, 2016; Hill et al., 2015; Michaud & Turgeon, 2013; van Noord et al., 2010). The majority of these studies focus on approved indications for the drug.

Both unmodifiable and modifiable risk factors can potentiate drug-induced QT prolongation as might occur with domperidone. Unmodifiable risk factors include independent risk factors, such as female gender, increasing age, genetic predisposition, and structural heart disease.

Many of the studies showing a link between domperidone and VA or SCD have been focused on older age groups (Johannes, 2010; van Noord et al., 2010). Between January 1985 and August 15, 1986, Health Canada received nine case reports of heart and rhythm disorders, including torsades de pointes, related to domperidone among patients, median age 42 (Djelouah & Scott, 2007). Most had used domperidone for approved indications, and the data did not establish causality. A summary safety alert published in 2015 by Health Canada stated that cases supporting the association between domperidone and serious abnormal heart rhythms were reported worldwide, including 342 reports of serious heart-related events in the manufacturer's database and 137 reports found in the World Health Organization database (Government of Canada, 2015a).

Hill et al. (2015) and Hill (2016) estimated domperidone to be the cause of 231 cardiac deaths per year in the French population age 18 years and older. The estimated exposure to domperidone was derived from national drug reimbursement claims, did not differentiate between on- and off-label uses, and included the reproductive age group. Domperidone is used off label in France, but these uses do not include using the drug to treat LMS.

Smolina et al. (2016) completed a study that examined the relationship between the cardiac outcomes of domperidone when used to treat LMS and VA. This retrospective, population-based cohort study looked at all women with a live birth in British Columbia between January 2002 and December 2011. The study estimated the rate of hospitalization for VA among women who were or were not exposed to domperidone.

This study (Smolina et al., 2016) concluded that the risk of VA requiring hospitalization was rare. There were no hospitalizations for cardiac arrest and 21 hospitalizations for VA during the postpartum period. The risk of VA was approximately double among those exposed to domperidone, although this association was not statistically significant. However, the study lacked power due to the small number of identified outcomes, an inability to conduct dose-response analyses, and a lack of access to emergency room records.

Hondeghem and Logghe (2017) report on recalculated data from a study by the European Medicines Agency on domperidone-associated cardiac events to determine the effects of age and sex. Using this and several other sources of data, the authors calculated SCD among women age 20 to 39 years treated 2 to 4 weeks with domperidone. This reanalysis estimated that the probability of SCD was about

112 SCDs per million treatments of domperidone (at 30 mg/day). At higher doses, this would increase to 635 SCDs per million treatments. The authors consider that there is a higher propensity in women to proarrhythmias by medications that block the hERG ion channels than in men. Other authors also suggest that gender is an independent risk factor for adverse drug reactions from drug-induced long QT syndrome (Drici & Clement, 2001; Vink et al., 2018).

Drici and Clement (2001) point out that two thirds of torades de pointes cases occur in women and that women are more likely to experience drug-induced adverse effects than men due to their "greater degree of polypharmacy, the increased bioavailability of drugs and a greater sensitivity of their target organs. Drug-induced LQTS with its associated torsade de pointes represents a particularly interesting model of female gender as a risk factor for adverse effects" (p. 582).

Modifiable risk factors associated with domperidone include the use of >1 QT-prolonging medication, dose levels of over 30 mg/day, and the concomitant use of medicines that affect the metabolism of other QT-prolonging medications or those that cause electrolyte abnormalities (New Zealand Medicines and Medical Devices, 2010).

The risk of using concurrent QT-prolonging drugs with domperidone is a concern because of the large number of drugs that are QT prolonging—some, such as antidepressants and antibiotics, which are commonly prescribed to women in the reproductive age group (Credible Meds, 2019). Some research indicates that it may be relatively common for patients to be concurrently prescribed more than one QT-prolonging drug, placing them at increased cardiac risk (Ehrenpreis et al., 2017).

The cardiac risks of domperidone are dose related with doses of over 30 mg/day associated with higher risks (Government of Canada, 2015b; Johannes et al., 2010; van Noord et al., 2010). Safety warnings about domperidone issued by national health regulators, such as Health Canada and the European Medicines Agency, recommend doses of no higher than 30 mg/day (European Medicines Agency, 2014; Government of Canada, 2012; Government of Canada, 2015b).

An additional safety concern is whether domperidone being transferred through human milk exposes the infant to risks. Although domperidone at small doses would be expected to produce low domperidone serum levels in babies, Hondeghem and Logghe (2017) suggest current studies on domperidone's effects are too limited to produce reliable information. In addition, they raise concerns that the blood–brain barrier in developing infants is less mature than in adults, potentially making them more vulnerable to the adverse effects of the drug.

In a review of the safety profile of domperidone, the authors conclude that the limitations of current research mean that the benefits of domperidone have not been established.

Both Health Canada and the European Medicines Agency have issued warnings about the approved indications for domperidone. The UK Medicines and Healthcare Products Regulatory Agency (MHRA) has also issued a "Dear Healthcare Professional Letter" regarding the risk of cardiac affects associated with the use of the drug and has recommended that its use be restricted to nausea and vomiting and that the dose and duration of use be minimal (Medicines and Healthcare Products Regulatory Agency, 2014). In a review of the safety of drugs prescribed in France, the journal *La revue Prescrire* described domperidone as a drug to avoid because of its limited efficacy and adverse effect profile (Prescrire Analysis, 2014, February 19).

Weighing the Benefits and Potential Harms of Domperidone to Treat LMS

In order to establish whether a drug should be taken, its potential benefits and harms must be weighed in relation to each other. For example, liver toxicity may be an acceptable risk in a drug approved to treat cancer but would be unacceptable if it was used for acne.

Some authors suggest that drugs prescribed for off-label indications should be subject to a more vigorous assessment of their risks and benefits because the degree to which they have been tested for other indications is unknown (Gazarian et al., 2006). Elements of this assessment would include determining the seriousness or life-threatening nature of the health condition, whether effective and safe treatments already exist to treat it, and the evidence base for its off-label use.

Clinical practices such as ensuring rooming-in, skin-to-skin contact, information on breastfeeding techniques, and support that helps women achieve breastfeeding success are well-established, effective, treatments for LMS that pose no or minimal risks. Domperidone is associated with increased cardiac risks and may act as a neuroleptic in some women. There is a lack of research on the potential harms of domperidone for women and their babies. Research is also lacking on the efficacy of doses over the recommended guidelines of 30 mg/day for increasing milk supply and the safety of these doses for mothers.

In addition, current research on domperidone has not measured a broader range of meaningful outcomes arising from the use of domperidone. These include measuring the drug's impact on the baby's weight over a specified time period or whether taking domperidone leads to a longer duration of breastfeeding. Considering these limitations, it may well be that using domperidone to treat LMS must be reexamined. A precautionary approach to using any prescription drug, particularly one that is being prescribed off label, should always be a guiding principle.

Key Points to Remember

1. Drugs that are prescribed off-label, in many cases, have not undergone the comprehensive testing protocols that are required for approved drugs and, for this reason, could potentially pose more harm. Research also indicates that most off-label uses lack strong evidence of their effectiveness.
2. Prior to prescribing any drug off label, a more systematic assessment of the drug's risks and benefits should be undertaken. This would include an evaluation of a drug's risks and benefits, the consideration of the seriousness of the health condition being addressed, and whether other safer treatments already exist.
3. Low milk supply (LMS) is one of the major reasons why mothers stop breastfeeding early and before they want to. More must be done to understand the complex factors that contribute to LMS, including early and over-diagnosis of the condition, early technological interventions, mother's own perceptions of her milk supply and inconsistent information, and support and encouragement available to women in the first few weeks postpartum.

Case Study

A new mother comes to see you with her one-week-old baby. She looks very tired and near tears and states, "My baby is crying all the time. I'm really worried I don't have enough milk. I read online that domperidone really helps. One of the hospital staff told me I might just be one of those women who can't produce enough milk. Can you help me?"

Case Study Questions

1. *What approach would you take to assist this mother?*
2. *What other information do you need specific to her past experience, pregnancy, and birth?*
3. *How might you incorporate relational practice communication techniques to illicit a mothers' fears and concerns, determine her goals for infant feeding, and identify where she is getting her information?*
4. *Consider factors important to the mother's breastfeeding self-efficacy. Are there strategies you might incorporate to enhance that and to evaluate her support systems? What effect might the hospital staff's comment have had on the mother?*

References

Ahluwalia, I. B., Morrow, B., & Hsia, J. (2005). Why do women stop breastfeeding? Findings from the Pregnancy Risk Assessment and Monitoring System. *Pediatrics, 116,* 1408–1412. https://doi.org/10.1542/peds.2005-0013

AlSahab, B., Lanes, A., Feldman, M., & Tamim, H. (2010). Prevalence and predictors of 6-month exclusive breastfeeding among Canadian women: a national survey. *BMC Pediatrics, 10*(1), 20. https://doi.org/10.1186/1471-2431-10-20

Apotex Inc. (2015, March 6). *Product monograph. Apo-Domperidone.* https://health-products.canada.ca/dpd-bdpp/index-eng.jsp

Arana, A., Johannes, C. B., McQuay, L. J., Varas-Lorenzo, C., Fife, D., & Rothman, K. J. (2015). Risk of out-of-hospital sudden cardiac death in users of domperidone, proton pump inhibitors, or metoclopramide: A population-based nested case-control study. *Drug Safety, 38*(12), 1187–1199. https://doi.org/10.1007/s40264-015-0338-0

Asztalos, E. V., Campbell-Yeo, M., daSilva, O. P., Ito, S., Kiss, A., & Knoppert, D. (2017). Enhancing human milk production with domperidone in mothers of preterm infants: Results from the EMPOWER trial. *Journal of Human Lactation, 33*(1),181–187. https://doi.org/10.1177/0890334416680176

Blank, C., Eaton, V., Esterman, A., & James, S. (2003). A double blind randomised controlled trial of domperidone and metoclopramide as pro-lactational agents in mothers of preterm infants. Department of Perinatology, Department of General Practice Flinders University of South Australia (unpublished).

Brockway, M., Benzies, K., & Hayden, K. A. (2017). Interventions to improve breastfeeding self-efficacy and resultant breastfeeding rates: A systematic review and meta-analysis. *Journal of Human Lactation, 33*(3), 486–499. https://doi.org/10.1177/0890334417707957

Buffery, P. J., & Strother, R. M. (2015). Domperidone safety: A mini-review of the science of QT prolongation and clinical implications of recent global regulatory recommendations. *New Zealand Medical Journal, 128*(1416), 66–74. https://pubmed.ncbi.nlm.nih.gov/26117678/

Campbell, S. H., Lauwers, J., Mannel, R., & Spencer, R. (2018). *Core curriculum for interdisciplinary lactation care.* Jones & Bartlett.

Campbell-Yeo, M. L., Allen, A. C., Joseph, K. S., Ledwidge, J. M., Caddell, K., Allen, V. M., & Dooley, K. C. (2010). Effect of domperidone on the composition of preterm human breast milk. *Pediatrics, 125*(1), e107–e114. https://doi.org/10.1542/peds.2008-3441

Champion, M. C., Hartnett, M., & Yen, M. (1986). Domperidone, a new dopamine antagonist. *CMAJ: Canadian Medical Association Journal, 135*(5), 457–461.

Credible Meds. (2019, May 13). *Risk categories for drugs that prolong QT and induce Torsade de Pointes (TdP).* https://www.crediblemeds.org/new-drug-list

daSilva, O. P., Knoppert, D. C., Angelini, M. M., & Forret, P. A. (2001). Effect of domperidone on milk production in mothers of premature newborns: A randomized, double-blind, placebo-controlled trial. *CMAJ: Canadian Medical Association Journal, 164*(1), 17–21.

Djelouah, I., & Scott, C. (2007). Domperidone: Heart rate and rhythm disorders. *Canadian Adverse Reaction Newsletter, 17*(1), 2.

DiTomasso, D., & Paiva, A. L. (2018). Neonatal weight matters: An examination of weight changes in full-term breastfeeding newborns during the first two weeks of life. *Journal of Human Lactation, 34*(1), 86–92. https://doi.org/10.1177/0890334417722508

Doggrell, S. A., & Hancox , J. C. (2014). Cardiac safety concerns for domperidone, an antiemetic and prokinetic and galactogogue medicine. *Expert Opinion on Drug Safety, 12*(1), 131–138.

Doyle, M., & Grossman, M. (2018). Case report: Domperidone use as a galactogogue resulting in withdrawal symptoms upon discontinuation. *Archives of Women's Mental Health, 21*, 461–463. https://doi.org/10.1007/s00737-017-0796-8

Drici, M. D., & Clement, N. (2001). Is gender a risk factor for adverse drug reactions: The example of drug-induced long QT Syndrome. *Drug Safety, 24*(8), 575–585. https://doi.org/10.2165/00002018-200124080-00002

Eguale, T., Buckeridge, D. L., Winslade, N. E., Benedetti, A., Hanley, J. A., Tamblyn, R. (2012). Drug, patient, and physician characteristics associated with off-label prescribing in primary care. *Archives of Internal Medicine, 172*, 781–788.

Eguale, T., Buckeridge, D. L., Verma, A., Winslade, N. E., Benedetti, A., Hanley, J. A., & Tamblyn, R. (2016). Association of off-label drug use and adverse drug events in an adult population. *JAMA Internal Medicine, 176*, 55–63. https://doi.org/10.1001/jamainternmed.2015.6058

Ehrenpreis, E. D., Roginsky, G., Alexoff, A., & Smith, D. G. (2017). Domperidone is commonly prescribed with QT-interacting drugs: Review of a community-based practice and a postmarketing adverse drug event reporting database. *Journal of Clinical Gastroenterology, 51*(1), 56–62. https://doi.org/10.1097/MCG.0000000000000543

European Medicines Agency. (2014, Septermber 1). *Restrictions on the use of domperidone-containing medicines.* https://www.ema.europa.eu/en/documents/referral/domperidone-article-31-referral-restrictions-use-domperidone-containing-medicines_en.pdf

Galipeau, R., Dumas, L., & Lepage, M. (2017). Perception of not having enough milk and actual milk production of first-time breastfeeding mothers: Is there a difference? *Breastfeeding Medicine, 12*(4), 211–217. https://doi.org/10.1089/bfm.2016.0183

Gatti, L. (2008). Maternal perceptions of insufficient milk supply in breastfeeding. *Journal of Neurosurgery, 40*, 355–363. https://doi.org/10.1111/j.1547-5069.2008.00234.x

Gazarian, M., Kelly, M., McPhee, J. R., Graudins, L. V., Ward, R. L., & Campbell, T. S. (2006). Off-label use of medicines: Consensus recommendations for evaluating appropriateness. *Medical Journal of Australia, 185*(10), 544–548.

Giudicessi, J. R., Ackerman, M. J., & Camgeri, M. (2018). Cardiovascular safety of prokinetic agents: A focus on drug-induced arrhythmias. *Neurogastroenterology & Motility, 30*(6), e13302.

Government of Canada. (2012, March 2). *Recalls and alerts: Domperidone maleate - association with serious abnormal heart rhythms and sudden death (cardiac arrest) - for health care professionals.* https://www.healthycanadians.gc.ca/recall-alert-rappel-avis/hc-sc/2012/15857a-eng.php.

Government of Canada. (2015a, January 20). *Recalls and safety alerts: Domperidone maleate - association with serious abnormal heart rhythms and sudden death (cardiac arrest) - for the public.* https://healthycanadians.gc.ca/recall-alert-rappel-avis/hc-sc/2015/43449a-eng.php

Government of Canada. (2015b, January 26). *Summary safety review - Domperidone - Serious abnormal heart rhythms and sudden death.* https://hpr-rps.hres.ca/reg-content/summary-safety-review-detail.php?lang=en&linkID=SSR00039

Herring, C., McManus, A., & Weeks, A. (2010). Off-label prescribing during pregnancy in the UK: An analysis of 18,000 prescriptions in Liverpool Women's Hospital. *International Journal of Pharmacy Practice, 18*, 226–229.

Hill, C. (2016). More on domperidone and sudden cardiac death. *Prescrire International, 25*(176), 278–279.

Hill, C., Nicot, P., Piette, C., LeGleut, K., Durand, G., & Toussaint, B. (2015). Estimating the number of sudden cardiac deaths attributable to the use of domperidone in France: Domperidone-attributable deaths in France. *Pharmacoepidemiology & Drug Safety, 24*(5), 543–547. https://doi.org/10.1002/pds.3771

Hondeghem, L. M., & Logghe, N. H. (2017). Should domperidone be used as a galactogogue? Possible safety implications for mother and child. *Drug Safety, 40,* 109–113. https://doi.org/10.1007/s40264-016-0478-x

Hookway L. (2016). An exploration of common infant behaviour misinterpretations that can lead to a perception of low milk supply. *Community Practice, 89*(1), 28–31.

Jolly, K., Gammage, M. D., Cheng, K. K., Bradburn, P., Banting, M. V., & Langman, M. J. S. (2009). Sudden death in patients receiving drugs tending to prolong the QT interval. *British Journal of Clinical Pharmacology, 68*(5), 743–751. https://doi.org/10.1111/j.1365-2125.2009.03496.x

Johannes, C. B., Varas-Lorenzo, C., McQuay, L. J., Midkiff, K. D., & Fife, D. (2010). Risk of serious ventricular arrhythmia and sudden cardiac death in a cohort of users of domperidone: A nested case-control study. *Pharmacoepidemiology & Drug Safety, 19,* 881–888. https://doi.org/10.1002/pds.2016

Kent, J., Prime, D., & Garbin, C. (2012). Principles for maintaining or increasing breast milk production. *JOGNN: Journal of Obstetric, Gynecologic & Neonatal Nursing, 41*(1), 114–121. https://doi.org/10.1111/j.1552-6909.2011.01313.x

Knoppert, D. C., Page, A., Warren, J., Seabrook, J. A., Carr, M., Angelini, M., Killick, D., & Orlando, P. D. (2013). The effect of two different domperidone doses on maternal milk production. *Journal of Human Lactation, 29*(1), 38–44. https://doi.org/10.1177/0890334412438961

Leurer, M., & Misskey, E. (2015). "Be positive as well as realistic": A qualitative description analysis of information gaps experienced by breastfeeding mothers. *International Breastfeeding Journal, 10,* 10. https://doi.org/10.1186/s13006-015-0036-7

Li, R., Fein, S. B., Chen, J., & Grummer-Strawn, L. M. (2008). Why mothers stop breastfeeding: Mothers' self-reported reasons for stopping during the first year. *Pediatrics, 122,* 69–76. https://doi.org/10.1542/peds.2008-1315i

Macdonald, P. D., Ross, S. R. M., Grant, L., & Young, D. (2003). Neonatal weight loss in breast and formula fed infants. *Archives of Disease in Childhood. Fetal and Neonatal Edition, 88*(6), F472–F476. https://doi.org/10.1136/fn.88.6.f472

Mannion, C., & Mansell, D. (2012). Breastfeeding self-efficacy and the use of prescription medication: A pilot study. *Obstetrics and Gynecology International,* 1–8. https://doi.org/10.1155/2012/562704

Marasco, L. A. (2014). Unsolved mysteries of the human mammary gland: Defining and redefining the critical questions from the lactation consultant's perspective. *Journal of Mammary Gland Biology and Neoplasia, 19,* 71. https://doi.org/10.1007/s10911-015-9330-7

McCarter-Spaulding, D. (2001). Parenting self-efficacy and perception of insufficient breast milk. *JOGNN: Journal of Obstetric, Gynecologic Neonatal Nursing, 30*(5), 515–522. https://doi.org/10.1111/j.1552-6909.2001.tb01571.x

Medicines and Healthcare Products Regulatory Agency. (2014, December 11). *Domperidone: Risks of cardiac side effects.* https://www.gov.uk/drug-safety-update/domperidone-risks-of-cardiac-side-effects

Mehrabadi, A., Reynier, P., Platt, R. W., & Filion, K. B. (2018). Domperidone for insufficient lactation in England 2002–2015: A drug utilization study with interrupted time series analysis. *Pharmacoepidemiol Drug Safety, 27,* 1316–1324. https://doi.org/10.1002/pds.4621

Michaud, V., & Turgeon, J. (2013). Domperidone and sudden cardiac death: How much longer should we wait? *Journal of Cardiovascular Pharmacology, 61*(3), 215–217. https://doi.org/10.1097/FJC.0b013e31827e2573

Moore, E. R., Bergman, N., Anderson, G. C., & Medley, N. (2016). Early skin-to-skin contact for mothers and their healthy newborn infants. *Cochrane Database of Systematic Reviews, 2016*(11). https://doi.org/10.1002/14651858.CD003519.pub4

Neifert, M., DeMarzo, S., Seacat, J., & Young, D. (1990). The influence of breast surgery, breast appearance, and pregnancy-induced breast changes on lactation sufficiency as measured by infant weight gain. *Birth, 17*(1), 31–38.

New Zealand Medicines and Medical Devices. (2010). Drug-induced QT prolongation and Torades de Pointes: The facts. *Prescriber Update, 3*(4), 27–29. https://medsafe.govt.nz/profs/PUArticles /DrugInducedQTProlongation.htm

Noel-Weiss, J., Courant, G., & Woodend, A. K. (2008). Physiological weight loss in the breastfed neonate: A systematic review. *OpenMed, 2*(4), e99.

Papastergiou, J., Adallah, M., Tran, A., & Folkins, C. (2013). Domperidone withdrawal in a breast-feeding woman. *Canadian Pharmacists Journal, 146*(4), 210–212.

Prescrire Analysis. (2014, February 19). *Domperidone: An indication of how many sudden deaths in France could be prevented by avoiding this low-efficacy drug.* https://english.prescrire.org/Docu /DownloadDocu/PDFs/domperidone_an_indication_of_how_many_sudden_deaths.pdf

Public Health Agency of Canada. (2009). *What mothers say: The Canadian maternity experiences survey 2009.* https://www.canada.ca/content/dam/phac-aspc/migration/phac--aspc/rhs-ssg/pdf /survey-eng.pdf

Puil, L., Mintzes B., Currie, J., Oberlander, T., & Hanley, G. (2016). *Post-partum domperidone use: What is the added value of observational data in an assessment of potential benefit versus harm?* (Poster) Cochrane International Colloquium.

Radley, D. C., Finkelstein, S. N., & Stafford, R. S. (2006). Off-label prescribing among office-based physicians. *Archives of Internal Medicine, 166,* 1021–1026. https://doi.org/10.1001/archinte .166.9.1021

Rai et al. (2016). Research letter. *Indian Journal of Pediatrics, 25,* 1–2.

Renfrew, M., McCormick, F., Wade, A., Quinn, B., & Dowswell, T. (2012). Support for healthy breastfeeding mothers with healthy term babies. *Cochrane Database for Systematic Reviews, 2012*(5), CD001141. https://doi.org/10.1002/14651858.CD001141.pub4

Scanlon, K. S., Alexander, M. P., Serdula, M. K., & Davis, M. K. (2002). Assessment of infant feeding: The validity of measuring milk intake. *Nutrition Reviews, 60*(8), 235–251. https://doi .org/10.1301/002966402320289368

Smolina, K., Mintzes, B., Hanley, G. E., Oberlander, T. F., & Morgan, S. G. (2016). The association between domperidone and ventricular arrhythmia in the postpartum period: Domperidone and arrhythmia postpartum. *Pharmacoepidemiol Drug Safety, 25*(10), 1210–1214. https://doi .org/10.1002/pds.4035

Straus, S., Sturkenboom, M., Bleumink, G, van der Lei, J., de Graeff, P., Kingma, J. H., & Stricker, B. H. Ch. (2005). Non-cardiac QTc-prolonging drugs and the risk of sudden cardiac death. *European Heart Journal,* (19), 2007–2012. https://doi.org/10.1093/eurheartj/ehi312

Tawia, S., & McGuire, L. (2014). Early weight loss and weight gain in healthy, full-term, exclusively-breastfed infants. *Breastfeeding Review, 22*(1), 31–42.

Torres, J. M. (2014). Medicalizing to demedicalize: Lactation consultants and the (de)medical-ization of breastfeeding. *Social Science & Medicine, 100,* 159–166. https://doi.org/10.1016/j .socscimed.2013.11.013

U.S. Food & Drug Administration (FDA). (2019, April 15). *How to request domperidone for limited access use.* https://www.fda.gov/drugs/investigational-new-drug-ind-application/how-request -domperidone-expanded-access-use

van Noord, C., Dieleman, J. P., van Herpen, G., Verhamme, K., & Sturkenboom, C. J. M. (2010). Domperidone and ventricular arrhythmia or sudden cardiac death: A population-based case-control study in the Netherlands. *Drug Safety, 33*(11), 1003–1014. https://doi.org/10 .2165/11536840-000000000-00000

Verd, S., de Sotto, D., Fernández, C., & Gutiérrez, A. (2018). Impact of in-hospital birth weight loss on short and medium term breastfeeding outcomes. *International Breastfeeding Journal, 13*(1), 25–27. https://doi.org/10.1186/s13006-018-0169-6

Vink, A. S., Clur, S. B., Wilde, A. A. M., & Blom, N. A. (2018). Effect of age and gender on the QTc-interval in healthy individuals and patients with long-QT syndrome. *Trends in Cardiovas-cular Medicine, 28*(1), 64–75. https://doi.org/10.1016/j.tcm.2017.07.012

Wan, E. W., Davey, K., Page-Sharp, M., Hartmann, P. E., Simmer, K., & Ilett, K. F. (2008). Dose-effect study of domperidone as a galactagogue in preterm mothers with insufficient milk supply, and its transfer into milk. *British Journal of Clinical Pharmacology, 66,* 283–289. https://doi .org/10.1111/j.1365-2125.2008.03207.x

Weda, M., Hoebert, J., Vervloet, M., Puigmarti, C. M., Damen, N., Marchange, S., Langedijk, J., Lisman, J., & van Dijk, . (2018, October 28). *Study on off-label use of medicinal products in the European Union.* https://ec.europa.eu/health/sites/health/files/files/documents/2017_02_28 _final_study_report_on_off-label_use_.pdf

CHAPTER 15

The Role of Physiotherapy in Breastfeeding Support

Mercedes Eustergerling, PT, IBCLC

LEARNING OBJECTIVES

1. Describe the physiotherapy scope of practice.
2. Apply physiotherapy principles to breastfeeding support.
3. Evaluate the role of physiotherapists in breastfeeding support across practice settings.
4. Design interdisciplinary breastfeeding support systems inclusive of physiotherapy.

KEY WORDS

- **Allodynia:** The experience of pain from non-nociceptive stimuli.
- **Alveoli:** The component of the mammary gland that synthesizes and stores milk; alveoli are lined with lactocytes and form a saclike structure.
- **Ankyloglossia (tongue tie):** An impairment in tongue function associated with a lingual frenulum that restricts tongue movement.
- **Biomedical model:** A conceptual model of health that attributes illness to biochemical and physiological factors.
- **Biopsychosocial model:** A conceptual model of health that encompasses biological, psychological, and social factors and how they overlap.
- **Blocked ducts (plugged ducts):** Localized inflammation of the breast that is noninfectious mastitis; characterized by redness, swelling, pain, heat, and/or loss of function.
- **Blood–breast barrier:** The lactocytes are connected by tight junctions, forming a barrier for substances moving between the milk in the alveoli and the bloodstream.
- **Breast crawl:** A series of reflex-driven movements to reach the breast, identify the nipple and areola, latch on, and suckle.
- **Central sensitization:** The increased response to stimuli from the central nervous system.

- **Congenital muscular torticollis:** A unilateral shortening of the sternocleidomastoid (SCM) muscle, resulting in ipsilateral cervical side flexion and contralateral cervical rotation.
- **Cryotherapy:** The use of cold for therapeutic benefit.
- **Frenotomy:** A procedure to cut a frenulum, often referring to the lingual frenulum if not otherwise specified.
- **Hypertonia:** Greater-than-normal resistance to passive stretch, describing one muscle or a group of muscles.
- **Hypotonia:** Less than normal resistance to passive stretch, describing one muscle or a group of muscles.
- **Lactocyte:** Cells that form the alveolar walls and synthesize milk.
- **Latch:** The way that an infant attaches to the breast, bottle, or feeding device.
- **Mastitis:** Inflammation of the breast, with or without an associated infection.
- **Milk ducts:** Canals that allow milk to flow from the alveoli to the nipple.
- **Milk ejection reflex:** The contraction of myoepithelial cells around the alveoli in response to oxytocin.
- **Nociception:** The detection of noxious stimuli and transmission of pertinent information through the nervous system.
- **Persistent pain (chronic pain):** Pain lasting more than 3 months or beyond the normal healing time of a condition.
- **Positioning:** The arrangement of the bodies and limbs of a dyad during feeds, with or without the use of props, pillows, or supports.
- **Spasticity:** Muscular resistance to passive movement that is velocity dependent.
- **Term infant:** An infant who is born between 37 weeks and 41 weeks and 6 days of gestation.
- **Therapeutic breast massage:** A manual technique that uses gentle massage toward the axilla and manual expression of milk to decrease symptoms associated with breast inflammation.
- **Therapeutic ultrasound:** The application of ultrasonic waves as an intervention, as opposed to diagnostic ultrasound.

Overview

Traditionally, physiotherapy is associated with the treatment of a person's movement and function. In fact, physiotherapy practice encompasses all of the body's systems, including integumentary, lymphatic, and urinary. Physiotherapists work in a variety of settings, including hospitals, schools, rehabilitation centers, private clinics, and more. This broad scope puts physiotherapists in a position to be involved throughout a health care system with an impact on a wide range of conditions, including breastfeeding support. This chapter presents breastfeeding as a functional activity for parent and infant and outlines the role of physiotherapists in this specialty area and the unique perspective they can bring.

An Overview of Physiotherapy

Physiotherapy (also called physical therapy) is a health profession that focuses on a person's movement and function. A physiotherapist views functional movement as integral to an individual's health and participation in society, and uses movement as a means to promote, maintain, and restore physical, psychological, and social function (World Confederation for Physical Therapy, 2017).

The profession is often associated with the treatment of the musculoskeletal, cardiorespiratory, and neurological body systems, since many university curricula are divided along these lines. However, physiotherapy practice encompasses all of the body's systems, including integumentary, lymphatic, and urinary. Physiotherapists work in a variety of settings, including hospitals, schools, rehabilitation centres, private clinics, and more. This broad scope puts physiotherapists in a position to be involved throughout a health care system with an impact on a wide range of conditions.

Maternal Conditions in Breastfeeding

A lactating individual can experience a variety of conditions, including those that are localized to the breast tissue and those that affect the entire body. Localized breast conditions, such as **mastitis** and nipple skin breakdown, arise as a direct result of breastfeeding dysfunction, and their management requires effective breastfeeding support. Other conditions, such as fibromyalgia, can impact one's ability to feed an infant, and exclusive breastfeeding similarly relies on their proper management. A physiotherapist with lactating individuals in their clinical practice has a responsibility to be informed on the unique anatomy and physiology of the lactating breast, the impact of breastfeeding dysfunction on a person's well-being, and the role of comorbidities in establishing or maintaining breastfeeding goals.

Local Breast Conditions

Within the lactating breast are unique anatomical and physiological features not found elsewhere in the body. **Lactocytes**—the cells that line the **alveoli** and produce milk are specific to breast tissue. **Milk ducts**, areolae, and nipples are other examples. The **blood–breast barrier** is analogous to other systems, such as the blood–brain barrier, but the understanding of one does not fully equate to an understanding of the other. For this reason, physiotherapists and other health care professionals must acquire breast-specific knowledge in order to assess and treat the conditions that affect it. Research demonstrating the efficacy of a treatment in another body part must be replicated in the lactating breast to be valid and applied in a clinical practice.

There are research studies, books, and continuing education courses, of course, to provide physiotherapists with an understanding of the unique properties of a lactating breast. This knowledge is necessary to carry out a complete assessment and gather the data that are needed to inform one's clinical decision making. In a survey of health care professionals, one participant noted that "mothers expected their health-care providers would have the knowledge and skills to assist them with common breastfeeding concerns" (Radzyminski & Callister, 2015, p. 103). The World Health Organization (WHO) recommends that health care professionals who advise pregnant women and mothers should have at least 18 hours of breastfeeding education (Ward & Byrne, 2011).

The lactating breast also has anatomical and physiological similarities with other body parts, and thus many of the fundamental principles of physiotherapy can be transferred to this population. This is how **therapeutic ultrasound** and low-level laser therapy came to be used for breast inflammation and nipple wounds, respectively. However, validation in the lactating breast is still necessary for evidence-based care.

Physiotherapy assessment and intervention can be applied to the tissue of a lactating breast when pathology arises. The following conditions involve inflammation, pain, and/or tissue damage of the breast.

Inflammation

Blocked or plugged milk ducts is a set of terms used to describe breast inflammation that is not infectious mastitis. In the literature, there is no clear differentiation between *blocked ducts* and *noninfectious mastitis*, though colloquially these terms typically represent different degrees of severity of breast inflammation. Symptoms of blocked ducts include localized tenderness, firmness, redness, and warmth (Campbell, 2006). Mastitis may also include systemic signs and symptoms, such as fever, chills, and aching (Amir et al., 2014).

Lactation mastitis need not involve an infection or pathogen, but by definition it always involves inflammation (WHO, 2000). Amir et al. (2014) outline the best practices for the treatment of breast inflammation, whether infectious or not. The first line of treatment is conservative (i.e., not pharmaceutical) in nature and can be carried out by a physiotherapist. The treatment of breast inflammation—blocked ducts and mastitis—involves frequent and effective milk removal from the affected breast, as well as supportive measures, such as rest, hydration, nutrition, and pain management. The WHO (2000) similarly recommends effective milk removal as a primary component of the treatment of breast inflammation.

Effective Milk Removal

Effective milk removal is dependent on three factors: feeding frequency, resistance to flow within the breast, and infant **latch** and suck mechanics. The latter will be discussed in a later section of this chapter.

Feeding frequency may or may not fall under the scope of practice of a physiotherapist. Valid arguments can be made on both sides, and each clinician will have to consult with their local legislators and regulatory bodies to guide their practice. On the one hand, feeding frequency can be viewed from the infant's perspective and belongs under the scope of dieticians, pediatricians, and family physicians. Physiotherapists do not typically make assessments or recommendations on nutritional needs, and interdisciplinary care is imperative to ensuring that changes in feeding frequency do not negatively impact the infant's growth and development.

On the other hand, feeding frequency can be viewed from the parent's perspective. One can consider recommendations on feeding frequency as managing the load on the tissues, limiting exposure to pro-inflammatory cytokines, and setting the parameters (volume, frequency, duration, etc.) of a home program for self-management. These are certainly within the scope of a physiotherapist, and they are necessary components of physiotherapy interventions throughout the body.

Thus, with an interdisciplinary approach to manage the infant's nutritional needs, a physiotherapist can implement the recommendations from the WHO (2000) and Amir et al. (2014) to breastfeed on demand—in other words, to feed infants as often as they desire, without restricting access to the breast. If the dyad is not exclusively breastfeeding or there are other factors limiting the infant's ability to remove milk from the breast, hand expression or a pump can be used.

The second factor in effective milk removal is resistance to milk flow within the breast. Human milk is made continuously and stored in the alveoli. If it is not removed, it distends the alveoli and opens the tight junctions between the lactocytes that line those alveoli. This allows pro-inflammatory cytokines—which protect the breast from infection—to enter the surrounding tissues and trigger an inflammatory response (WHO, 2000). Swelling is a component of inflammation, and if the tissues around the alveoli and ducts swell, this can impact the milk ducts, which are easily compressed (Hassiotou & Geddes, 2013). Compression of a milk duct increases the resistance to flow and therefore impedes milk removal from that part of the breast.

Cryotherapy

Physiotherapists have many techniques and options for managing inflammation. One of the most well-known modalities is **cryotherapy**: the use of cold for therapeutic benefit. Ice, a common component of acute injury management, is part of the RICE mnemonic (Rest, Ice, Compress, Elevate). However, in recent years there has been a push to question this tried-and-true approach.

It is reasonable to postulate that if ice reduces or interrupts inflammation, then the benefits of this natural process will not be realized. In acute injury, inflammation is followed by repair (scarring) and then tissue remodeling. The argument can then be made that using ice to limit inflammation will negatively impact the healing process. This argument is countered by studies that demonstrate no negative effect on healing despite reduced inflammation (Collins, 2008; Ramos et al., 2016).

A key difference between these cryotherapy studies and the lactating population is that breast engorgement, blocked ducts, and mastitis do not involve an acute tissue injury analogous to an ankle sprain or orthopaedic surgery. There is no known need for tissue repair and remodeling on the same scale in breast conditions. However, there is a need for swelling and pain management. The use of cold can play a role in the treatment of symptoms since it reduces both swelling and pain (Nadler, 2004). The breast tissue may have an advantage in pain management via cryotherapy because topical application affects the tissues 2 cm to 4 cm below the skin (Nadler, 2004), and breast tissue innervation is predominantly superficial (Hassiotou & Geddes, 2013).

Manual Therapy

A second modality for inflammation management is manual therapy. Swelling can be reduced by moving fluid from the breast and into the lymphatic system. Lymphatic drainage massage is a technique that is used in the breast cancer population to treat lymphedema (Williams et al., 2002). It has not specifically been tested in people with breast inflammation secondary to lactation, but aside from active infection in mastitis, there are no other contraindications in this population.

Therapeutic breast massage has been studied in lactating individuals with engorgement, plugged ducts, and mastitis. Researchers found positive results in the reduction of pain, engorgement, and plugged ducts (Witt et al., 2016). The technique involves gentle massage toward the axilla and hand expression of milk. In this way, it is similar to lymphatic drainage massage, but it is simpler for an individual to do independently and incorporates milk removal.

Box 15-1 Trauma-violence-informed Care

It is important to note here that breast palpation can be re-traumatizing for some individuals. Trauma-violence-informed care:

1. *Realizes the widespread impact of trauma and understands potential paths for recovery.*
2. *Recognizes the signs and symptoms of trauma in clients, families, staff, and others involved with the system.*
3. *Responds by fully integrating knowledge about trauma into policies, procedures, and practices.*
4. *Resists re-traumatization.*

(Substance Abuse and Mental Health Services Administration [SAMHSA], 2014)

Therapeutic Ultrasound

A brief internet search for "physiotherapy for mastitis" or "physiotherapy for blocked ducts" reveals page upon page of clinics offering therapeutic ultrasound for the treatment of these conditions. In a study of Australian physiotherapists in hospitals and private practices, 91% of interventions for mastitis involved therapeutic ultrasound (Diepeveen et al., 2019). Ultrasound parameters were variable, and their efficacies were not noted.

Despite its widespread use, there is no evidence to support therapeutic ultrasound as a treatment for breast inflammation. Two studies document the effectiveness of a multimodal treatment regimen, including therapeutic ultrasound, by physiotherapists (Cooper & Kowalsky, 2015) and chiropractors (Lavigne & Gleberzon, 2012). Neither study isolates therapeutic ultrasound as a variable nor uses a control group. When examining therapeutic ultrasound versus sham ultrasound (control) in breast engorgement, both groups had improvements in pain and hardness, with no significant benefit to the true ultrasound (McLachlan et al., 1991). Furthermore, a pilot study found no significant difference in outcomes between individuals treated by physiotherapists, with or without ultrasound, for blocked ducts (Campbell & Smillie, 2003).

It is worth noting that ultrasound parameters provided by the International Breastfeeding Centre (2017) are cited throughout these studies and widely used in clinical practice. They do not appear to be based on research, and it is not evident why ultrasound is recommended at all, given the available literature. Some physiotherapists may opt to use this modality for its placebo effect (McLachlan et al., 1991). However, with the amount of time an ultrasound treatment takes, it offsets other components, such as therapeutic breast massage, infant evaluation, history taking, and feed observation. Ultrasound is also a passive treatment that does not contribute to self-efficacy, and it is not accessible in all geographic areas.

Tissue Damage and Wound Care

When an individual sustains an ankle sprain, a physiotherapist will employ treatment techniques to minimize secondary tissue damage and to promote tissue healing. Likewise, for someone with osteoarthritis, the physiotherapist will adapt motor patterns and improve muscle strength to reduce compressive and shear stresses on the cartilage, while using modalities and movement to manage pain and encourage tissue remodeling.

For wound care, physiotherapists may receive training in this area at the entry-level programs and/or in continuing education, depending on their local curricula. The principles are much the same for injuries that are inside the body or at its surface. In the multidisciplinary wound care team, physiotherapists are underutilized, given that they can address many facets of wound care in a cost-effective way (O'Sullivan-Drombolis & Orr, 2011; Woelfel & Gibbs, 2017; Zhou et al., 2015).

Breastfeeding wounds on the nipple can arise from poor infant latch and **positioning**, oral anomalies, and suck disorders (Tait, 2000). Likewise, pump problems can contribute to nipple injury (Qi et al., 2014). The wounds are typically in the form of cracks, fissures, or abrasions, and they can be painful (Tait, 2000). Open skin provides an entry point for pathogens. Nipple pain is one of the leading causes of exclusive breastfeeding cessation (Kent et al., 2015).

In the management of any wound, it is imperative to minimize the stresses on the tissue that have formed the wound. This is often attempted in breastfeeding by changing the infant's positioning and latch, thereby altering the suck mechanics as well as the pressure or friction on the nipple. However, one study found incomplete resolution of nipple pain in cases where positioning and latch were contributors, and parents were given advice on positioning and latch (Kent et al., 2015). This suggests that nipple pain and nipple wounds may be complex. The study's authors suspect that nipple pain arises from a cascade of events and that early intervention is key. The role of a physiotherapist in latch and positioning is discussed later in this chapter.

In addition to nipple wound prevention by addressing positioning, latch, and suck mechanics, physiotherapists can also treat existing wounds. In multidisciplinary wound care teams, physiotherapists employ the use of biophysical agents (O'Sullivan-Drombolis & Orr, 2011). This is an aspect of infant feeding support that is not done by lactation consultants. It is a unique way in which physiotherapists can contribute their skills and knowledge. There is evidence for the effectiveness of low-level laser therapy (LLLT) and light-emitting diodes (LEDs) in this population (Chaves et al., 2012; Coca et al., 2016).

Pain

The management of acute and chronic pain requires interdisciplinary collaboration. Pain is a phenomenon that can deeply impact an individual's quality of life and functional capacity in many ways, and physiotherapists play a role in the prevention, screening, diagnosis, and treatment of pain-related conditions.

Until recently, pain education across health professions curricula was lacking. For physiotherapists specifically, a 1991 study of orthopaedic physiotherapists found that 72% reported their pain education as inadequate, and 96% preferred not to work with people with chronic pain (Wolff et al., 1991). In 2001, North American physiotherapy programs included 4 hours of pain education (Scudds et al., 2001).

The profession has since increased the number of contact hours in pain education to 37.5 in the United Kingdom in 2011, 45 in Norway in 2014, and 31 in the United States in 2015 (Bement & Sluka, 2015; Briggsl et al., 2011; Leegaard et al., 2014). In Australia, an innovative physiotherapy curriculum embeds pain education in all years, throughout the subjects (Hush et al., 2018). Canadian stakeholders in physiotherapy pain education identified and began to address barriers to pain education in that country (Wideman et al., 2018). In fact, the Canadian group proposed helping physiotherapists to identify as pain practitioners.

Applying the Current Understanding of Pain Science

The trend toward physiotherapists as leaders in pain education and pain practice is promising for both health care providers and those experiencing pain. Physiotherapists have a broad scope of practice, allowing them to incorporate many elements of pain science into their patient interactions.

Pain was traditionally seen as arising from human body tissue, and in many people's understanding of the topic, that paradigm persists. It was the gate control theory that first implicated the brain in the pain experience decades ago (Melzack & Wall, 1965). The theory placed the spinal cord at the center of pain processing, with bottom-up influences coming from afferent nerve fibers and top-down modulation from the brain. Different factors could either open or close the metaphorical gate in the spinal cord that allowed nerve signals to go through. Those signals would eventually reach the areas that determined responses, behaviors, and experiences.

The gate control theory continues to be the primary explanation for the use of transcutaneous electrical nerve stimulation (TENS) in physiotherapy today. Its publication also facilitated a shift from surgical pain management to pain modulation through the brain (Melzack & Katz, 2004). The trend away from a **biomedical model** of pain, and toward one that encompasses the whole person, was bolstered by the publication of the **biopsychosocial model** (Engel, 1977). In the biopsychosocial approach to health and disease, three facets of an individual's experience are considered, as are their overlapping properties. The biological facet encompasses genetic and tissue factors; the psychological facet involves thoughts, behaviors, and moods; and the social facet includes cultural, socioeconomic, and support systems.

Pain Science in Breastfeeding Support

The use of current pain science in breastfeeding literature is sparse and mixed. Few papers address pain from a perspective other than a biomedical one, resulting in a divide in the field of breastfeeding support. There is research on tissue-based causes of breast and nipple pain and separate research on psychosocial factors in breastfeeding. For the clinician, it can be challenging to apply scattered information to the whole person in front of them. Likewise, pain research from other populations may not easily translate to breastfeeding-related pain because of the unique aspects of breast tissue, postpartum psychological factors, and breastfeeding-specific social and cultural contexts.

The Academy of Breastfeeding Medicine **persistent pain** protocol (Berens et al., 2016) is a positive step in the recognition of parental pain during lactation, and it identifies gaps in the literature on breast and nipple pain. It does, however, employ a largely tissue-based approach to pain. This protocol defines persistent pain as lasting longer than 2 weeks. Typically, the definition of persistent pain is based on a longer time frame (3 to 6 months) or on the normal healing time of a condition (Treede et al., 2015). Several of the proposed causes of pain in the protocol are acute in nature, and they can be resolved with a biomedical treatment approach. Examples include breast pump trauma and bacterial infections.

The protocol does promote the consideration of the individual's psychological health and the link between breastfeeding-related pain and depression. The only listed condition that is not tissue based, however, is **allodynia**/functional pain. Recommended treatments include medications (nonsteroidal anti-inflammatory, beta blocker, and antidepressant) and trigger point massage, all of which are passive and tissue based. The authors recognize the role of psychological therapy for chronic pain but do not include it in the table of conditions.

A key gap in this protocol is the differentiation of **nociception**, acute pain, and persistent pain. Nociception is the ascending message from the sensory nerves to the central nervous system. Pain is an output of the central nervous system, and it can occur in the absence of the involved body part (e.g., phantom limb pain). Acute pain can be managed by tissue healing or treating the underlying condition. Persistent pain requires a comprehensive approach that addresses the facilitative and inhibitory inputs on the central nervous system, utilizes neuroplasticity, and encompasses the multifactorial nature of the pain experience.

Perhaps the clearest example of this in the protocol is the inclusion of herpes zoster infection and the omission of postherpetic neuralgia. The latter is a neuropathic pain condition lasting longer than 3 months (Sampathkumar et al., 2009). It is associated with **central sensitization** and anxiety (Schlereth et al., 2015). Central sensitization is the increased response to stimuli from the central nervous system, and allodynia is a characteristic component. It is this type of condition that is lacking from the Academy of Breastfeeding Medicine's protocol: the very conditions that physiotherapists and other team members are equipped to assess and treat.

The authors recommend more study in central sensitization, neuropathic pain, mood disorders, catastrophization, and dysautonomias in breastfeeding-related pain. While this would add to the understanding of breastfeeding-specific aspects of pain, the argument can be made that a health professional experienced in persistent pain can assess and treat an individual with current knowledge. Personal experience supports that the use of the biopsychosocial model allows for individualized pain management, treating pain as the condition itself. An example is included in the case study at the end of this chapter.

One theoretical paper addresses the need for modern neuroscience in breastfeeding-related nipple pain. Amir et al. (2014) "believe the understanding of nipple pain in lactation has been overly simplistic" (p. 127) and propose the application of a biopsychosocial lens to this population. They present a Breastfeeding Pain Reasoning Model that facilitates a comprehensive assessment of an individual experiencing pain. Following from the assessment, they provide evidence-based management recommendations. This model opens the door for physiotherapists—who are already assessing and managing chronic pain through a biopsychosocial lens—to apply their skills to the lactation population.

The Breastfeeding Pain Reasoning Model includes trauma history as a predisposing factor for nipple and breast pain. It is worth revisiting the principles of trauma-violence-informed care in the context of an individual with pain. Refer to the boxed content in the manual therapy section.

Summary of Physiotherapy for Maternal Conditions in Breastfeeding

The scope of practice of physiotherapists encompasses many of the challenges of lactation. In the case of wound care, a physiotherapist brings unique skills to the interdisciplinary team. With increasing pain education in physiotherapy curricula around the world, the physiotherapist provides a crucial biopsychosocial perspective to breastfeeding pain. Physiotherapists can make significant contributions if they become knowledgeable about breast anatomy, physiology, and pathology.

Infant Conditions in Breastfeeding

Maternal breast conditions are directly linked to the function of the infant during feeds. In the first part of this chapter, for example, nipple wounds were related to the infant's oral mechanics. Breast inflammation was tied to effective milk removal, in which the infant plays a crucial role. This section of the chapter will describe the infant components that may be assessed and managed by physiotherapy.

Neonatal breastfeeding is a neurological event. It is a sequence of behaviors that are reflex driven and occur in the same way across cultures and geography. From that biological norm, there are factors that can impact the process and, ultimately, breastfeeding function. For example, an infant can have abnormal reflexes, high or low tone, structural anomalies, or functional limitations.

Breastfeeding is an infant's first motor milestone. A healthy, **term infant** placed skin to skin on a lactating parent will use a series of reflex-driven movements to reach the breast, identify the nipple and areola, latch on, and suckle. This process, often called the **breast crawl**, was first described by Widström et al. in 1987. Motor components of the first feed are outlined in **Table 15-1**, and while the neonatal reflexes are intact, the process is similar for subsequent feeds.

Any impairment of these motor tasks will impact the infant's ability to reach the breast and transfer milk. These impairments may be modifiable, such as a reflex that's inhibited by maternal handling, or they may be inherent. Adaptations can be made for inherent impairments, such as low tone or limb injury. A physiotherapist can observe the breastfeed from start to finish, identify barriers to infant motor function, and modify or adapt as needed.

Cardiorespiratory Factors

Above all else, an infant will prioritize airway protection and breathing. This is a survival instinct that takes precedence over feeding. Disruption of normal breathing during feeds can require the infant to compensate, either by altering the suck-swallow-breathe mechanics or by unlatching from the breast, both of which can reduce the volume of transferred milk.

The swallowing reflex involves the coordination of muscles to move food from the oral cavity and into the esophagus, without any diversion into the airway. It is a complex motor task that will not be fully described here since that is not the primary focus of this chapter. Comprehensive resources for understanding the infant swallow exist (Geddes & Sakalidis, 2016; Genna, 2016). Of note, when the bolus reaches the pharynx, it must be directed into the digestive tract without compromising the airway.

Table 15-1 Reflex and Motor Components of the First Breastfeed

Behavior	Leg & Foot	Trunk	Arm & Hand	Neck	Jaw	Tongue
Rooting				x	x	
Hand to mouth			x	x	x	
Stepping	x	x				
Moving horizontally		x	x			
Reaching		x	x	x		
Looking		x	x	x		
Head bobbing		x		x		
Licking				x	x	x
Gaping				x	x	
Sucking					x	x
Swallowing					x	x

© Mercedes Eustergerling.

One way that airway access is closed off during swallowing is by elevation of the soft palate (Kramer, 1985). This prevents milk from going up and into the nasal cavity. Next, the vocal folds close, and the hyoid bone and larynx move upward (Geddes, 2016). This prevents milk from going into the trachea. Physiotherapists who work in a cardiorespiratory setting may have experience helping individuals following aspiration, when this mechanism did not function properly.

Blocking off the airway during a swallow means that breathing and swallowing do not occur simultaneously. Therefore, during each swallow, there is a momentary pause in breathing. The effect of this over time is seen in lower oxygen saturation levels after a feed, whether at the breast or bottle (Hammerman & Kaplan, 1995). (Notably, feeding at the breast results in a smaller oxygen saturation decrease.) For infants with existing cardiorespiratory compromise, the hypoxia can impact feeding function.

Cardiac Factors

Signs of congenital heart disease in an infant include increased hypoxia with effort, breathlessness, and an elevated resting respiratory rate (Genna, 2016). These infants may take frequent breaks or stop feeding as a compensation (Sadowski, 2009). It is important for the physiotherapist to recognize the signs of an infant with cardiorespiratory-related feeding difficulties.

Much like the management of aerobic exercise for adults with heart disease, the physiotherapist can play a role in adapting the activity to match an infant's cardiac function. Short, frequent feeds in this population help to avoid hypoxia and decrease the risk of aspiration (Genna, 2016). Parents and caregivers can also be educated on allowing breaks during breastfeeds to occur and incorporating breaks into bottle feeds. For infants recovering from cardiac surgery, a longer delay to oral feeding is associated with poorer oral feeding outcomes at discharge (Sables-Baus et al., 2012). Physiotherapists can help these infants not only from a cardiorespiratory perspective but also with any neurological or musculoskeletal barriers to oral feeding.

Respiratory Factors

The interruption of breathing during swallows can impact an infant with an existing respiratory dysfunction. During breastfeeding, the **milk ejection reflex** pushes milk from the breast alveoli and into the ducts, making it available to the infant at the nipple. The positive pressure of the milk ejection lasts 45 seconds to 3.5 minutes (Cannon, 2019). During that time, a burst of suck-swallow activity takes place, and the infant requires sufficient respiratory reserves to accommodate the reduced breathing. Between milk ejections, respiration can recover.

Examples of conditions that impact the respiratory function of an infant include cystic fibrosis, asthma, acute bronchiolitis, pneumonia, tuberculosis, lung cancer, congenital respiratory disorders, such as a hernia of the diaphragm, and upper respiratory tract infections, such as the common cold. In premature infants, conditions, such as apnea of prematurity, bronchopulmonary dysplasia, and respiratory distress syndrome, also impact the respiratory function.

Physiotherapists optimize the function of individuals with a variety of cardiopulmonary conditions—acute or chronic, congenital or acquired, and young or old. Indeed, the physiotherapy profession in the United States saw tremendous growth as a result of the polio epidemics of the early 20th century (Neumann, 2004). In the context of infant feeding, the physiotherapist can educate parents, caregivers, and the health team on the impact of feeding mechanics on respiratory function. Much like the use of short, frequent feeds for infants with cardiac conditions, the physiotherapist can employ paced feeding in cases of respiratory dysfunction.

The breast naturally paces a feed with its short bursts of milk ejection followed by a recovery phase. A physiotherapist who is working with an infant with cystic fibrosis, for example, can ask to observe a breastfeed as part of the functional evaluation of the infant. If the parent is using breast compressions or other methods to create a steady flow of milk, the physiotherapist can provide education and recommend a hands-off approach. For a bottle-fed infant, the breaks must be intentionally created. A physiotherapist can work with the parents of an infant experiencing respiratory difficulties with feeds, recommending pulling the bottle out after 45 seconds (the equivalent of a short milk ejection reflex). The timing can be adjusted according to the infant's needs. Note that the total milk volume is not adjusted by the physiotherapist; rather, it is the work of feeding that is reduced.

Box 15-2 Study Exercise

Think about your own swallow-breathe patterns. When you drink water out of an open cup, at which point in the breathing pattern do you swallow? What strategies do you employ to pause the influx of water during the swallow? Does it change if you use a straw? How might a different milk delivery method require adaptations in the suck-swallow-breathe mechanics? Consider the breast, a bottle with a slow flow rate, a bottle with a fast flow rate, a syringe, and cup feeding. What would you expect to see?

Table 15-2 Swallow and Respiratory Patterns in the Majority of Infants, Separated by Mode of Feeding

Group	I-I	I-E	E-I	E-E
Bottle Fed		x		x
Breastfed			x	x

© Mercedes Eustergerling.

In a healthy term infant, the role of the physiotherapist in cardiopulmonary function is to understand normal feeding mechanics and convey evidence-based care. Much of the literature on infant suck-swallow-breathe patterns is based on bottle feeding or extrapolated from adult biomechanics. For example, bottle-fed infants are more likely to swallow before an exhalation, whereas breastfed infants are more likely to swallow after an exhalation (Cannon, 2019). These trends are visualized in **Table 15-2**. The reason for one third of swallows occurring between expiration and inspiration is not well understood. It is possible that this is a mechanism for maintaining higher oxygen saturation during feeds, and certainly less hypoxia is seen in breastfeeding infants than in their bottle-fed counterparts (Hammerman & Kaplan, 1995). It is up to the physiotherapist to understand the evidence as it pertains to the biological norm of breastfeeding, and then to evaluate and address any barriers in individual cases.

Neurological Factors: Reflexes and Tone

A term baby is born with a set of primitive reflexes that help with performing essential tasks with limited motor abilities. Many of the reflexes involved in feeding are outlined in Table 15-1. The basis of a reflex—at any stage of life—is a simple process:

- A stimulus signal is conducted by the afferent nerves.
- Interneurons perform basic information processing 'that' takes place at a subconscious level.
- A response signal is conducted by the efferent nerves.
- The response is carried out by muscles, glands, and other tissues.

It is easy to see how a reflex can be inhibited or facilitated by looking at this process. First, each reflex has a specific stimulus that initiates the cascade. If the stimulus is not present, the reflexive behavior will not be observed. The physiotherapist or parent can elicit a desired motor response by introducing the corresponding stimulus. Conversely, the motor response may not be desirable during an activity, and it can be inhibited by removing the reflex-specific stimulus. Many of the recommendations that lactation consultants make to improve infant positioning and latch are based on this principle.

Second, the infant's nervous system needs optimal function to carry ascending and descending signals. If the reflex involves any processing, for example at the spinal cord, those structures are also susceptible to pathology and dysfunction. There are many conditions that can impact neurological function in an infant. These include chromosomal abnormalities (such as Down syndrome), congenital neurological disorders (such as spina bifida and cerebral palsy), and injuries (such as brachial plexus and spinal cord injuries). Physiotherapists are able to help with optimal function in these individuals by utilizing neuroplasticity and by adapting the activity.

Third, a motor response requires the proper function of the neuromuscular junction and muscle. Conditions that impact these structures will affect infant feeding. Examples of neuromuscular junction conditions include congenital myasthenia and infantile botulism. Muscle impairments, such as **congenital muscular torticollis**, are described in the Torticollis, Latch, and Tongue Tie section of this chapter.

What is immediately visible in many of these conditions is the impact of the neurological system on motor outputs. On a global scale, this can manifest as high tone (**hypertonia**) or low tone (**hypotonia**) of the muscles. Infants with high muscle tone or **spasticity** (two different but similar terms) demonstrate resistance to passive stretch. The muscles restrict the normal movement of their joints, including the limbs, trunk, neck, and jaw. Infants with low muscle tone present with weakness and difficulty executing motor tasks, especially against resistance or gravity. In both cases, compensatory strategies may be employed that are inefficient or fatiguing.

Physiotherapists evaluate the impairments that contribute to altered feeding function and create an intervention plan to address them. Neurological physiotherapy is highly individualized and dependent on the person's condition and context. Traditionally, this area of physiotherapy has divided itself into camps, with practitioners ascribing to schools of thought. Many still practice this way today. However, there is a shift toward the framework of the International Classification of Funtioning, Disability and Health (ICF) (WHO, 2001). This approach highlights that an individual's functional abilities are tied to tissue impairments and the environment, more so than the diagnosis. As neurological physiotherapy moves toward this model, practitioners are free to utilize the most appropriate interventions for an individual, regardless of the school of thought from which they originated (Barnes, 2003; Dimitriadis et al., 2016).

In the context of breastfeeding as the functional activity, physiotherapists can use any or all of the following approaches. These can be applied to an infant with a neurological condition or one whose neuromuscular function can be improved for the desired feeding outcomes.

1. *Breaking the task down into its components.* The physiotherapist may practice head-righting with an infant in order to assist with feeding equally from both breasts. Other examples are light touch at the chin to practice gape for a deep latch and prone activities (tummy time) for trunk stability and neck extension.
2. *Practicing the entire task with adaptations or modifications.* The infant can be positioned on pillows or props to compensate for weakness in postural muscles. Other examples include the dancer hold, which is often taught by lactation consultants for infants with hypotonia, and changing the parent's position to reduce the work against gravity.
3. *Using hands-on techniques to provide targeted sensory input.* Approaches in infant handling can serve as sensory input to alter the subsequent motor patterns and muscle tone. Facilitatory and inhibitory techniques include tapping, brushing, quick stretch, slow stretch, and ice. Increasing proprioceptive input facilitates the postural muscles (Metcalfe & Lawes, 1998).

© Mercedes Eustergerling.

Musculoskeletal Factors: Torticollis, Latch, and Tongue Tie

Muscles can restrict the range of motion of a joint if they are hypertonic or short. In the context of an infant's breastfeeding function, there are two primary mechanisms of muscle impairment in the absence of neurological conditions: congenital muscular torticollis (hereafter referred to as torticollis) and muscle overuse resulting from abnormal motor patterns.

Torticollis is a unilateral shortening of the sternocleidomastoid (SCM) muscle, resulting in ipsilateral cervical side flexion and contralateral cervical rotation. The incidence of torticollis is 4% to 16% of newborns (Kaplan et al., 2018). The condition may present with thickening or masses in the SCM, and its etiology is not completely understood. There are several subtypes within the torticollis population, making it difficult to study infants with the condition as a homogeneous group. Researchers have identified three main subtypes: postural (Boere-Boonekamp & van der Linden-Kuiper, 2001), muscular, and SCM mass (Cheng et al., 2001), but these categories are based on severity, and not etiology. Therefore, blanket statements about torticollis should be appraised with caution. It is possible, for example, that the documented associations with cranial deformation, hip dysplasia, brachial plexus injury, and lower-extremity anomalies (Kaplan et al., 2018) are related to the subtypes that have longer bodies, breech presentation, or forceps use during delivery. Much research does not separate samples into subtypes, instead looking at infants with torticollis as a whole.

Researchers studying torticollis agree that early intervention significantly improves outcomes for infants (Carenzio et al., 2015; Lee et al., 2017; Petronic et al., 2010). Current physiotherapy treatment recommendations are described in detail by Kaplan et al. (2018) in a freely available guideline. In this guideline, the first two days after birth are identified as a window when health care providers and parents can identify risk factors for torticollis and employ prevention strategies for postural preference. At present, very few birth centers across the world have physiotherapists on staff in the postpartum units. Infants who are not admitted to the neonatal intensive care unit may not see a physiotherapist for weeks or months, if at all. Incorporating infant-feeding support into the core competencies of a physiotherapist could create opportunities for the early identification of torticollis, reducing the episode of care and saving resources from more invasive interventions (Kaplan et al., 2018).

The association of torticollis and feeding function is well documented (Genna, 2015; Lal et al., 2011; Wall & Glass, 2006). Research indicates a potential bidirectional relationship, where torticollis can impact feeding preferences and abilities, and positions during feeding can lead to the development of torticollis. Interestingly, in a survey of physiotherapists in New Zealand, 95% of respondents almost or always asked about feeding status or feeding difficulties when assessing torticollis (Hale & Piggot, 2009). However, the objective assessments of these physiotherapists did not include an observed feed, with no mention of functional interventions for feeding. This is a valuable insight into physiotherapists' understanding of infant feeding as a functional motor activity, combined with their limited knowledge of how to assess and treat feeding difficulties.

Of note, the most immediately obvious mechanism of musculoskeletal feeding dysfunction may not tell the full story. It is reasonable to assume that muscular asymmetries make it difficult to maintain an optimal latch, either by pulling the head toward a directional preference or by restricting the range of motion of the neck and jaw. Certainly, torticollis can contribute to asymmetry of jaw, cheek, and lip function during breastfeeding (Genna, 2016). It may be tempting for the physiotherapist to focus on the mechanics of suck and swallow, as a physiotherapist with some knowledge of infant feeding can competently assess these areas. However, a lactation consultant may point out that effective feeding mechanics begin before the infant's mouth makes contact with the parent.

Genna (2016) outlines the phases of infant feeding, starting with an active phase of nonlocomotive movement and ending with sleep. A look at the earlier phases highlights the other impacts of musculoskeletal impairments on feeding function. For example, Brimdyr et al. (2003) found that the infant's chin, nose, and head position; cheekline; lip flange; angle of mouth opening; and body rotation were not associated with maternal nipple pain. There was, however, a slight association between nipple pain and rooting, gaping, sealing, and sucking behaviors. If torticollis and its related spinal and hip asymmetries impact the infant's abilities to express normal reflex motor patterns, then reaching the breast (the breast crawl) and latching on can also be affected. Recommendations for feeding the infant with torticollis highlight the role of infant-led latching and provide positional adaptations to accommodate the asymmetries (Genna, 2016). Allowing infants to use their hands for feeding helps with neck and shoulder stability (Genna & Barak, 2010).

Physiotherapists understand that asymmetries and repetitive maladaptive motor patterns can lead to the overuse and underuse of muscle groups. For example, tennis players may develop hypertrophy of the arm muscles in their dominant arm, with relative weakness in their nondominant arm. Unilateral inattention following a stroke can similarly result in muscle overload in one limb and underuse in the other. Torticollis intervention is important for the establishment of effective motor patterns in the infant.

Likewise, decreased surface electromyography activity is observed in the suprahyoid muscles of infants with a greater degree of **ankyloglossia** (França et al., 2020). In other words, a thicker tongue tie, with more anterior attachments and associated with few sucks/long breaks, inadequate coordination, nipple biting, and tongue snapping, is related to decreased activation of muscles that lift the hyoid bone. Hyoid elevation happens concurrently with elevation of the larynx during swallowing. Two suprahyoid muscles (the mylohyoid and the anterior belly of the digastric) also have attachments on the mandible and help to pull down the jaw. The electromyography study did not examine other muscle groups that may have increased activity to compensate for impaired tongue movements. However, in an older population, masseter activity during jaw protrusion decreased after

frenotomy (Tecco et al., 2015). Begnoni (2018) identifies that masseter activity can either increase or decrease, depending on the type of atypical swallow.

There is no question that ankyloglossia (tongue tie) can impact infant feeding. The key is to properly assess and diagnose the condition in order to determine the best course of treatment. It is true that a visible frenulum that does not alter feeding function is not a pathology that requires surgery. As with all other conditions that a physiotherapist evaluates, it is the function of the tongue that should inform the diagnosis of a tongue tie. Hazelbaker (1993) developed an assessment tool for ankyloglossia that includes functional and appearance items. This tool and its subsequent versions have been used in studies of tongue tie and frenotomy. Though it may have some limitations, it has good interrater reliability (Amir et al., 2006) and can serve as a consistent measure of ankyloglossia to compare across research studies. In infants with feeding dysfunction from ankyloglossia, a frenotomy improves milk intake, maternal nipple pain, and nipple compression with the tongue (Ballard et al., 2002; Geddes et al., 2008). Infants with tongue dysfunction in the absence of ankyloglossia should be evaluated by a physiotherapist or occupational therapist.

It is an interesting trend within the culture of breastfeeding support that musculoskeletal or biomechanical issues are referred to craniosacral therapists, osteopaths, and chiropractors (Genna et al., 2017; Haleryn & Mohr, 2019). These professions are defined differently across the world, and they range from unregulated practice to the equivalent of a medical doctor. What is missing from this group of so-called bodyworkers is physiotherapy. One has to wonder, why is a physiotherapist only considered for torticollis management (Genna et al., 2017)? What skills, knowledge, and research does the profession need to facilitate infant feeding beyond the sternocleidomastoid?

Infant Factors: Summary

Breastfeeding is the first motor milestone for many infants. It is a complex function that involves the cardiorespiratory, neurological, and musculoskeletal systems working together toward the common goal of milk transfer. For infants with pathology or medical conditions, the physiotherapist should assess this functional activity and use evidence-based interventions. For infants with biomechanical impairments, physiotherapists play a role in facilitating normal movement in all phases of feeding.

Breastfeeding as Public Health

The benefits of breastfeeding to both parent and infant are well documented, and the other chapters in this book describe them in detail. Effective breastfeeding support requires interdisciplinary collaboration (Campbell et al., 2019). Until now, the role of the physiotherapist on this team has not been outlined. With breastfeeding-specific knowledge and skills, physiotherapists can contribute to meeting individual and organizational goals for breastfeeding.

Looking at the role of physiotherapy on the parental feeding experience, the link between breastfeeding and pain is key. Nipple pain is one of the top reasons for cessation of breastfeeding, and it is a common reason for seeking breastfeeding support (Kent et al., 2015). Parents are often given contradictory information on pain with feeding: that breastfeeding is not supposed to hurt, and that some pain is normal. Improvements to the understanding of normal sensations in breastfeeding, the whole-person assessment of pain in this population, and acute pain management can help to minimize persistent pain. It is known that well-managed acute postsurgical pain can prevent subsequent persistent pain (Gordon et al., 2005; Kehlet et al., 2006; McGreevy et al., 2011).

One of the difficulties in addressing parts of the pain experience—as opposed to a whole-person approach—is that it can create unintended public health consequences. Opioid prescription for pain management is cited as one example, as it has led to opioid misuse on a tremendous scale (Carr, 2016). Persistent pain itself is a public health issue, and it is increasingly being framed as such by policy makers and researchers (Carr, 2016; Goldberg & McGee, 2011; Interagency Pain Research Coordinating Committee, 2016). As research continues to focus on postoperative, cancer, and neuropathic pain, the impact of pain on breastfeeding should not be forgotten. The sequelae of chronic pain include depression, inability to work, and use of health care resources. The impacts of breastfeeding-related pain include depression, less time between pregnancies, and use of health care resources. Brown et al. (2016) found that pain-related breastfeeding cessation increased the risk of depressive symptoms.

Physiotherapists receive more pain education than most other health professions, and that amount continues to increase. They are well-positioned to address breastfeeding pain from a biopsychosocial perspective, and they can address many feeding issues in the parent and in the infant. From the perspective of persistent pain management as a public health issue, the physiotherapist belongs on an interdisciplinary breastfeeding support team.

For the infant, breastfeeding is the first motor milestone. Feeding dysfunctions can provide insights into impairments that might not be immediately obvious. For example, the first sign of torticollis may be a preference to feed from one breast over the other. Functional movement is the cornerstone of physiotherapy, and much like persistent pain, participation in physical activity is a public health issue. Addressing barriers to movement in the early days of life can allow an infant to continue with normal motor development. For those with pathology or medical conditions, providing the foundation for physical activity may be even more important. About half of adults with disabilities are inactive, and they are 50% more likely to have a chronic disease than adults with disabilities who are physically active (Carroll et al., 2014). Martin Ginis et al. (2016) provide several recommendations for increasing participation in physical activity for people with physical disabilities. Among the recommendations is increasing self-efficacy. For the parents of infants with physical disabilities, seeing their child succeed at a task, such as breastfeeding, may be helpful for their belief that physical activity is feasible.

Gaps in Existing Physiotherapy Care for Breastfeeding

The inclusion of physiotherapists in breastfeeding support relies on the practitioners having sufficient knowledge and on the health system's willingness to utilize them in that role. Several gaps exist between the current roles of physiotherapists and the full integration of the profession into feeding support.

An opportunity for adding breastfeeding support into existing physiotherapy practice is in the context of women's health physiotherapy. This is sometimes known as pelvic physiotherapy. Pelvic physiotherapists ask about breastfeeding status during the assessment, since the hormones that are involved in lactation have an impact on pelvic health. These physiotherapists often help people with persistent pain, history of trauma, and intimate topics. They would be ideal candidates for learning how to support breastfeeding. Likewise, pediatric physiotherapists work with infants who have cardiorespiratory and neuromusculoskeletal impairments. Again, in parallel to pelvic physiotherapists, pediatric physiotherapists ask about breastfeeding status but may not have the knowledge to assess or manage feeding issues. It is worth noting that some physiotherapists have completed lactation-specific training, such as certificiation as an International Board Certified Lactation Consultant (IBCLC). Such physiotherapists are currently the exception and few in number. Education opportunities are needed for physiotherapists to learn breastfeeding-specific anatomy, physiology, assessments, and interventions. Since feeding involves the interaction of parent and infant, women's health physiotherapists will have the opportunity to take a step into paediatrics, and pediatric physiotherapists will have the opportunity to take a step into women's health.

Primarily in Australia and the United States of America, some physiotherapists are already providing treatments for breast inflammation. The vast majority involve therapeutic ultrasound, followed by education and advice, and manual therapy (Diepeveen et al., 2019). The gaps here involve knowledge translation about the efficacy of therapeutic ultrasound in breast inflammation, the inclusion of infant factors, and the assessment of a feed. A whole-person, biopsychosocial approach to the breastfeeding person's experience is necessary over the biomedical model of tissue-based assessment and treatment. Current practice appears to overemphasize the tissues (Cooper & Kowalsky, 2015), and this is a gap that can be addressed by applying physiotherapy principles to this population.

The U.S. Surgeon General's call to action to support breastfeeding notes that "there are few opportunities for future physicians and nurses to obtain education and training on breastfeeding, and the information on breastfeeding in medical texts is often incomplete, inconsistent, and inaccurate" (U.S. Department of Health and Human Services, 2011, p. 26). Certainly, there is little to no attention given to breastfeeding as a functional activity in physiotherapy textbooks. Breastfeeding is a nearly universal activity, and its evaluation should be given the same weight as the assessment of gait and ambulation in physiotherapy education.

Physiotherapists are well positioned to incorporate breastfeeding support into their existing practices. With sufficient knowledge in the area, it is possible that more infant feeding research will incorporate a physiotherapy perspective and that interdisciplinary teams will include the profession.

Key Points to Remember

1. Physiotherapists have a broad scope of practice that focuses on movement and function.
2. Breastfeeding is a functional activity for both the parent and the infant.

3. A biopsychosocial approach is appropriate to address the multifactorial nature of pain in this population.
4. For the infant, breastfeeding is a motor milestone that involves the cardiorespiratory, neurological, and musculoskeletal systems, among others.
5. Physiotherapy education should incorporate the assessment and optimization of breastfeeding as a functional activity.
6. Many of the common barriers to breastfeeding can be addressed by physiotherapy, and the physiotherapist's unique skills and knowledge should be utilized to improve public health via breastfeeding.

Case Study

Eskarne is a 31-year-old woman who presents to the outpatient physiotherapy clinic with mastitis. She has a 3-week-old daughter named Berezi. Eskarne's pregnancy was uncomplicated. She went into labor spontaneously at 39 weeks 5 days, and her labor was long. Pain management interventions included nitrous oxide gas and an epidural. During the pushing phase, Berezi's shoulder got stuck, and after a few attempts to get the shoulder out, the physician performed an episiotomy. Mother and child tried feeding right away, but Eskarne was inexperienced and Berezi wouldn't latch. She didn't want to ask for help because the physician and nurse were busy.

Over the past 3 weeks, they have gotten some help from friends and family members, and they are now exclusively breastfeeding. Berezi now has a shallow latch and falls asleep after 10 minutes. She wants to feed every 1.5 hours, and Eskarne thinks the shallow latch and frequent feedings are causing her nipple pain. Eskarne has wounds on both nipples that bleed after breastfeeding. She is taking oral antibiotics and does not have a fever. The underside of her right breast is red, hot, and firm.

Berezi's assessment reveals full range of motion in her neck with no palpable masses in the muscles. Her skin color appears normal, and she is breathing quietly without signs of distress. Her reflexes are normal except for the right upper limb, which has a weak palmar grasp and low tone. Berezi startles, and her arm goes into internal rotation with elbow extension and wrist flexion. Her tongue lateralization, elevation, and extension are normal. She sucks on a gloved finger with a cupped tongue and peristaltic rhythm. Her palate is a normal shape without a cleft. There is a highly elastic, thin lingual frenulum.

At the breast, Eskarne places her baby in the cross-cradle position with the help of a U-shaped pillow. She tucks Berezi's arms down and out of the way so she won't scratch her face. Berezi latches onto the nipple, moves her head quite a bit during the feed, and gums the nipple. She has loud swallows (gulps) and falls asleep after 10 minutes. Eskarne reports that Berezi is easy to burp and that her family thinks that she is a fussier baby than others.

Case Study Questions

1. What does a trauma-violence-informed approach look like in this situation? Are there specific parts of Eskarne's story that she may consider traumatic? How is pain affected by trauma?
2. Is this case appropriate for physiotherapy intervention? What other team members should be involved?

3. What is your working hypothesis for Berezi's feeding difficulties? Are there other conditions that you would want to rule out? If so, what information would you need?

4. What is the role of the shoulder in breastfeeding?

5. How would you help Berezi to attain a deeper latch and more effective suck at the breast?

6. What techniques or tools would you use to treat Eskarne's breast inflammation and nipple wounds?

7. How would you apply the biopsychosocial model to Eskarne's pain experience? What education would you provide about nipple pain?

© Mercedes Eustergerling.

Additional Resources

Therapeutic breast massage and hand expression of milk
https://player.vimeo.com/video/65196007
Physical therapy management of congenital muscular torticollis: Clinical practice guideline
https://rccinc.ca/wp-content/uploads/2019/02/Clinical-Practice-Guideline-for-Physical-Therapy
-Management-of-Congenital-Muscular-Torticollis.pdf
World Confederation of Physical Therapy, scope of practice overview
https://www.wcpt.org/node/29535
Trauma-Informed Care
https://store.samhsa.gov/system/files/sma14-4884.pdf
https://www.health.harvard.edu/blog/trauma-informed-care-what-it-is-and-why-its-important
-2018101613562
http://www.traumainformedcareproject.org
Breast Pain Model
https://pubmed.ncbi.nlm.nih.gov/25770578
International Association for the Study of Pain
https://www.iasp-pain.org
Supporting Sucking Skills in Breastfeeding Infants
Genna, C. W. (Ed.). (2016). *Supporting sucking skills in breastfeeding infants* (3rd ed.). Jones & Bartlett.

References

Amir, L. H., & Academy of Breastfeeding Medicine Protocol Committee. (2014). ABM clinical protocol #4: Mastitis, revised March 2014. *Breastfeeding Medicine, 9*(5), 239–243. https://doi .org/10.1089/bfm.2014.9984

Amir, L. H., James, J. P., & Donath, S. M. (2006). Reliability of the Hazelbaker assessment tool for lingual frenulum function. *International Breastfeeding Journal, 1*(1), 3. https://doi.org/10.1186 /1746-4358-1-3

Ballard, J. L., Auer, C. E., & Khoury, J. C. (2002). Ankyloglossia: Assessment, incidence, and effect of frenuloplasty on the breastfeeding dyad. *Pediatrics, 110*(5), e63–e63. https://doi.org/10.1542 /peds.110.5.e63

Barnes, M. P. (2003). Principles of neurological rehabilitation. *Journal of Neurology, Neurosurgery & Psychiatry, 74*(suppl 4), iv3–iv7. http://dx.doi.org/10.1136/jnnp.74.suppl_4.iv3

Begnoni, G. (2018). *Electromyographic evaluation of the efficacy of myofunctional therapy in patients with atypical swallowing.* University of Milan, Italy. https://air.unimi.it/retrieve/handle /2434/618978/1153101/phd_unimi_R11261.pdf

Bement, M. K. H., & Sluka, K. A. (2015). The current state of physical therapy pain curricula in the United States: A faculty survey. *The Journal of Pain, 16*(2), 144–152. https://doi.org/10.1016/j .jpain.2014.11.001

Berens, P., Eglash, A., Malloy, M , & Steube, A. M. (2016). ABM clinical protocol #26: Persistent pain with breastfeeding. *Breastfeeding Medicine, 11*(2), 46–53. https://doi.org/10.1089/bfm.2016.29002.pjb

Boere-Boonekamp, M. M., & van der Linden-Kuiper, L. T. (2001). Positional preference: Prevalence in infants and follow-up after two years. *Pediatrics, 107*(2), 339–343. https://doi.org/10.1542/peds.107.2.339

Briggsl, E. V., Carrl, E. C., & Whittakerl, M. S. (2011). Survey of undergraduate pain curricula for healthcare professionals in the United Kingdom. *European Journal of Pain, 15*(8), 789–795. https://doi.org/10.1016/j.ejpain.2011.01.006

Brimdyr, K., Blair, A., Cadwell, K., & Turner-Maffei, C. (2003). The relationship between positioning, the breastfeeding dynamic, the latching process and pain in breastfeeding mothers with sore nipples. *Breastfeeding Review, 11*(2), 5.

Brown, A., Rance, J., & Bennett, P. (2016). Understanding the relationship between breastfeeding and postnatal depression: The role of pain and physical difficulties. *Journal of Advanced Nursing, 72*(2), 273–282. https://doi.org/10.1111/jan.12832

Campbell, S. H. (2006). Recurrent plugged ducts. *Journal of Human Lactation, 22*(3), 340–343. https://doi.org/10.1177/0890334406290362

Campbell, S. H., & Smillie, C. M. (2003, August). Recurrent plugged ducts: The effect of traditional therapy versus ultrasound therapy. In *Health Care Conference and Annual Meeting of the International Lactation Consultant Association, Milk, Mammals & Marsupials: An International Perspective*, Sydney, Australia.

Campbell, S. H., Lauwers, J., Mannel, R., & Spencer, B. (2019). *Core curriculum for interdisciplinary lactation care.* Jones & Bartlett.

Cannon, A. (2019). Suck swallow breathe coordination in exclusively breastfed infants and those with oral anomalies [Doctoral dissertation, The University of Western Australia]. The University of Western Australia Research Repository. https://doi.org/10.26182/5dea0d3501790

Carenzio, G., Carlisi, E., Morani, I., Tinelli, C., Barak, M., Bejor, M., & Dalla Toffola, E. (2015). Early rehabilitation treatment in newborns with congenital muscular torticollis. *European Journal of Physical and Rehabilitation Medicine, 51*(5), 539–545.

Carr, D. B. (2016). "Pain is a public health problem"—What does that mean and why should we care? *Pain Medicine, 17*(4), 626–627. https://doi.org/10.1093/pm/pnw045

Carroll, D. D., Courtney-Long, E. A., Stevens, A. C., Sloan, M. L., Lullo, C., Visser, S. N., Fox, M. H., Armour, B. S., Campbell, V. A., Brown, D. R., & Dorn, J. M. (2014). Vital signs: Disability and physical activity—United States, 2009–2012. *MMWR. Morbidity and Mortality Weekly Report, 63*(18), 407.

Chaves, M. E. D. A., Araújo, A. R., Santos, S. F., Pinotti, M., & Oliveira, L. S. (2012). LED phototherapy improves healing of nipple trauma: A pilot study. *Photomedicine and Laser Surgery, 30*(3), 172–178. https://doi.org/10.1089/pho.2011.3119

Cheng, J. C. Y., Wong, M. W. N., Tang, S. P., Chen, T. M. K., Shum, S. L. F., & Wong, E. M. C. (2001). Clinical determinants of the outcome of manual stretching in the treatment of congenital muscular torticollis in infants: A prospective study of eight hundred and twenty-one cases. *The Journal of Bone & Joint Surgery, 83*(5), 679–687.

Coca, K. P., Marcacine, K. O., Gamba, M. A., Corrêa, L., Aranha, A. C. C., & de Vilhena Abrão, A. C. F. (2016). Efficacy of low-level laser therapy in relieving nipple pain in breastfeeding women: A triple-blind, randomized, controlled trial. *Pain Management Nursing, 17*(4), 281–289. https://doi.org/10.1016/j.pmn.2016.05.003

Collins, N. C. (2008). Is ice right? Does cryotherapy improve outcome for acute soft tissue injury? *Emergency Medicine Journal, 25*(2), 65–68. https://doi.org/10.1136/emj.2007.051664

Cooper, B. B., & Kowalsky, D. (2015). Physical therapy intervention for treatment of blocked milk ducts in lactating women. *Journal of Women's Health Physical Therapy, 39*(3), 115–126. https://doi.org/10.1097/jwh.0000000000000037

Diepeveen, L. C., Fraser, E., Croft, A. J. E., Jacques, A., McArdle, A. M., Briffa, K., & McKenna, L. (2019). Regional and facility differences in interventions for mastitis by Australian physiotherapists. *Journal of Human Lactation, 35*(4), 695–705. https://doi.org/10.1177/0890334418812041

Dimitriadis, Z., Skoutelis, V., & Tsipra, E. (2016). Clinical reasoning in neurological physiotherapy. *Archives of Hellenic Medicine/Arheia Ellenikes Iatrikes, 33*(4), 447–457.

Engel, G. L. (1977). The need for a new medical model: A challenge for biomedicine. *Science, 196*(4286), 129–136. https://doi.org/10.1126/science.847460

França, E. C. L., Albuquerque, L. C. A., Martinelli, R. L. C., Gonçalves, I. M. F., Souza, C. B., & Barbosa, M. A. (2020). Surface electromyographic analysis of the suprahyoid muscles in infants based on lingual frenulum attachment during breastfeeding. *International Journal of Environmental Research and Public Health, 17*(3), 859. https://doi.org/10.3390/ijerph17030859

Geddes, D. T., & Sakalidis, V. S. (2016). Breastfeeding: How do they do it? Infant sucking, swallowing and breathing. *MIDIRS Midwifery Digest, 26*(1), 95.

Geddes, D. T., Langton, D. B., Gollow, I., Jacobs, L. A., Hartmann, P. E., & Simmer, K. (2008). Frenulotomy for breastfeeding infants with ankyloglossia: Effect on milk removal and sucking mechanism as imaged by ultrasound. *Pediatrics, 122*(1), e188–e194. https://doi.org/10.1542/peds.2007-2553

Genna C. W. (2015). Breastfeeding infants with congenital torticollis. *Journal of Human Lactation: Official Journal of International Lactation Consultant Association, 31*(2), 216–220. https://doi.org/10.1177/0890334414568315

Genna, C. W. (Ed.). (2016). Supporting sucking skills in breastfeeding infants (3rd ed.). Jones & Bartlett.

Genna, C. W., & Barak, D. (2010). Facilitating autonomous infant hand use during breastfeeding. *Clinical Lactation, 1*(1), 15–20. https://doi.org/10.1891/215805310807011846

Genna, C. W., Murphy, J., Kaplan, M., Hazelbaker, A. K., Baeza, C., Smillie, C., Martinelli, R., Marchesan, I., & Douglas, P. (2017). Complementary techniques to address tongue-tie. *Clinical Lactation, 8*(3), 113–117. https://doi.org/10.1891/2158-0782.8.3.93

Goldberg, D. S., & McGee, S. J. (2011). Pain as a global public health priority. *BMC Public Health, 11*(1), 770. https://doi.org/10.1186/1471-2458-11-770

Gordon, D. B., Dahl, J. L., Miaskowski, C., McCarberg, B., Todd, K. H., Paice, J. A., Lipman, A. G., Bookbinder, M., Sanders, S. H., Turk, D. C., & Carr, D. B. (2005). American pain society recommendations for improving the quality of acute and cancer pain management: American pain society quality of care task force. *Archives of Internal Medicine, 165*(14), 1574–1580. https://doi.org/10.1001/archinte.165.14.1574

Hale, L., & Piggot, J. (2009). The physiotherapy management of infants with congenital muscular torticollis: A survey of current practice in New Zealand. *New Zealand Journal of Physiotherapy, 37*(3), 128.

Haleryn, J., & Mohr, J. (2019, October). *Structure and function: How the infant's structure affects the infant's function.* Session presented at the meeting of Canadian Lactation Consultant Association, Vancouver, Canada.

Hammerman, C., & Kaplan, M. (1995). Oxygen saturation during and after feeding in healthy term infants. *Neonatology, 67*(2), 94–99. https://doi.org/10.1159/000244149

Hassiotou, F., & Geddes, D. (2013). Anatomy of the human mammary gland: Current status of knowledge. *Clinical Anatomy, 26*(1), 29–48. https://doi.org/10.1002/ca.22165

Hazelbaker, A. K. (1993). *The assessment tool for lingual frenulum function: Use in a lactation consultant private practice.* (Master's Thesis). Pacific Oaks College, Pasadena, CA. https://doi.org/10.1186/1746-4358-1-3

Hush, J. M., Nicholas, M., & Dean, C. M. (2018). Embedding the IASP pain curriculum into a 3-year pre-licensure physical therapy program: Redesigning pain education for future clinicians. *Pain Reports, 3*(2), e645. https://doi.org/10.1097/PR9.0000000000000645

Interagency Pain Research Coordinating Committee. (2016). *National pain strategy: A comprehensive population health-level strategy for pain.* Department of Health and Human Services.

International Breastfeeding Centre. (2017). *Blocked ducts and mastitis.* https://ibconline.ca/information-sheets/blocked-ducts-mastitis

Kaplan, S. L., Coulter, C., & Sargent, B. (2018). Physical therapy management of congenital muscular torticollis: A 2018 evidence-based clinical practice guideline from the APTA Academy of Pediatric Physical Therapy. *Pediatric Physical Therapy, 30*(4), 240–290. https://doi.org/10.1097/PEP.0000000000000544

Kehlet, H., Jensen, T. S., & Woolf, C. J. (2006). Persistent postsurgical pain: Risk factors and prevention. *The Lancet, 367*(9522), 1618–1625. https://doi.org/10.1016/s0140-6736(06)68700-x

Kent, J. C., Ashton, E., Hardwick, C. M., Rowan, M. K., Chia, E. S., Fairclough, K. A., Menon, L. L., Scott, C., Mather-McCaw, G., Navarro, K., & Geddes, D. T. (2015). Nipple pain in breastfeeding mothers: Incidence, causes and treatments. *International Journal of Environmental Research and Public Health, 12*(10), 12247–12263. https://doi.org/10.3390/ijerph121012247

Kramer, S. S. (1985). Special swallowing problems in children. *Gastrointestinal Radiology, 10*(1), 241–250.

Lal, S., Abbasi, A. S., & Jamro, S. (2011). Response of primary torticollis to physiotherapy. *Journal of Surgery Pakistan (International), 16*(4), 153–156.

Lavigne, V., & Gleberzon, B. J. (2012). Ultrasound as a treatment of mammary blocked duct among 25 postpartum lactating women: A retrospective case series. *Journal of Chiropractic Medicine, 11*(3), 170–178. https://doi.org/10.1016/j.jcm.2012.05.011

Lee, K., Chung, E., & Lee, B. H. (2017). A comparison of outcomes of asymmetry in infants with congenital muscular torticollis according to age upon starting treatment. *Journal of Physical Therapy Science, 29*(3), 543–547. https://doi.org/10.1589/jpts.29.543

Leegaard, M., Valeberg, B. T., Haugstad, G. K., & Utne, I. (2014). Survey of pain curricula for healthcare professionals in Norway. *Vård i Norden, 34*(1), 42–45. https://doi.org/10.1177/010740831403400110Martin Ginis, K. A., Ma, J. K., Latimer-Cheung, A. E., & Rimmer, J. H. (2016). A systematic review of review articles addressing factors related to physical activity participation among children and adults with physical disabilities. *Health Psychology Review, 10*(4), 478–494. https://doi.org/10.1080/17437199.2016.1198240

McGreevy, K., Bottros, M. M., & Raja, S. N. (2011). Preventing chronic pain following acute pain: Risk factors, preventive strategies, and their efficacy. *European Journal of Pain Supplements, 5*(2), 365–376. https://doi.org/10.1016/j.eujps.2011.08.013

McLachlan, Z., Milne, E. J., Lumley, J., & Walker, B. L. (1991). Ultrasound treatment for breast engorgement: A randomised double blind trial. *Australian Journal of Physiotherapy, 37*(1), 23–28. https://doi.org/10.1016/S0004-9514(14)60531-6

Melzack, R., & Katz, J. (2004). The gate control theory: Reaching for the brain. In T. Hadjistavropoulos & K. D. Craig (Eds.), *Pain: Psychological perspectives* (pp. 13–34). Lawrence Erlbaum.

Melzack, R., & Wall, P. D. (1965). Pain mechanisms: A new theory. *Science, 150*(3699), 971–979. https://doi.org/10.1126/science.150.3699.971

Metcalfe, A. B., & Lawes, N. (1998). A modern interpretation of the Rood Approach. *Physical Therapy Reviews, 3*(4), 195–212. https://doi.org/10.1179/ptr.1998.3.4.195

Nadler, S. F., Weingand, K., & Kruse, R. J. (2004). The physiologic basis and clinical applications of cryotherapy and thermotherapy for the pain practitioner. Pain physician, 7(3), 395–400.

Neumann, D. A. (2004). Historical perspective—polio: Its impact on the people of the United States and the emerging profession of physical therapy. *Journal of Orthopaedic & Sports Physical Therapy, 34*(8), 479–492. https://doi.org/10.2519/jospt.2004.0301

O'Sullivan-Drombolis, D., & Orr, L. (2011). Underutilization of physiotherapists and biophysical agents in wound care. *Wound Care Canada, 9*(3), 8–14.

Petronic, I., Brdar, R., Cirovic, D., Nikolic, D., Lukac, M., Janic, D., Pavicevic, P., Golubovic, Z., & Knezevic, T. (2010). Congenital muscular torticollis in children: Distribution, treatment duration and out come. *European Journal of Physical and Rehabilitation Medicine, 46*(2), 153–157.

Qi, Y., Zhang, Y., Fein, S., Wang, C., & Loyo-Berríos, N. (2014). Maternal and breast pump factors associated with breast pump problems and injuries. *Journal of Human Lactation, 30*(1), 62–72. https://journals.sagepub.com/doi/10.1177/0890334413507499

Radzyminski, S., & Callister, L. C. (2015). Health professionals' attitudes and beliefs about breastfeeding. *The Journal of Perinatal Education, 24*(2), 102–109. https://doi.org/10.1891/1058-1243.24.2.102

Ramos, G. V., Pinheiro, C. M., Messa, S. P., Delfino, G. B., de Cássia Marqueti, R., de Fátima Salvini, T., & Durigan, J. L. Q. (2016). Cryotherapy reduces inflammatory response without altering muscle regeneration process and extracellular matrix remodeling of rat muscle. *Scientific Reports, 6*, 18525. https://doi.org/10.1038/srep18525

Sables-Baus, S., Kaufman, J., Cook, P., & Da Cruz, E. (2012). Oral feeding outcomes in neonates with congenital cardiac disease undergoing cardiac surgery. *Cardiology in the Young, 22*(1), 42–48. https://doi.org/10.1017/S1047951111000850

Sadowski, S. L. (2009). Congenital cardiac disease in the newborn infant: Past, present, and future. *Critical Care Nursing Clinics of North America, 21*(1), 37–48. https://doi.org/10.1016/j.ccell.2008.10.001

Sampathkumar, P., Drage, L. A., & Martin, D. P. (2009). Herpes zoster (shingles) and postherpetic neuralgia. *Mayo Clinic Proceedings, 84*(3), 274–280. https://doi.org/10.4065/84.3.274

Schlereth, T., Heiland, A., Breimhorst, M., Féchir, M., Kern, U., Magerl, W., & Birklein, F. (2015). Association between pain, central sensitization and anxiety in postherpetic neuralgia. *European Journal of Pain, 19*(2), 193–201. https://doi.org/10.1002/ejp.537

Scudds, R. J., Scudds, R. A., & Simmonds, M. J. (2001). Pain in the physical therapy (pt) curriculum: A faculty survey. *Physiotherapy Theory and Practice, 17*(4), 239–256. https://doi.org/10.1080/095939801753385744

Substance Abuse and Mental Health Services Administration (SAMHSA). (2014). SAMHSA's concept of trauma and guidance for a trauma-informed approach. https://store.samhsa.gov/system/files/sma14-4884.pdf

Tait, P. (2000). Nipple pain in breastfeeding women: Causes, treatment, and prevention strategies. *Journal of Midwifery & Women's Health, 45*(3), 212–215. https://doi.org/10.1016/s1526-9523(00)00011-8

Tecco, S., Baldini, A., Mummolo, S., Marchetti, E., Giuca, M. R., Marzo, G., & Gherlone, E. F. (2015). Frenulectomy of the tongue and the influence of rehabilitation exercises on the sEMG activity of masticatory muscles. *Journal of Electromyography and Kinesiology, 25*(4), 619–628. https://doi.org/10.1016/j.jelekin.2015.04.003

Treede, R. D., Rief, W., Barke, A., Aziz, Q., Bennett, M. I., Benoliel, R., Cohen, M., Evers, S., Finnerup, N. B., First, M. B., Giamberardino, M. A., Kaasa, S., Kosek, E., Lavand'homme, P., Nicholas, M., Perrot, S., Scholz, J., Schug, S., Smith, B. H., . . . & Wang, S. J. (2015). A classification of chronic pain for ICD-11. *Pain, 156*(6), 1003–1007. https://www.ncbi.nlm.nih.gov/pmc/articles/PMC4450869/

https://pubmed.ncbi.nlm.nih.gov/25844555/

U.S. Department of Health and Human Services. (2011). The surgeon general's call to action to support breastfeeding. https://www.ncbi.nlm.nih.gov/books/NBK52682/pdf/Bookshelf_NBK52682.pdf

van Vlimmeren, L. A., van der Graaf, Y., Boere-Boonekamp, M. M., L'Hoir, M. P., Helders, P. J., & Engelbert, R. H. (2007). Risk factors for deformational plagiocephaly at birth and at 7 weeks of age: A prospective cohort study. *Pediatrics, 119*(2), e408–e418. https://doi.org/10.1542/peds.2006-2012

Wall, V., & Glass, R. (2006). Mandibular asymmetry and breastfeeding problems: Experience from 11 cases. *Journal of Human Lactation, 22*(3), 328–334. https://doi.org/10.1177/0890334406290096

Ward, K. N., & Byrne, J. P. (2011). A critical review of the impact of continuing breastfeeding education provided to nurses and midwives. *Journal of Human Lactation, 27*(4), 381–393. https://doi.org/10.1177/0890334411411052

Wideman, T. H., Miller, J., Bostick, G., Thomas, A., & Bussières, A. (2018). Advancing pain education in Canadian physiotherapy programmes: Results of a consensus-generating workshop. *Physiotherapy Canada, 70*(1), 24–33. https://doi.org/10.3138/ptc.2016-57

Widström, A. M., Ransjö-Arvidson, A. B., Christensson, K., Matthiesen, A. S., Winberg, J., & Uvnäs-Moberg, K. (1987). Gastric suction in healthy newborn infants: Effects on circulation and developing feeding behaviour. *Acta Paediatrica, 76*(4), 566–572. https://doi.org/10.1111/j.1651-2227.1987.tb10522.x

Williams, A. F., Vadgama, A., Franks, P. J., & Mortimer, P. S. (2002). A randomized controlled crossover study of manual lymphatic drainage therapy in women with breast cancer-related lymphoedema. *European Journal of Cancer Care, 11*(4), 254–261. https://doi.org/10.1046/j.1365-2354.2002.00312.x

Witt, A. M., Bolman, M., Kredit, S., & Vanic, A. (2016). Therapeutic breast massage in lactation for the management of engorgement, plugged ducts, and mastitis. *Journal of Human Lactation, 32*(1), 123–131. https://doi.org/10.1177/0890334415619439

Woelfel, S., & Gibbs, K. A. (2017). *The role of physical therapists in wound management: An update.* https://www.acewm.org/uploads/content_files/files/The_Role_of_Physical_Therapists_in_Wound_Management.pdf

Wolff, M. S., Michel, T. H., Krebs, D. E., & Watts, N. T. (1991). Chronic pain—Assessment of orthopedic physical therapists' knowledge and attitudes. *Physical Therapy, 71*(3), 207–214. https://doi.org/10.1093/ptj/71.3.207

World Confederation for Physical Therapy. (2017). Policy statement: Description of physical therapy. https://www.wcpt.org/policy/ps-descriptionPT#appendix_1

World Health Organization (WHO). (2000). Mastitis: Causes and management (No. WHO/FCH/CAH/00.13). https://www.who.int/maternal_child_adolescent/documents/fch_cah_00_13/en

World Health Organization (WHO). (2001). International classification of functioning, disability and health: ICF. https://apps.who.int/iris/handle/10665/42407

Zhou, K., Krug, K., & Brogan, M. S. (2015). Physical therapy in wound care: A cost-effectiveness analysis. *Medicine, 94*(49), e2202. https://doi.org/10.1097/MD.0000000000002202

Glossary

Advocacy for Health Inequity "A deliberate attempt to influence decision makers and other stakeholders to support or implement policies that contribute to improving health equity using evidence" (Farrer et al., 2015, p. 396).

AIDED A framework including 22 enabling factors and 15 barriers to breastfeeding promotion that served as the building blocks for the breastfeeding gear model (BFGM) (Pérez-Escamilla et al., 2012).

Allodynia The experience of pain from non-nociceptive stimuli.

Allyship "[A]n active, consistent, and ongoing practice of unlearning and re-evaluating, in which a person in a position of privilege and power seeks to operate in solidarity with a targeted group. Practicing Allyship is not linear or constant and requires ongoing self-reflection and learning" (Anti-Oppression Network, n.d.).

Alveoli The component of the mammary gland that synthesizes and stores milk; alveoli are lined with lactocytes and form a saclike structure.

Ankyloglossia (tongue tie) An impairment in tongue function associated with a lingual frenulum that restricts tongue movement.

Artificial foods Foods that caused sickness in infants at the end of the 19th century. They included raw cow's milk; homemade concoctions of pureed table scraps, cow's milk, and water; and the commercial infant foods.

Augmentation Used when ongoing labor is determined not to be effective.

Baby-friendly Hospital Initiative A global initiative that began in 1991 to protect, promote, and support breastfeeding in facilities that provide maternity and newborn services. (Nyqvist et al., 2013; World Health Organization [WHO], 2018a)

Biomedical model A conceptual model of health that attributes illness to biochemical and physiological factors.

Biopsychosocial model A conceptual model of health that encompasses biological, psychological, and social factors and how they overlap.

Birthing practices Based on cultural influences, science, personal references, and health history, birth practices are how a pregnant individual gives birth to another human being.

Blocked ducts (plugged ducts) Localized inflammation of the breast that is noninfectious mastitis; characterized by redness, swelling, pain, heat, and/or loss of function.

Blood–breast barrier The lactocytes are connected by tight junctions, forming a barrier for substances moving between the milk in the alveoli and the bloodstream.

Body mass index (BMI) A weight-to-height ratio used to measure underweight, normal weight, overweight, and obesity. Measured in kg/m^2, BMI is an imperfect measure but is used in international research.

Breast crawl A series of reflex-driven movements to reach the breast, identify the nipple and areola, latch on, and suckle.

Breastfeeding Also called nursing, it is the feeding of young babies with milk from a mother's breast.

Breastfeeding dyad The infant and the human source of their nutrition. Often this is the biological mother, but this can also be a primary caregiver/nonbiological parent feeding directly at the breast or through a supplemental feeding system at the breast.

Breastfeeding Gear Model (BFGM) A model that identifies the key areas, or "gears," that need to be coordinated for synchronization of efforts to enhance (scale up) breastfeeding health promotion programs globally (Pérez-Escamilla et al., 2012).

Center their story A way of providing context and meaning to their experience through careful listening and relational practice, a main goal of the relational framework of breastfeeding support.

Central sensitization The increased response to stimuli from the central nervous system.

Cervix The opening between the uterus and vagina in a female.

Cesarean Birth Surgical removal of a fetus through the abdominal cavity.

Chestfeeding The feeding of young babies with human milk from a person's chest, often used by transgender and nonbinary people (Spalding, 2020).

Children's Rights The United Nations Convention on the Rights of the Child (United Nations General Assembly, 1989) sets out 18 human rights for all children around the world that define the standards in international law for how children must be treated to survive and thrive.

Collective Impact (CI) "The commitment of a group of important actors from different sectors to a common agenda for solving a specific social problem" (Kania & Kramer, 2011, p. 36)

Colonialism A controlling or governing influence of a nation acquiring full or partial political control of a dependent country, territory, or people, occupying it with settlers, and exploiting it economically.

Community Coalition Action Theory (CCAT) Provides a contextual understanding of inter-organizational collaboration related to community health promotion (Butterfoss & Kegler, 2009)

Congenital muscular torticollis A unilateral shortening of the sternocleidomastoid (SCM) muscle, resulting in ipsilateral cervical side flexion and contralateral cervical rotation.

Criminalization The social, political, and economic process through which interaction with the (in)justice system occurs.

Cryotherapy The use of cold for therapeutic benefit.

Cultural humility A process of self-reflection to understand personal and systemic biases and to develop and maintain respectful interactions and relationships based on mutual trust. Cultural humility involves humbly acknowledging oneself as a learner when it comes to understanding another's experience (First Nations Health Authority, n.d.).

Delayed lactogenesis II The onset of copious milk production later than 72 hours postpartum.

Depuration The removal of impurities from bodily fluids or tissues. Toxins are depurated from breast adipose tissue during weight loss.

Discrimination A prejudicial or unjust treatment of individuals based on a specific characterization, such as race, age, or sex.

Electronic fetal monitoring Use of instruments to monitor the fetal heartbeat and uterine contractions during labor.

Emergency An emergency is any situation with the potential to cause life-threatening or significant harm to an individual, household, community, nation or multiple nations and which does or could outstrip the capacity of local resources to respond. Emergencies can take many forms and typically do not impact all members of affected groups equitably. The term *emergency* is often used interchangeably with the term *disaster*, though the latter more often refers to a sudden-onset emergency affecting a specific geographic area, such as a tornado.

Endorphins Hormones secreted by the body in response to pain, extreme exertion, or high stress.

Epidural Regional anesthesia that can block pain receptors and numb specific areas in the lower region of the body. Epidural catheters are placed in the epidural space of the spinal column. Epidurals are frequently used during labor.

Exclusive breastfeeding A process wherein the infant receives only human milk and no other liquids or solids (WHO, 2019).

Feeding cues The deliberate body movements and sounds to communicate with caregivers when the infant is ready to feed or is hungry. There are three levels of feeding cues. These include early cues, such as lip smacking and bringing hands to mouth; mid cues such as more body movements, sucking on hands and rooting; and late signals, such as crying, fussiness, and becoming red in the face.

Feeding on cue Parent responsiveness to infant feeding cues.

Formula industry The industrial sector that manufactures infant formula.

Formula The word used to refer to standardized human milk substitutes.

Frenotomy A procedure to cut a frenulum, often referring to the lingual frenulum if not otherwise specified.

Global Strategy Infant and Young Child Feeding (GSIYCF) Aims to revitalize efforts to promote, protect, and support appropriate infant and young child feeding

Global Strategy on Infant and Young Child Feeding (GSIYCF) (2003) The Global Strategy on Infant and Young Child Feeding, jointly created by the World Health Organization (WHO) and the United National International Children's Emergency Fund (UNICEF), is a global guidance document with the aim of promoting, protecting, and supporting IYCF. It has been adopted by the World Health Assembly (WHA), the decision-making body of the WHO, and forms the basis for IYCF policy globally, with the objective of raising awareness of the importance of IYCF, increasing government commitment to funding IYCF programs and services, and creating an enabling environment for parents and caregivers.

Globalization A term used to describe the increasing connectedness and interdependence of world cultures and economies.

Going home Discharge from a setting that is not home by origination.

Health belief model A framework for health promotion that motivates individuals to change lifestyle and health behaviors related to their perception of risk of negative health consequences if they do not change their behavior

Health communication Process of communicating health promotion information to influence personal health choices and improve health literacy (Rimal & Lipinski, 2009).

Health Equality A state of being equal, in status and opportunities, with an aim to ensure that everyone gets fair and just access to enjoy full, healthy lives. Does not take into consideration privileges and rights afforded given one's race, gender, or social standing and that everyone does not start from the same place (EQUIP Health Care, 2017).

Health Equity Being fair and impartial takes into consideration that not everyone has similar privileges and contexts, so focuses on ensuring and treating those requiring care to have access to *what they need* to enjoy full, healthy lives. It aims to remove differences that may be unjust or unnecessary so resources or social institutions and policies can accommodate the needs of those requiring care (EQUIP Health Care, 2017).

Health promotion Social and environmental activities or processes to enhance health and well-being, by addressing and preventing the root causes of illness, not just treatment and cure (World Health Organization [WHO], 2016).

Hydrotherapy The use of warm water to help with pain management.

Hypertonia Greater-than-normal resistance to passive stretch, describing one muscle or a group of muscles.

Hypotonia Less than normal resistance to passive stretch, describing one muscle or a group of muscles.

IFE Core Group The Infant Feeding in Emergencies Core Group is a collaborative interagency expert group created to review and issue guidance on IYCF-E for policy makers and program managers.

Implicit bias Associations outside of conscious awareness that lead to negative evaluation of a person on the basis of irrelevant characteristics, such as race or gender, and are known to contribute to systemic inequities in healthcare service delivery, both broadly in healthcare and specifically in lactation care (Fitzgerald & Hurst, 2017; Thomas, 2018).

Incarceration The state of being confined in jail, prison, or another carceral facility, including immigration and youth detention.

Indigenous Native to or originating from a particular region or place.

Induction of labor Use of medications or natural methods to initiate labor contractions.

Industrialization The period of the development of the industries on a large scale; the transformation of an economy from an agricultural-based one to an industrial one.

Infant and Young Child Feeding (IYCF) Global term for nutrition guidance and programs from pregnancy through 23 months of age. IYCF includes breastfeeding, complementary feeding and nutrition for the non-breastfed child, and maternal nutrition through pregnancy and lactation. In some documents, Maternal, Infant & Young Child Nutrition (MIYCN) is also used to refer to similar guidance and programs.

Infant and Young Child Feeding in Emergencies ("IYCF-E") Global term for nutrition guidance and programs from pregnancy through 23 months of age during emergencies.

Infant and Young Child Feeding in Emergencies: Operational Guidance for Emergency Relief Staff and Programme Managers v 3.0 (Ops Guidance) Resource developed for policy makers, program managers, and staff providing support to children 0 to 23 months of age and their parents and caregivers in emergencies. This is the core reference document for the development and implementation of evidence-based IYCF-E policies and practices.

Infant behavior The cues, actions, and sounds an infant makes to communicate his or her needs to caregivers.

Infant feeding The act of supplying food and nourishment to an infant.

Initial latch The first latch after birth.

Innocenti Declaration A document capturing the renewed commitment on the 15th anniversary of the 1990 Innocenti Declaration, which added five operational targets as part of the ongoing global strategy on Infant and Young Child Feeding. Endorsed by the Standing Committee on Nutrition on March

17, 2006. The World Health Assembly welcomed the Call to Action made in the declaration on May 27, 2006

International Baby Food Action Network (IBFAN) Consists of public interest groups around the world working to safeguard infant and young child health and to reduce morbidity and mortality. It calls for laws to end predatory marketing and ensure food safety and monitoring so that systems are free from commercial influence (https://www.ibfan.org)

International Code of Marketing of Breast-milk Substitutes Passed as a resolution of the WHA in 1981 and updated periodically through subsequent WHA resolutions, the Code is a key mechanism for preventing the inappropriate distribution and promotion of human milk substitutes (formula) in emergency and humanitarian settings. Resolutions WHA49.15, WHA55.25, WHA59.21, and WHA63.23 are of particular relevance to emergency and humanitarian settings.

International Code of Marketing of Breast-milk Substitutes (the Code) A short hand reference to the international code developed by the WHO and United Nations International Children's Emergency Fund (UNICEF) and signed by the majority of countries worldwide to minimize marketing of human milk substitutes.

Interprofessional communication "Occurs when health providers/students communicate with each other, with people and their families, and with the community in an open collaborative and responsible manner" (Winnipeg Regional Health Authority, n.d., para 1).

Intersectionality A theoretical framework which posits that multiple social categories (e.g., race, ethnicity, gender, sexual orientation, socioeconomic status) intersect at the micro level of individual experience to reflect multiple interlocking systems of privilege and oppression at the macro, social–structural level (e.g., racism, sexism, heterosexism) (Bowleg, 2012).

Lactational programming Programming that stems from an exposure that occurs during the period when the mother is nursing her infant, which may lead to changes in the nutrients, hormones, or bioactive components in the milk and epigenetic changes in the infant.

Lactocyte Cells that form the alveolar walls and synthesize milk.

Latch The way that an infant attaches to the breast, bottle, or feeding device.

Listening from the heart Listening in a deep way that includes letting go of oneself and one's own agenda.

Low milk supply (LMS) A perceived or physiologically based deficit of human milk that is considered to be insufficient to meet a baby's needs.

Mastitis Inflammation of the breast, with or without an associated infection.

Milk ducts Canals that allow milk to flow from the alveoli to the nipple.

Milk ejection reflex The contraction of myoepithelial cells around the alveoli in response to oxytocin.

Mothers A woman in relation to her child; a female parent.

Motivational interviewing (MI) "A counselling technique designed to meet clients at their point of willingness to change and to support clients in incremental steps towards a goal" (Scherer & Love-Zaranka, p. 427).

Neo-BFHI A core document created to provide three guiding principles and Ten Steps to protect, promote, and support breastfeeding in neonatal intensive care units and for parents of premature infants. The Nordic and Quebec working groups prepared this document based on the Baby-friendly Hospital Initiative (BFHI; Hedberg-Nyqvist et al., 2015; WHO, 2018).

Nociception The detection of noxious stimuli and transmission of pertinent information through the nervous system.

Obesity A chronic, relapsing, multifactorial, neurobehavioral disease, wherein an increase in body fat promotes adipose tissue dysfunction and abnormal fat mass physical forces, resulting in adverse metabolic, biomechanical, and psychosocial health consequences. Obesity is measured by a body mass index of >30.

Off-label prescribing Occurs when a drug is prescribed for an indication, patient group, dose level, or method of administration that has not been approved by a national health regulator such as Health Canada. The use of domperidone to treat LMS is an off-label use.

PAHO/WHO Pan American Health Organization/World Health Organization.

Patient-centered care A framework that supports patients to make informed decisions and retain control over their health care choice. The Institute of Medicine defines it as "providing care that is respectful of, and responsive to, individual patient preferences, needs, and values, and ensuring that patient values guide all clinical decisions" (IOM, 2001, p. 6).

Pediatricians Medical practitioners specializing in the treatment of children and disease specific to this population.

Persistent pain (chronic pain) Pain lasting more than 3 months or beyond the normal healing time of a condition.

Physiological Birth Labor is allowed to begin on its own, and there are no routine or medical interventions that alter the course of the labor or birth.

Pitocin Synthetic oxytocin. Used to augment labor or reduce risk of postpartum hemorrhage.

Placenta Essential organ of pregnancy. Attached to the wall of the uterus. The role is to allow for nutrient uptake by and removal of waste from the fetus.

Policy A set of ideas or a plan of what to do in particular situations that has been agreed to officially by a group of people, a business organization, a government, or a political party. (Cambridge University Press, 2020)

Positioning The arrangement of the bodies and limbs of a dyad during feeds, with or without the use of props, pillows, or supports.

Postpartum weight retention The difference in prepregnancy weight and weight at 1 year postpartum.

Prolongation of the QT interval An alteration of the electrical activity in the ventricular chambers of the heart which can lead to fatal arrhythmias.

Public health The health of the population in its entirety; the branch of medicine dealing with public health (includes hygiene, epidemiology, and disease prevention).

Racism Discrimination, prejudice, or antagonism directed against a person or people based on their membership in a particular ethnic or racial group, typically a minority or marginalized group.

Reasoned action approach A theory that emerged from the theory of planned behavior and reasoned action, which integrated and redefined initial constructs to create a framework that better predicts human behaviors incorporating attitude; subjective norm; and perceived behavioral control—capacity (e.g., self-efficacy) and autonomy (individual control) (Fishbein & Ajzen, 2011)

Reflective practice A way of being that involves both an examination of experiences to understand situations for improvement of practice and the deeper process of questioning assumptions and interrogating the power and morality infused in practice to raise one's awareness and critical conscience (Wigginton et al., 2019).

Renewed understanding of the situation During a lactation consult, integrating the parent's story, goals and information gathered during the history and/or assessment to arrive at a new more holistic understanding of the issue.

Reproductive Health The World Health Organization (WHO, n.d.) defines reproductive health as a state of complete physical, mental, and social well-being and not merely the absence of disease or infirmity, in all matters relating to the reproductive system and to its functions and processes.

Rooming-in From birth to discharge, the infant remains in the room with the birthing parent and family members. The infant is only removed from the room for procedures or testing that cannot occur in the parent's birthing suite or hospital room. .

Scaling Up Public Health Initiatives Specific interventions to increase the quality of and improve specific programs and initiatives, taking into consideration the political, social, economic, and legislative actions necessary and the context to support public health initiatives.

Self-efficacy The confidence individuals have in their ability to enact a behavior or complete a task, a manipulable concept that targeted interventions can affect and explain changes in behavior. According to social cognitive theory (SCT), self-efficacy as a construct within it explains one's confidence in one's ability and is a product of experience in performing the behavior, vicarious experience (observation), persuasion, and emotional response.

Settlers Persons who move with a group of others to live in a new area, country. May be co-conspirators with the powerful colonizing group, or consider themselves a visitor to the area or in allyship with the indigenous peoples inhabiting the new area.

Shared decision making (SDM) "Form of nondirective counselling where the professional and patient come together as experts, in clinical evidence and lived experience to help the family reach their goals" (Munro et al., 2019, p. 394).

Shared Decision Making a key component of patient-centered care that represents a collaborative process in which clinicians and patients work together to make decisions about health care, balancing risks and expected outcomes and considering patients' preferences and values (National Learning Consortium, 2013).

Skin-to-Skin Placing an infant with only a diaper on, or naked, stomach down, between the breasts or on the anterior chest of an awake and alert adult. The premise of skin-to-skin is to promote bonding, help an infant self-regulate, and, if applicable, promote breastfeeding.

Social cognitive theory A learning theory developed by Albert Bandura that incorporates practice, observational learning, modelling, and self-efficacy, which allows enhancement of knowledge, attitudes, and behaviors to positively reinforce one's performance (Bandura, 1986).

Social Determinants of Health (SDOH) Effects of gender, poverty, trauma, race, status (immigrant, refugee), sexual orientation, and health literacy on one's ability to attain health and general well-being.

Social Justice Justice in terms of wealth, opportunities, and privileges in a society may represent the political–philosophical concept centered on equality among people along various social dimensions.

Socio-ecological model (SEM) Multilevel framework of health promotion recognizing the interaction of the environment and individual within a social system (Bronfenbrenner, 1977).

Spasticity Muscular resistance to passive movement that is velocity dependent.

Sphere Standards The Sphere Standards are the most commonly recognized set of minimum humanitarian standards, which are widely used by nongovernmental organizations in humanitarian response.

Stigma A mark of disgrace associated with a specific quality, circumstance, or person.

Sustainable food Food that has a positive impact on health, climate, economy, and the earth.

Systemic racism Racism resulting from the inherent biases and prejudices of policies and practices of social and political organizations, groups, or institutions (The Free Dictionary, 2015); systemic racist practices (e.g., residential schools, continued influence today).

Term infant An infant who is born between 37 weeks and 41 weeks and 6 days of gestation.

The theory of planned behavior A theory linking one's beliefs and behaviors, taking into consideration the individual's attitude, perception of subjective norms, and perceived behavioral control of the behavior that shapes the individual's behavioral intentions and behaviors (Ajzen, 1985).

Therapeutic breast massage A manual technique that uses gentle massage toward the axilla and manual expression of milk to decrease symptoms associated with breast inflammation.

Therapeutic ultrasound The application of ultrasonic waves as an intervention, as opposed to diagnostic ultrasound.

Trauma-and-Violence-Informed care Takes into consideration the need for a complete picture of a patient's life situation, past and present, to provide effective care and healing; practices that promote a culture of safety, empowerment, and healing. Care is tailored to address interrelated forms of violence.

UNICEF A United Nations agency that is responsible for humanitarian and developmental aid being provided to children worldwide. With a presence in 192 countries and territories, it is one of the most widespread and recognizable social welfare organizations in the world (https://en.wikipedia.org/wiki/UNICEF)

United Nations Convention on the Rights of the Child One of the most widely ratified human rights treaties in history. An international agreement on childhood created in 1990 as a commitment to the world's children to protect and transform their lives. The goal is to be sure that children enjoy a full childhood by garnering leaders from government, business, and community to fulfill their commitments to the convention (https://www.unicef.org/crc)

Uterus A pear-shaped organ of the female reproductive system. The uterus is located in the lower pelvis and plays a significant role in reproduction.

The WHO Code A short hand reference to the international code developed by the WHO and United Nations International Children's Emergency Fund (UNICEF) and signed by the majority of countries worldwide to minimize marketing of human milk substitutes (see International Code of Marketing of Breast-milk Substitutes; Gray, 2017).

WHO/UNICEF Baby-friendly Hospital Initiative (BFHI) World Health Organization/United Nations Children's Fund Baby-friendly Hospital Initiative.

World Alliance for Breastfeeding Action (WABA, 2020) A global network of individuals and organizations dedicated to the protection, promotion, and support of breastfeeding worldwide (https://waba.org.my)

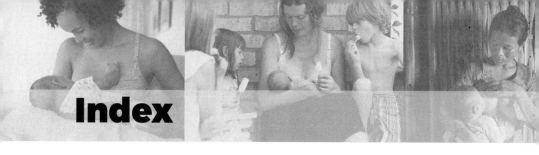

Index

Note: Page numbers followed by 'b', 'f' and 't' indicate material in boxes, figures and tables respectively.